A FRESH LOOK AT ANXIETY DISORDERS

Edited by **Federico Durbano**

A Fresh Look at Anxiety Disorders
http://dx.doi.org/10.5772/59525
Edited by Federico Durbano

Contributors

Guillem Pailhez, Antonio Bulbena, Juan Castaño, Cristina Vendrell, Maria Del Mar Ballester, Silvia Rosado, Núria Mallorquí, Carolina Baeza, Cicek Hocaoglu, Anna Boyajyan, Diana Avetyan, Lilit Hovhannisyan, Gohar Mkrtchyan, Audrey McKinlay, Michelle Albicini, J. Landeira-Fernandez, Daniel Mograbi, Vitor Castro-Gomes, Elie Cheniaux, Malgorzata Dabkowska, Agnieszka Dabkowska, Delia Marina Podea, Aurora Sabau, Karol Julien Wild, Sarosh Khalid-Khan, Dorte M. Christiansen, Lei Zhang, Floriana Irtelli, Federico Durbano, Stefania Doria, Roberto Sanlorenzo, Juan Francisco Rodríguez-Landa, Abraham Puga-Olguin, León Jesús Germán-Ponciano, Rosa Isela García-Ríos, Cesar Soria-Fregoso, Blandina Bernal-Morales, Frank Pulido-Criollo, Claude Belanger, Theodora Katerelos, Michel Perreault, Marie-Christine Payette, Ghassan El-Baalbaki, André Marchand, David Gratzer, Faiza Khalid-Khan

Published by InTech
Janeza Trdine 9, 51000 Rijeka, Croatia

Publishing Process Manager Ivona Lovric
Technical Editor InTech DTP team
Cover InTech Design team

First published September, 2015
Printed in Croatia

Additional hard copies can be obtained from orders@intechopen.com

A Fresh Look at Anxiety Disorders, Edited by Federico Durbano
p. cm.
ISBN 978-953-51-2149-7

Meet the editor

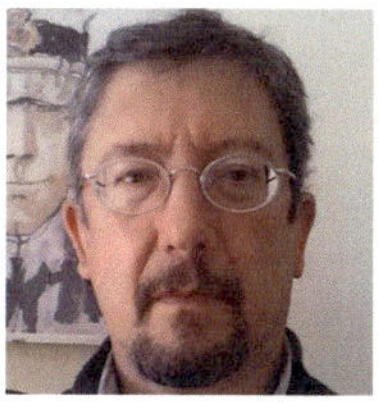

Dr Federico Durbano was born in Genua, Italy, in 1963. He received a degree in Medicine at the University of Milan, Italy, and at the same University, he did a specialization in Psychiatry. Soon after, he became a specialist in Forensic Psychiatry, giving his contribution in different Italian courts. Since 2001, he has been working in Fatebenefratelli and Ophtalmic Hospital in Milan, Italy, formerly as Chief Coordinator of the Emergency Psychiatric Service, and since 2012, as Chief Coordinator of Community Psychiatric Services. In addition, he is responsible for quality processes and risk management of the Mental Health Department, producing local guidelines on different topics. As a teacher, he collaborates with the University of Milan Nursing School, and he is the course director of a number of courses on aggressivity, prevention of violence, and self-defense for nurses and other health operators. He has been a speaker at more than 100 national congresses and a teacher at more than 50 national training courses. So far, Dr Durbano published about 150 papers on psychiatric issues, with a particular focus on psychosomatics, general psychiatry, and community psychiatry.

Contents

Preface

Two years after the preceding book on anxiety (New Insight into Anxiety Disorders, InTech, 2013) but also following others published by InTech in the previous years, here we are again with some updates on anxiety disorders. Someone will ask why we speak again of anxiety, considering anxiety disorders as "secondary disorders." Let us describe some epidemiological data, showing the vastity of the phenomenon and suggesting the social impact of it.

According to WHO epidemiological data, mental disorders account for the third leading cause of disability-adjusted life years (DALYs), with a 15.2% of prevalence, following cancer (15.4%) and cardiovascular diseases (26.6%). The global burden of these noncommunicable diseases comprises 81.3% of all disease burden [1]. In the mental health domain, anxiety disorders rank sixth (4% of all years lived with disability, YLD) in the contribution to chronic conditions in Europe, neuropsychiatric disorders being the first in the whole cause of all YLD [2].

The economic consequences of these health losses are equally large; a recent study estimated that the cumulative global impact of mental disorders in terms of lost economic output will amount to US$ 16.3 million between 2011 and 2030 (data from the World Economic Forum, the Harvard School of Public Health, The global economic burden of non-communicable diseases, Geneva, World Economic Forum, 2011).

There are more facts that account for the importance attributed to mental illnesses, in particular, their very early ages of onset (AOO) compared to other medical illnesses [3]. WMH analyses show that early-onset mental disorders are significant predictors of the subsequent onset and persistence of a wide range of physical disorders and that mental disorders beginning in childhood-adolescence have significant adverse effects on subsequent role transitions, being associated with high levels of role impairment [4,5].

According to the recent WHO global survey of 26 countries, anxiety disorders as a whole are the most common among mental disorders, with a 12-month prevalence of 2.4%–18.2% (depending on the country surveyed), much greater than mood disorders (ranging from 0.8% to 9.6%) which are ranked second.

In a 2004 European epidemiological survey, anxiety accounted for 13.6% prevalence (versus 13.9% for mood disorders), being a leading cause of psychiatric morbidity [6]. In a similar study, average prevalence estimates for any anxiety disorder in the 12 months prior to assessment are 10.6% and, in a lifetime, 16.6%; women have generally higher prevalence rates than men, the magnitude of the difference varying in different contexts [7].

The USA data are more impressive than European ones; anxiety disorders accounted for 28.8% lifetime prevalence, much greater than mood disorders (20.8%) [8].

In more recent works, anxiety disorders are ranked first in epidemiological surveys all over the world, ranging from 4.8% to 31% lifetime prevalence and from 3% to 19% 12-month prevalence estimates [9].

Even if a recent meta-analysis showed a significant data dispersion mainly due to methodological bias and different survey instruments, the data globally confirmed that anxiety disorders are common, early-onset, and very debilitating [10].

These data are sufficient to maintain clinical attention to anxiety as a disorder. In the previous book, we described the evolutionary importance of anxiety and some other "normal" aspects of it and also the neurobiological basis of its pathological manifestations and some other clinical aspects.

In this new book, we were oriented in giving some more neurobiological data of specific anxiety disorders, in particular, PTSD, which is growing in interest due to its relation to modern civilization problems (terrorism, local wars, natural and unnatural disasters). But our interest being a clinical one, we selected representative works on psychosomatic (the relationship of psychological function/dysfunction and the body dysfunctions), in particular, the ones related with immunology.

It is well described how anxiety heightens cardiovascular morbidity risks [11], cardiovascular mortality (well more than depression alone) [12], but less known to lay public are the data linking anxiety to specific psychosomatic aspects.

This new book is not organized in sections as the preceding one, but the chapters have a logical path. Beginning from the recent evidence on risk factors (neurobiological but also environmental and developmental), not forgetting sex differences in clinical expression of anxiety disorders, the contributing authors put some remarks on psychobiology of panic and give some new issues on genetics of PTSD (with a possible future clinical application of genetic screening) and on neurophysiology of anger in PTSD – a forgotten but impressively important dimension of this pathology.

Anxiety disorders are highly comorbid, the comorbidity being the norm rather than the exception, with a mean co-morbidity index of 74.1%, not only fulfilling different anxiety disorders criteria but also a significant and strong relation with affective disorders (OR 6.6) and substance use disorders (OR 2.4) [13]. From the contributing authors of this book, there emerges also a significant link of anxiety to heightening of suicide risk and with the dramatically worsening of psychosis.

Following these chapters, we present some data on psychosomatic: a promising linkage between anxiety and some immunological dysfunctions (joint hypermobility syndrome), some clinical data on the association between anxiety and menopause (in particular, the one following surgical procedures), and a particularly interesting feature on the link between infantile cranial trauma and subsequent anxiety syndromes. In the pre-adult aspects of anxiety, there is a contribution on the influence that anxiety has on scholarly performance.

Finally, the last five chapters are centered on non-pharmacological interventions, specifically on alternative complementary medicine; a contribution is centered on expectancies of psychotherapies and their role in clinical response (or better, outcome); then a chapter on the review of some alternative approaches to anxiety treatment and their outcomes in specific anxiety syndromes; a chapter on yoga for the treatment of stress in the workplace, which is particularly interesting since the authors present their experiences in applying yoga directly in the workplace; a chapter on the usefulness of mindfulness in treating some forms of anxiety; and the very interesting last chapter, on the modern approach to psychological treatment using a mobile app.

So, thanking all the contributing authors, we think we have done a pretty good job to give some up-to-date and useful clinical contributions to anxiety study and treatment.

Hoping to have other books following this, I wish you a good reading.

References

[1] Global Health Estimates 2014 Summary Tables: DALY by cause, age and sex, by WHO Region, 2000–2012.

[2] Global Health Estimates 2014 Summary Tables: YLD by cause, age and sex, by WHO Region, 2000–2012.

[3] Kessler RC, Amminger GP, Aguilar-Gaxiola S, et al. (2007). Age of onset of mental disorders: a review of recent literature. Curr Opin Psychiatry. 20(4):359–64.

[4] He Y, Zhang M, Lin EH, et al. (2008). Mental disorders among persons with arthritis: results from the World Mental Health Surveys. Psychol Med. 38(11):1639–50.

[5] Ormel J, Von Korff M, Burger H, et al. (2007). Mental disorders among persons with heart disease – results from World Mental Health surveys. Gen Hosp Psychiatry. 29(4):325–34.

[6] Alonso J, Angermeyer MC, Bernert S et al. (2004). Prevalence of mental disorders in Europe: results from the European Study of the Epidemiology of Mental Disorders (ESEMeD) project. Acta Psychiatr Scand Suppl. 109(420):21–7. doi:10.1111/j.1600-0047.2004.00327.x. PMID 15128384.

[7] Somers JM, Goldner EM, Waraich P, Hsu L (2006). Prevalence and incidence studies of anxiety disorders: a systematic review of the literature. Can J Psychiatry. 51(2):100–13. PMID 16989109.

[8] Kessler RC, Berglund P, Demler O, et al. (2005). Lifetime prevalence and age-of-onset distributions of DSM-IV disorders in the National Comorbidity Survey Replication. Arch Gen Psychiatry. 62(6):593–602. doi:10.1001/archpsyc.62.6.593. PMID 15939837.

[9] Kessler RC, Aguilar-Gaxiola S, Alonso J, et al. (2009). The global burden of mental disorders: an update from the WHO World Mental Health (WMH) Surveys. Epidemiol Psichiatr Soc. 18(1):23–33.

[10] Steel Z, Marnane C, Iranpour C, et al. (2014). The global prevalence of common mental disorders: a systematic review and meta-analysis 1980–2013. Int. J. Epidemiol. 43(2):476–93. doi:10.1093/ije/dyu038.

[11] Roest AM, Martens EJ, de Jonge P, Denollet J. (2010). Anxiety and risk of incident coronary heart disease: a meta-analysis. J Am Coll Cardiol. 56(1):38–46. doi:10.1016/j.jacc.2010.03.034.

[12] Martens EJ, de Jonge P, Na B, Cohen BE, Lett H, Whooley MA. (2010). Scared to death? Generalized anxiety disorder and cardiovascular events in patients with stable coronary

heart disease: the Heart and Soul Study. Arch Gen Psychiatry. 67(7):750–8. doi:10.1001/archgenpsychiatry.2010.74.

[13] Michael T, Zetsche U, Margraf J. (2007). Epidemiology of anxiety disorders. Psychiatry. 6(4):136–42.

Dr. Federico Durbano
SS Psichiatria Territorio e Comunità
Dipartimento di Salute Mentale e Neuroscienze
A.O. Fatebenefratelli e Oftalmico
Milano, Italy

Chapter 1

Risk Factors of Anxiety Disorders in Children

Malgorzata Dabkowska and Agnieszka Dabkowska-Mika

Additional information is available at the end of the chapter

http://dx.doi.org/10.5772/61169

Abstract

Anxiety disorders are common; lifetime prevalence for the group of disorders is estimated to be as high as 25%. The main question is What is the relative contribution of genetics and environment to etiology of anxiety disorders? The anxiety disorders are not, from a genetic perspective, etiologically homogeneous. Structural equation modeling provides estimates of variance in liability to a disorder that is attributable to additive genetic, common familial environmental, and individual-specific environmental factors. Familial aggregation that largely results from genetic risk factors has been documented for all of the major anxiety disorders. Genes predispose to two broad groups of disorders dichotomized as panic-generalized-agoraphobic anxiety versus specific phobias. The candidate genes are the ones encoding the central and peripheral nervous system receptors and transporters. Trauma in childhood disposes to further anxiety disorders through the hyperactivity of the HPA axis and the hypersecretion of CRF. Traumatic experience in developmental age leads to neurobiochemical changes in brain, typical for panic disorder or PTSD. Behavioral inhibition in early childhood is a predictor of further anxiety disorders. Some types of parental behaviors and family environment can lead to them, as well as improper interactions between parents and child.

Keywords: Anxiety disorders, children, risk factors, environmental, genes

1. Introduction

Anxiety disorders are among the most common psychological disorders in younger patients, affecting 6% to 20% of developed countries children and adolescents [1]. In the etiology of anxiety disorders there is a complex interplay of biological and genetic vulnerabilities, temperamental qualities, negative environmental influences and negative attachment experiences, parental psychopathology, and disadvantageous sociocultural factors [2].

Biological risk factors include genetics and child temperament. Anxiety disorders are highly comorbid with each other and with mood disorders. There is a growing number of studies searching for candidate genes of anxiety disorders through human genome scan. Studies of environmental risk factors in the development of childhood anxiety disorders have focused on parent–child interactions and parental anxiety.

2. Environmental risk factors

2.1. Gender

Girls are more vulnerable than boys for anxiety. Female sex consistently emerges as a risk factor for the development of anxiety disorders. Females are about twice as likely as males to develop each of the anxiety disorders [3]. The female preponderance emerges early in life, and retrospective data indicate that at age 6, females are already twice as likely to have experienced an anxiety disorder as are males [4].

2.2. Age

There is a typical age of onset for different kinds of anxiety disorders—separation anxiety disorder and some specific phobias usually start before age of 12 years [5]; social phobia in late childhood, adolescence, and very rarely after 25 years [5,6]. Agoraphobia, panic disorder, and general anxiety disorder usually emerge later in adolescence or early adulthood, with some cases starting even before 12 [5, 7].

2.3. Temperament

The importance of emotional deregulation is emphasized in anxiety disorders. Negative emotional responses are more frequent and intensive in anxious children, as well as difficulties in reappraisal according to negative emotional situations. These children trust more on emotion regulation strategies. All of that can lead to functional impairment, intensive negative emotions, and disturbing in emotion regulation self-efficacy [8]. The vigilance–avoidance attention pattern is found in anxious adults and children, who initially gaze more at threatening pictures than nonanxious adults and children (vigilance) but subsequently gaze less at them than nonanxious adults and children (avoidance) [9]. Children and adolescents with anxiety disorders could have different temperaments and character profiles in accordance with diagnostic groups, which imply the specific pathophysiological mechanism of each anxiety disorder [10]. Behavioral inhibition in early childhood is a predictor of further anxiety disorders. Some types of parental behaviors and family environment can lead to them, as well as improper interactions between parents and child. Both parental acceptance and parental overcontrol are related to anxiety. It is confirmed that the overcontrolling behavior of parents can be a predictor of anxiety in a child and is connected with constant fear in adolescence. What is more, an absence of maternal overcontrol can diminish the significance of high behavioral inhibition on further social anxiety symptoms. It has occurred that there is a significant connection between parents' avoiding behavior and symptoms of anxiety in child. Some studies indicate that among environmental risk factors, an inhibited temperament has the greatest impact and can moderate others' factors influence. Some results suggest that the association between behavioral inhibition and anxiety disorder is accounted for by children who have stable behavioral inhibition. Children who remained inhibited at 4, 5 1/2, and 7 1/2 years had higher rates of anxiety disorders than children who were not consistently inhibited. With few exceptions, behavioral inhibition was shown to be a risk factor for the development of anxiety disorders [11–13]. There are also indications for specificity in this association within anxiety disorders (strong associations particularly to social phobia). Toddlers and preschoolers with behavioral inhibition and a family history of anxiety disorder and stable inhibition have an increased risk of anxiety disorders, particularly social phobia, and may benefit from preventative parenting interventions. Avoidant personality disorder is reported to be especially prevalent in people with anxiety disorders. Approximately 10–50% of people who have panic disorder with agoraphobia have avoidant personality disorder, as well as about 20–40% of people who have social phobia; 45% among people with generalized anxiety disorder have avoidant personality disorder [14].

2.4. Parental factors

Infants who were anxiously attached in infancy develop more anxiety disorders during childhood and adolescence than infants who were securely attached [15]. Parents affected by anxiety disorders usually cannot learn how to manage anxiety in their children because they do not have this ability themselves. These children develop anxiety disorders more often, sometimes as early as in toddlerhood [16]. Anxiety disorders are common among offspring of anxious and depressed parents. Offspring of anxious parents were significantly more likely to have only anxiety disorders. Offspring of depressed or mixed anxious/depressed parents had a broader range of disorders and more comorbid disorders [17]. A large body of work has demonstrated that parent anxiety disorders increase the risk for similar problems in children. Parent anxiety symptoms moderated the relationship between parent- and child-externalizing symptoms, such that the strength of this relationship was reduced in the presence of high levels of parent anxiety symptoms [18]. Parental psychopathology and rearing were associated with offspring social phobia, independently as well as in their interaction. The examination the role of parental psychopathology and family environment for the risk of social phobia in a large sample of adolescents showed that parental social phobia was associated with offspring's risk to develop social phobia. Other parental anxiety disorders, depression, and alcohol use disorders were also associated with offspring social phobia. Parental rearing styles of overprotection, rejection, and lack of emotional warmth were associated with offspring social phobia. Observations suggested a continued graded relationship between familial risk factors and offspring SAD [19,20]. The risk factor of anxiety disorders during childhood is parenting behavior as a possible factor in the transmission of anxiety from parent to child. The emotions in families with an anxious parent differed significantly from families without an anxious parent [21].

Environmental mechanisms (e.g., maternal anxious attachment perceptions, maladaptive parenting practices, parental modeling of anxiety, and avoidance) may account for the observed association between parent and child anxiety [22]. The potential role of learning from parents in the development of child anxiety has three specific mechanisms: parental modeling, information transfer, and parental reinforcement of anxious/avoidant behavior. A variety of parenting practices (i.e., parental overcontrol, parental overprotection, parental emotional warmth/positivity, parental rejection/criticism, and parenting styles) could be factors that may pose risk for the development of child anxiety [23]. Both parental use of aversive control and nonresponsiveness were directly related to overall levels of child anxiety disorder-related behavior [24]. Parenting stress, parental psychopathology, and family functioning are associated with child anxiety [25,26]. Anxious attachment may lead to separation anxiety. Children with temperamental vulnerability may develop anxiety disorders, when their mastery and autonomy are restricted by overcontrolling, overprotective, and overly critical parenting styles. Parental rejection and control may lead to later anxiety and depression [27]. Anxiety disorders in children may be caused by insecure (especially anxious/resistant) attachment relationships with caregivers [27, 15]. Different attachment patterns (secure, ambivalent, avoidant, and disorganized) may relate to different types of anxiety symptoms and that behavioral inhibition may moderate these relations.

2.5. Culture factors

The culture-specific expression of anxiety is a risk factor for anxiety disorders, for example, Asian cultures typically show the lowest rates, whereas Russian and US samples show the highest rates of social anxiety disorder. The prevalence and expression of social anxiety depends on the particular culture. Social anxiety is assumed to be related to cultural norms across countries. In some works, researchers compared individualistic and collectivistic countries and found higher social anxiety and more positive attitudes toward socially avoidant behaviors in collectivistic rather than in individualistic countries [28–30].

2.6. Toxic environment

Patients with environmental illness experience a large number of psychiatric symptoms. Anxiety disorders were significantly more frequent in patients with environmental illness [31]. Organic brain damage with cognitive and behavioral impairment can be caused by acute and toxic exposure. Even low-to-moderate exposure, when it is chronic, may lead to anxiety and mood disturbances. Lead exposure particularly can result in anxiety and depression [32, 33].

2.7. A unique environmental factor and common shared environmental factor

It is said that two groups of disorders (specific phobias versus generalized/panic anxiety and agoraphobia, with social phobia between them) are associated with two genetic factors. Common and (in a greater degree) unique environmental factors shared across the disorders can explain remaining associations between the disorders. In the results of analyses from more than 5000 members of male–male and female–female twin pairs from the Virginia Adult Twin Study of Psychiatric and Substance Use Disorders, it occurred that shared environmental influences do not play a major role, as a single common factor was calculated below 12% of the total variance for any disorder. Researchers describe unique environmental factors as single common factor plus effects, which are characteristic for a disease [34]. During a lifetime, life experiences (unique for the patient or shared with other family members) may further influence the risk for anxiety disorders. It would have different significance, depending on the disorder. Something called a "set of unique environmental factors" can lead to one or another anxiety disorder [34].

2.8. Life experience/childhood adversities

The experience of a traumatic event may influence the development of anxiety disorders. Trauma in childhood disposes to further anxiety disorders through the hyperactivity of the HPA axis and the hypersecretion of CRF. Traumatic experience in developmental age leads to neurobiochemical changes in brain, typical for panic disorder or PTSD. Because of early trauma, there is change of genes and increase in anxiety sensitivity.

Experience of childhood trauma (e.g., sexual abuse) increases the risk of psychiatric or substance use disorder in maturity. Exposure of children to early adverse experiences is a risk factor for developing anxiety disorders. Early life stress, causing the chronic sensitization of those central nervous system circuits, which regulate stress and emotion, may be a biological explanation of increased vulnerability to stress and further development of anxiety. Childhood maltreatment has been linked to a variety of changes in brain structure and function and stress-responsive neurobiological systems. Deprivation of developmentally appropriate experience may reduce neuronal activity, resulting in a generalized decrease in neurotrophin production, synaptic connectivity, and neuronal survival, resulting in profound abnormalities in brain organization and structure [35]. Thus, childhood abuse and exposure to domestic violence can lead to numerous differences in the structure and physiology of the brain that expectedly would affect multiple human functions and behaviors [36, 37]. Neurobiological evidence supports the hypothesis of dysfunction in hippocampus, amygdala, medial prefrontal cortex, and other limbic structures believed to mediate anxiety and mood dysregulation following early abuse [37]. There are similarities in neurobiological results between some studies on early life stress in children and in animals. For example, children who suffer from generalized anxiety disorders and anticipated a laboratory stress task had increased levels of ACTH and normal levels of cortisol [38]. Altered behavioral and hormonal responses to central noradrenergic stimulation have been observed in children with several anxiety disorders. Neurobiological alterations are also present in children with PTSD related to early trauma. It may be that early life stress affects neurobiological function in children with other anxiety disorders as well, similar to findings in early-onset depression [39]. The adverse childhood experiences including abuse, witnessing domestic violence, and serious household dysfunction had a strong, graded relationship to the prevalence and risk of affective disturbances. For children with more than four experiences, the risk of panic reactions and anxiety was increased 2.5- and 2.4 -fold, respectively [40]. There is an etiological relation between stressful life events (unique to the individual or common to other members of the family) and anxiety disorders. Its effects on disorders are probably nonspecific, as many kinds of childhood adversity (loss events—

e.g., parental divorce; parental psychopathologies—e.g., maternal depression; interpersonal traumas—e.g., rape and natural disaster) are associated with adult psychiatric outcomes with little specificity, including anxiety disorders [41, 42]. These adversities were consistently associated with onset, but not persistence, of anxiety disorders [41].

2.9. Parental loss

Childhood parental loss or separation has been linked to various forms of adult psychopathologic characteristic [43, 44]. The study evaluating the relationship between parental loss prior to age 17 years and adult psychopathology in 1018 pairs of female twins from a population-based registry has shown the impact of parent death or separation for the risk of anxiety disorders. Researchers found association between parental separation (but not parental death) and increased risk for generalized anxiety disorders. Parental death and separation from mother (but not father) were related to panic disorder. A higher probability of developing phobia due to parental death (but no parental separation) was described. A model that includes parental loss as a form of specified family environment shows if it is truly an environmental risk factor for adult psychopathologic conditions [44]. Not only loss of parent has a relationship with affective disorders but also lack of adequate parental care takes important role in the increased risk of psychiatric disorders in adulthood. Studies on caregiving arrangements indicate that lack of care (characterized as neglecting rather than adverse behavior of parent) is associated with higher risk of depression. It is loss of mother rather than father that has impact more frequent [45].

2.10. Sexual abuse

Childhood sexual abuse is a strong risk factor of anxiety disorders. A study about the consequences of childhood sexual abuse in a birth cohort of more than 1,000 New Zealand children studied at the age of 18 years showed that children reporting sexual abuse had higher rates of anxiety disorder than those not reporting. The findings suggest that sexual abuse, particularly severe childhood sexual abuse, was associated with increased risk of psychiatric disorder in young adults even when due allowance was made for prospectively measured confounding factors [46]. Childhood sexual abuse has been found to elevate the risk for adult GAD and panic disorder, as well as other psychiatric and substance use disorders [46, 47]. Studies of the impact of traumatic events on health have shown that the history of childhood sexual or physical abuse was significantly more frequent in patients with panic disorder than those with social phobia. Rates of abuse of patients with generalized anxiety disorder were between results of these other groups, without significant differences [42]. Women with childhood sexual abuse have a substantially increased risk for developing a wide range of psychopathology. Most of this association is due to more severe forms of sexual abuse. The significant ORs for GAD and panic disorder were all approximately 1.9 [47]. In a group of 1411 women who report childhood sexual abuse (three levels: nongenital, genital, and intercourse), association with psychiatric disorders was assessed. Self-reported childhood sexual abuse was positively associated with all disorders, the most with genital and especially intercourse sexual abuse.

2.11. Peer violence

Bullying behavior is a frequent risk factor of anxiety disorder among adolescents. Twenty-percent of victims scored within the clinical range on a standard depression and anxiety measure [48].

Peer victimization was positively related to child-reported anxiety, social physique anxiety, and loneliness [49]. Bullying experiences are connected not only to concurrent psychiatric symptoms but also to future psychiatric symptoms, especially anxiety disorders [50, 51].

Bullying should be seen as an indicator of risk of various mental disorders in adolescence. Finnish adolescents taking part in the School Health Promotion Study were surveyed about bullying and victimization in relation to several psychiatric disorders. Anxiety was most frequent among bully victims and equally common among bullies and victims [52]. The relationship among bullying, victimization, and anxiety may be connected with sex. Sex differences were noted on measures of peer victimization and anxiety with boys reporting more victimization but less anxiety than girls [53].

2.12. Economical factors

Most children with anxiety disorders are from middle- to upper-middle class families; however, 50–75% of those with separation anxiety disorder come from low socioeconomic status homes [54–56]. Rates of anxiety disorders are greater for those with socioeconomic status disadvantage [57]. Socioeconomic status is one of many possible antecedents in the development of social anxiety disorder [58].

3. Genetic factors

Genetic factors play a significant role in etiology of anxiety disorders; for example, inherited risk factor for social phobia is estimated as 47% [59].

Increased risk for anxiety disorder in children occurs if at least one parent has anxiety disorder [60], or if both parents are affected [61, 62]. Common genetic risk factors for major depression and anxiety disorder have been described as "bidirectional"; both parental major depression increased the risk of anxiety disorder in child [63, 64], and parental anxiety disorder increased risk of depression in child [62, 65].

3.1. Twin studies

Torgersen [66] found that anxiety disorders (in total) are two times more frequent in MZ than in DZ co-twins; GAD is two times more frequent in MZ than in DZ co-twins. In a group with panic disorders and agoraphobia with panic attacks, anxiety disorders with panic attacks were even more than five times as frequent in MZ as in DZ.

There was research on 1030 pairs of twins about interrelationship between genetic and environmental risk factors for pairs of anxiety disorders and other mental diseases. The researchers found that anxiety disorders are genetically heterogeneous. However, there is one common genetic risk factor (with great impact) for phobia, panic disorder, and bulimia nervosa and another factor for major depression and generalized anxiety disorder [67].

A cohort study on 1412 pairs of MZ and DZ twins, ages 8–16 years [68], suggested that genetic influences on anxiety in childhood differ according to sex (greater extent in girls than in boys). Additive genetic effects play a moderate role in the etiology of manifest anxiety among females, but a more modest role for males. Moderate additive genetic effects were reported in another study on adult patients with generalized anxiety [69].

A significant familial aggregation according to panic disorder, GAD, and phobias was shown in meta-analysis based on family and twin studies [70].

Quite often, there is a comorbidity of anxiety disorder and another anxiety disorder or mood disorder [71]. It is consistent with the results indicating the same genetic factors for GAD and major depression [72, 73].

It is shown that polymorphism in the serotonin transporter gene regulatory region is associated with anxiety-related traits (3–4% of total variation and 7–9% of inherited variance in patients and their sibships) [74].

Through human scan genome, chromosomes 1, 7, 9, and 11 were linked to panic attacks and chromosome 3 to agoraphobia [75–77]. Analysis of links exhibits loci for panic attacks on chromosome 9q [77].

There is a growing number of studies about the significant role of FK506-binding protein 51 (FKBP5), a co-chaperone of steroid hormone receptors. It regulates stress-induced GR-mediated effects. Polymorphism in this gene is related with GR sensitivity and can regulate stress hormone system. Specific alleles of FKBP5 are associated with major depression, bipolar disorder, and posttraumatic stress disorder, as well as with faster response to antidepressant treatment [78]. It can lead to increased risk of stress-related psychiatric disorders when its genetic variation interacts with early life stress (ELS) to epigenetically program GR-induced transcription of FKBP5 [79].

Demethylation of allele-specific FKBP5 DNA interacts between childhood trauma and gene transcription, leading to dysfunction of the stress hormone system, immune cells, and those brain areas, which are associated with stress regulation [80].

4. Summary

An anxiety disorder during adolescence confers a strong risk for recurrent anxiety disorders during early adulthood [81]. In the future, adolescents with anxiety disorders are at an increased risk of subsequent anxiety, depression, illicit drug dependence, and educational underachievement as young adults.

Clinical features of anxiety (e.g., higher severity, duration, and avoidance) as well as comorbid other mental disorders are particularly useful for predicting an unfavorable course of anxiety disorders [82]. Early psychoeducation program for parents could decrease risk for anxiety disorder. As environmental risk factors are already well known, the next step is to distinguish what predictors have the greatest impact and how to moderate them. Vantage sensitivity hypothesis said that some genetic variants moderate outcome of positive intervention [83]. Through studies on trajectories of behaviorally inhibited children, it occurred that some inhibited infants and toddlers develop into normal children [84].

Knowledge of risk factors enables preventive actions with respect to the developing anxiety disorders in children. It seems important to undertake actions to increase the resilience capacity of individuals to cope with traumatic events. Donovan and Spence [85] present the results of research regarding the prevention of anxiety disorders. The main protective factors are social support in the presence of traumatic experiences and coping skills in the resilience to anxiety. Methods of prevention of childhood anxiety disorders could be divided to child, parent, and environment strategies.

Author details

Malgorzata Dabkowska[1*] and Agnieszka Dabkowska-Mika[2*]

*Address all correspondence to: gosiadab@interia.pl doagnieszki@interia.pl

1 Collegium Medicum, Nicolaus Copernicus University, Torun, Bydgoszcz, Poland

2 Psychiatry Clinic, Clinical Hospital of K. Jonscher, Poznan, Poland

References

[1] Walkup JT, Albano AM, Piacentini J, Birmaher B, Compton SN, Sherrill JT, Ginsburg GS, Rynn MA, McCracken J, Waslick B, Iyengar S, March JS, Kendall PC. Cognitive behavioral therapy, sertraline, or a combination in childhood anxiety. New England Journal of Medicine. 2008; 359,26:2753–2766. DOI: 10.1056/NEJMoa0804633.

[2] Pine DS, Grun J. Childhood anxiety: integrating developmental psychopathology and affective neuroscience. Journal of Child and Adolescent Psychopharmacology. 1999;9,1:1–12. DOI: 10.1089/cap.1999.9.1.

[3] Costello EJ, Mustillo S, Erkanli A, et al. Prevalence and development of psychiatric disorders in childhood and adolescence. Archives of General Psychiatry. 2003;60:837–844. DOI:10.1001/archpsyc.1996.01830110071009.

[4] Lewinsohn PM, Gotlib IH, Lewinsohn M, Seeley JR, Allen NB. Gender differences in anxiety disorders and anxiety symptoms in adolescents. Journal of Abnormal Psychology. 1998;107, 1:109–117. DOI.org/10.1037/0021-843X.107.1.109.

[5] Kessler RC, Berglund P, Demler O, et al. Lifetime prevalence and age-of-onset distributions of DSM-IV disorders in the National Comorbidity Survey Replication. Archives of General Psychiatry. 2005; 62:593–602. DOI: 10.1001/archpsyc.62.6.593.

[6] Wittchen HU, Fehm L. Epidemiology and natural course of social fears and social phobia. Acta Psychiatrica Scandinavica. 2003; 108(Suppl 417):4–18. DOI: 10.1034/j.1600-0447.108.s417.1.x.

[7] Wittchen HU, Nocon A, Beesdo K, et al. Agoraphobia and panic: prospective-longitudinal relations suggest a rethinking of diagnostic concepts. Psychotherapy and Psychosomatics. 2008; 77:147–157. DOI: 10.1159/000116608.

[8] Carthy T, Horesh N, Apter A, Gross JJ. Patterns of emotional reactivity and regulation in children with anxiety disorders. Journal of Psychopathology and Behavioral Assessment. 2010;32,1(March 2010b):23–36. DOI: 10.1007/s10862-009-9167-8.

[9] In-Albon T, Kossowsky J, Schneider S. Vigilance and avoidance of threat in the eye movements of children with separation anxiety disorder. Journal of Abnormal Child Psychology. 2010;38,2:225–235. DOI:10.1007/s10802-009-9359-4.

[10] Soo-churl C, Sun-woo J, Boong-nyun K, Jun-won H, Min-sup S, Jae-won K, Dong-seon C, Hyo-won K. Temperament and character among Korean children and adolescents with anxiety disorders. European Child and Adolescent Psychiatry. 2009; 18:60–64. DOI: 10.1007/s00787-008-0699-3.

[11] Caspi A, Moffitt TE, Newman DL, et al. Behavioral observations at age 3 years predict adult psychiatric disorders. Archive of General Psychiatry.1996;53:1033–1039.

[12] Hayward C, Killen JD, Kraemer HC, et al. Linking self-reported childhood behavioral inhibition to adolescent social phobia. Journal of the American Academy of Child and Adolescent Psychiatry. 1998;37:1308–1316. DOI: 10.1097/00004583-199812000-00015.

[13] Biederman J, Hirshfeld-Becker DR, Rosenbaum JF, et al. Further evidence of association between behavioral inhibition and social anxiety in children. American Journal of Psychiatry. 2001;158,10:1673–1679. DOI:10.1176/appi.ajp.158.10.1673.

[14] Van Velzen CJM. Social Phobia and Personality Disorders: Comorbidity and Treatment Issues. Groningen: University Library Groningen. 2002. Available from: http://irs.ub.rug.nl/ppn/240921941.

[15] Warren SL, Huston L, Egeland B, Sroufe LA. Child and adolescent anxiety disorders and early attachment. Journal of the American Academy of Child and Adolescent Psychiatry. 1997; 36,5:637–644.

[16] Hirshfeld-Becker DR, Biederman J. Rationale and principles for early intervention with young children at risk for anxiety disorders. Clinical Child and Family Psychology Review. 2002;5,3:161–172. DOI:10.1023/A:1019687531040.

[17] Beidel DC, Turner SM. At risk for anxiety: I. Psychopathology in the offspring of anxious parents. Journal of the American Academy of Child & Adolescent Psychiatry. 1997;36,7:918–924. DOI 10.1097/00004583-199707000-00013.

[18] Burstein M, Ginsburg GS, Jenn-Yun Tein JY. Parental anxiety and child symptomatology: an examination of and interactive effects of parent psychopathology. Journal of Abnormal Child Psychology. 2010;38,7:897–909. DOI: 10.1007/s10802-010-9415-0.

[19] Knappe S, Beesdo K, Fehm L, Lieb R, Wittchen HU. Associations of familial risk factors with social fears and social phobia: evidence for the continuum hypothesis in social anxiety disorder? Journal of Neural Transmission. 2000a;1166:639–648. DOI: 10.1007/s00702-008-0118-4.

[20] Knappe S, Lieb R, Beesdo K, Fehm L, Low NC, Gloster AT, Wittchen HU. The role of parental psychopathology and family environment for social phobia in the first three decades of life. Depression and Anxiety. 2009b;26,4:363–370. DOI: 10.1002/da.20527.

[21] Turner SM, Beidel DC, Roberson-Nay R, Tervo K. Parenting behaviors in parents with anxiety disorders. Behaviour Research and Therapy. 2003; 41,5:541–554. DOI: http://dx.doi.org/10.1016/S0005-7967(02)00028-1.

[22] Fisak B, Grills-Taquechel. Parental modeling, reinforcement, and information transfer: risk factors in the development of child anxiety? Clinical Child and Family Psychology. 2007;10:213–231. DOI:10.1007/s10567-007-0020-x.

[23] Ginsburg GS, Schlossberg MC. Family-based treatment of childhood anxiety disorders. International Review of Psychiatry. 2002;14:143–154. DOI: 10.1080/09540260220132662.

[24] Mellon RC, Moutavelis AG. Parental educational practices in relation to children's anxiety disorder-related behavior. Journal of Anxiety Disorders. 2011;25,6:829–834.

[25] Victor AM, Bernat DH, Bernstein GA, Layne AE. Effects of parent and family characteristics on treatment outcome of anxious children. Journal of Anxiety Disorders. 2007; 21,6:835–848. DOI: 10.1016/j.janxdis.2006.11.005.

[26] Manassis K, Hood J. Individual and familial predictors of impairment in childhood anxiety disorders. Journal of the American Academy of Child and Adolescent Psychiatry. 1998;37:428–434. DOI: 10.1097/00004583-199804000-00021.Rapee RM. Potential role of childrearing practices in the development of anxiety and depression. Clinical Psychology Review. 1997;17,1:47–67. DOI: 10.1016/S0272-7358(96)00040-2.

[27] Rapee RM. Potential role of childrearing practices in the development of anxiety and depression. Clinical Psychology Review. 1997;17,1:47–67. DOI: 10.1016/S0272-7358(96)00040-2.

[28] Hofmann SG, Anu Asnaani MA, Hinton D. Cultural aspects in social anxiety and social anxiety disorder. Depression and Anxiety. 2010;27,12:1117–1127. DOI: 10.1002/da.20759.

[29] Hong JJ, Woody SR. Cultural mediators of self-reported social anxiety. Behaviour Research and Therapy. 2007;45,8:1779–1789. DOI: 10.1016/j.brat.2007.01.011.

[30] Heinrichs N, Rapee RM, Alden LA, Bogels S, Hofman SG, Oh KJ, et al. Cultural differences in perceived social norms and social anxiety. Behaviour Research and Therapy. 2006;44:1187–1197. DOI: 10.1016/j.brat.2005.09.006.

[31] Bornschein S, Hausteiner C, Konrad F, Förstl H, Zilker T. Psychiatric morbidity and toxic burden in patients with environmental illness: a controlled study. Psychosomatic Medicine. 2006;68,1:104–109. DOI: 10.1097/01.psy.0000195723.38991.bf.

[32] Morrow LA, Gibson C, Bagovich GR, Stein L, Condray R, Scott A. Increased incidence of anxiety and depressive disorders in persons with organic solvent exposure. Psychosomatic Medicine. 2000;62,6:746–750. DOI: 10.1097/00006842-200011000-00002.

[33] Morrow LA, Stein L, Bagovich GR, Condray R, Scott A. Neuropsychological assessment, depression, and past exposure to organic solvents. Applied Neuropsychology. 2001; 2:65–73. DOI: 10.1207/S15324826AN0802_1.

[34] Hettema JM, Prescott CA, Myers JM, Neale MC, Kendler KS. The structure of genetic and environmental risk factors for anxiety disorders in men and women. Archives of General Psychiatry. 2005;62,2:182–189. DOI:10.1001/archpsyc.62.2.182.

[35] Perry BD. Childhood experience and the expression of genetic potential: what childhood neglect tells us about nature and nurture. Brain and Mind. 2002;3:79–100. DOI: 10.1023/A:1016557824657.

[36] Teicher MH. Wounds that time wouldn't heal: the neurobiology of childhood abuse. Cerebrum. 2000; 2:50–67. www.dana.org.

[37] Teicher MH, Andersen SL, Polcari A, Anderson CM, Navalta CP. Developmental neurobiology of childhood stress and trauma. Psychiatric Clinics of North America. 2002; 25:397–426. DOI: 10.1016/S0193-953X(01)00003-X.

[38] Gerra G, Zaimovic A, Zambelli U, Timpano M, Reali N, Bernasconi S, et al. Neuroendocrine responses to psychological stress in adolescents with anxiety disorder. Neuropsychobiology. 2000; 42:82–92. DOI:10.1159/000026677.

[39] Heim C, Nemeroff CB. The role of childhood trauma in the neurobiology of mood and anxiety disorders: preclinical and clinical studies. Biological Psychiatry. 2001;49,12:1023–1039. DOI: 10.1016/S0006-3223(01)01157-X.

[40] Anda RA, Felitti VJ, Bremner JD, Walker JD, Whitfield C, Perry BD, Dube SR, Giles WH. The enduring effects of abuse and related adverse experiences in childhood. A convergence of evidence from neurobiology and epidemiology. European Archives of Psychiatry and Clinical Neuroscience. 2006;256,3:174–186. DOI:10.1007/s00406-005-0624-4.

[41] Kessler RC, Davis CG, Kendler KS. Childhood adversity and adult psychiatric disorder in the US National Comorbidity Survey. Psychological Medicine. 1997;27:1101–1119. DOI: http://dx.doi.org/10.1017/S0033291797005588.

[42] Safren SA, Gershuny BS, Marzol P, Otto MW, Pollack MH. History of childhood abuse in panic disorder, social phobia, and generalized anxiety disorder. Journal of Nervous and Mental Disease. 2002; 190:453–456. DOI: 10.1097/00005053-200207000-00005.

[43] Lindesay J. Phobic disorders in the elderly. British Journal of Psychiatry. 1991;159:531–541. DOI: 10.1192/bjp.159.4.531.

[44] Kendler KS, Neale MC, Kessler RC, Heath AC, Eaves LJ. Childhood parental loss and adult psychopathology in women: a twin study perspective. Behaviour Research and Therapy. 1992;49:109–116. DOI: 10.1001/archpsyc.1992.01820020029004.

[45] Harris T, Brown GW, Bifulco A. Loss of parent in childhood and adult psychiatric disorder: the role of lack of adequate parental care. Psychological Medicine. 1986;16:641–659. DOI: http://dx.doi.org/10.1017/S0033291700010394.

[46] Fergusson DM, Horwood LJ, Lynskey MT. Childhood sexual abuse and psychiatric disorder in young adulthood, II: psychiatric outcomes of childhood sexual abuse. Journal of the American Academy of Child and Adolescent Psychiatry. 1996; 35:1365–1374. DOI: 10.1097/00004583-199610000-00024.

[47] Kendler KS, Bulik CM, Silberg J, Hettema JM, Myers J, Prescott CA. Childhood sexual abuse and adult psychiatric and substance use disorders in women: an epidemiological and cotwin control analysis. Archives of General Psychiatry. 2000;57:953–959. DOI: 10.1001/archpsyc.57.10.953.

[48] Espelage DL, Holt MK. Bullying and victimization during early adolescence. Peer influences and psychosocial correlates. Journal of Emotional Abuse. 2001;2,2–3:123–142. DOI: 10.1300/J135v02n02_08.

[49] Storch EA, Milsom VA, DeBraganza N, Lewin AB, Geffken GR, Silverstein JH. Peer victimization, psychosocial adjustment, and physical activity in overweight and at-risk-for-overweight youth. Journal of Pediatric Psychology. 2007; 32,1:80–89. DOI: 10.1093/jpepsy/jsj113.

[50] Kumpulainen K., Räsänen E. Children involved in bullying at elementary school age: their psychiatric symptoms and deviance in adolescence: an epidemiological sample. Child Abuse & Neglect. 2000;24,12:1567–1577. DOI:10.1016/S0145-2134(00)00210-6.

[51] Craig WM. The relationship among bullying, victimization, depression, anxiety, and aggression in elementary school children. Personality and Individual Differences. 1998;24,1:123–130. DOI: 10.1016/S0191-8869(97)00145-1.

[52] Kaltiala-Heino RA, RIMPELÄ M, Rantanen P, Rimpela A. Bullying at school—an indicator of adolescents at risk for mental disorders. Journal of Adolescence. 2000;23,6:661–674. DOI: 10.1006/jado.2000.0351.

[53] Grills AE, Ollendick TH. Peer victimization, global self-worth, and anxiety in middle school children. Journal of Clinical Child & Adolescent Psychology. 2002;31,1:59–68. DOI:10.1207/S15374424JCCP3101_08.

[54] Last CG, Francis G, Hersen M, et al. Separation anxiety and school phobia: a comparison using DSM III criteria. American Journal of Psychiatry. 1987;144,5:653–657. DOI.org/10.1176/ajp.144.5.653.

[55] Last CG, Perrin S, Hersen M, et al. DSM-III-R anxiety disorders in children: sociodemographic and clinical characteristics. Journal of the American Academy of Child and Adolescent Psychiatry. 1992; 31,6:1070–1076. DOI: 10.1097/00004583-199211000-00012.

[56] Velez CN, Johnson J, Cohen P. A longitudinal analysis of selected risk factors for childhood psychopathology. Journal of the American Academy of Child and Adolescent Psychiatry. 1989; 28,6:861–864. DOI: 10.1097/00004583-198911000-00009.

[57] Merikangas KR. Vulnerability factors for anxiety disorders in children and adolescents. Child and Adolescent Psychiatric Clinics of North America. 2005;14,4:649–6-79. DOI: 10.1016/j.chc.2005.06.005.

[58] Brook ChA, Schmidt LA. Social anxiety disorder: a review of environmental risk factors. Neuropsychiatric Disease Treatment. 2008;4,1:123–143. DOI: http://dx.doi.org/10.2147/NDT.S1799

[59] Skre l, Onstad S, Torgersen S, Philos DR, Lygren S, Kringlen E. The heritability of common phobic fear: a twin study of a clinical sample. Journal of Anxiety Disorders. 2000; 14 (6):549–562.

[60] Wittchen HU, Kessler RC, Pfister H, Lieb M. Why do people with anxiety disorders become depressed? A prospective-longitudinal community study. Acta Psychiatrica Scandinavica. Supplementum. 2000; 406:14–23. DOI: 10.1111/j.0065-1591.2000.acp29-03.x

[61] Merikangas KR, Avenevoli S, Dierker L, Grillon C. Vulnerability factors among children at risk for anxiety disorders. Biological Psychiatry. 1999 Dec 1;46(11):1523–1535. DOI: 10.1016/S0006-3223(99)00172-9.

[62] Johnson JG, Cohen P, Kasen S, Brook JS. Parental concordance and offspring risk for anxiety, conduct, depressive, and substance use disorders. Psychopathology. 2008; 41(2):124–128. DOI: 10.1159/000112028.

[63] Lieb R, Isensee B, Höfler M, Pfister H, Wittchen HU. Parental major depression and the risk of depression and other mental disorders in offspring: a prospective-longitu-

dinal community study. Archives of General Psychiatry. 2002 Apr;59(4):365–374. DOI: 10.1001/archpsyc.59.4.365.

[64] Weissman MM, Wickramaratne P, Nomura Y, Warner V, Pilowsky D, Verdeli H. Offspring of depressed parents: 20 years later. American Journal of Psychiatry. 2006 Jun; 163(6):1001–1008. DOI: 10.1176/appi.ajp.163.6.1001.

[65] Kendler KS, Davis CG, Kessler RC. The familial aggregation of common psychiatric and substance use disorders in the National Comorbidity Survey: a family history study. British Journal of Psychiatry. 1997; 170(June 1997):541–548. DOI: 10.1192/bjp. 170.6.541.

[66] Torgersen S. Genetic factors in anxiety disorders. Archives of General Psychiatry. 1983;40(10):1085–1089. DOI: 10.1001/archpsyc.1983.01790090047007.

[67] Kendler KS, Walters EE, Neale MC, Kessler RC, Heath AC, Eaves LJ. The structure of the genetic and environmental risk factors for six major psychiatric disorders in women: phobia, generalized anxiety disorder, panic disorder, bulimia, major depression, and alcoholism. Archives of General Psychiatry. 1995;52(5):374–383. DOI: 10.1001/archpsyc.1995.03950170048007.

[68] Topolski TD, Hewitt JK, Eaves LJ, Silberg JL, Meyer JM, Rutter M, Pickles A, Simonoff E. Genetic and environmental influences on child reports of manifest anxiety and symptoms of separation anxiety and overanxious disorders: a community based twin study. Behavior Genetics. 1997 Jan;27(1):15–28. DOI: 10.1023/A:1025607107566.

[69] Kendler KS, Neale MC, Kessler RC, Heath AC, Eaves LJ. Major depression and generalized anxiety disorder: same genes, (partly) different environments? Archives of General Psychiatry. 1992;49(9):716–722. DOI:10.1001/archpsyc.1992.

[70] Hettema JM, Neale MC, Kendler KS. A review and meta-analysis of the genetic epidemiology of anxiety disorders. American Journal of Psychiatry. 2001; 158:1568–1578. DOI: 10.1176/appi.ajp.158.10.1568.

[71] Maser JD, Cloninger CR (eds.). Comorbidity of Mood and Anxiety Disorders. Washington, DC, American Psychiatric Press, 1990.

[72] Roy MA, Neale MC, Pedersen NL, Mathé AA, Kendler KS. A twin study of generalized anxiety disorder and major depression. Psychological Medicine. 1995 Sep;25(5): 1037–1049. DOI: http://dx.doi.org/10.1017/S0033291700037533.

[73] Kendler KS. Major depression and generalised anxiety disorder. Same genes, (partly) different environments—revisited. British Journal of Psychiatry. Supplement. 1996 Jun;(30):68–75.

[74] Lesch KP, Bengel D, Heils A, Sabol SZ, Greenberg BD, Petri S, Benjamin J, Müller CR, Hamer DH, Murphy DL. Association of anxiety-related traits with a polymorphism in the serotonin transporter gene regulatory region. Science. 1996 Nov 29;274(5292): 1527–1531. DOI: 10.1126/science.274.5292.1527.

[75] Gelernter J, Bonvicini K, Page G, Woods SW, Goddard AW, Kruger S, Pauls DL, Goodson S. Linkage genome scan for loci predisposing to panic disorder or agoraphobia. Am T Med Genet 2001; 105 (6):548–557. DOI: 10.1002/ajmg.1496.

[76] Crowe RR, Goedken R, Samuelson S, Wilson R, Nelson J, Noyes R Jr. Genomewide survey of panic disorder. American Journal of Medicinal Genetics. 2001; 105 (I):105–109. DOI: 10.1002/1096-8628(20010108).

[77] Thorgerisson TE, Oskarsson H, Desnica N, Kostic JP, Stefansson JG, Kolbeinsson H, Lindal E, Gagunashvili N, Frigge ML, Kong A, Stefansson K, Gulcher JR. Anxiety with panic disorder linked to chromosome 9q in Iceland. American Journal of Human Genetics. 2003; 72 (5):1221–1230. DOI: 10.1086/375141.

[78] Binder EB. The role of FKBP5, a co-chaperone of the glucocorticoid receptor in the pathogenesis and therapy of affective and anxiety disorders. Psychoneuroendocrinology. 2009 Dec;34(Suppl 1):S186–S195. DOI: 10.1016/j.psyneuen.2009.05.021.

[79] Klengel T, Binder EB. Gene-environment interactions in major depressive disorder. Canadian Journal of Psychiatry. 2013 Feb;58(2):76–83.

[80] Klengel T, Mehta D, Anacker C, Rex-Haffner M, Pruessner JC, Pariante CM, Pace TW, Mercer KB, Mayberg HS, Bradley B, Nemeroff CB, Holsboer F, Heim CM, Ressler KJ, Rein T, Binder EB. Allele-specific FKBP5 DNA demethylation mediates gene-childhood trauma interactions. Nature Neuroscience. 2013 Jan;16(1):33–41. DOI: 10.1038/nn.3275.

[81] Pine DS, Cohen P, Gurley D, Brook J, Ma Y. The risk for early-adulthood anxiety and depressive disorders in adolescents with anxiety and depressive disorders, archives of general psychiatry. 1998;55,1:56–64. DOI: 10.1001/archpsyc.55.1.56.

[82] Asselmann E, Katja Beesdo-Baum K. Predictors of the course of anxiety disorders in adolescents and young. Current Psychiatry Reports. 2015;17:7. DOI: 10.1007/s11920-014-0543-z.

[83] Pluess M, Belsky J. Vantage sensitivity: individual differences in response to positive experiences. Psychological Bulletin. 2013; 139,4:901–916. DOI: 10.1037/a0030196.

[84] Degnan KA, Fox NA. Behavioural inhibition and anxiety disorders: multiple levels of a resilience process. Development and Psychopathology. 2007; 19:729–746. DOI: 10.1017/S0954579407000363.

[85] Donovan CL, Spence SH. Prevention of childhood anxiety disorders. Clinical Psychology Review. 2000; 20:509–531. DOI:10.1016/S0272-7358(99)00040-9.

Chapter 2

Examining Sex and Gender Differences in Anxiety Disorders

Dorte M. Christiansen

Additional information is available at the end of the chapter

http://dx.doi.org/10.5772/60662

Abstract

Several studies have examined sex differences in different anxiety disorders. Females are repeatedly found to be more likely than males to suffer from anxiety in general and to be diagnosed with most anxiety disorders, including agoraphobia (AG), panic disorder (PD), separation anxiety (SA), specific phobia (SP), social anxiety disorder (SAD), generalised anxiety disorder (GAD), obsessive-compulsive disorder (OCD), and acute and posttraumatic stress disorder (ASD and PTSD), although the latter three are technically no longer categorised as anxiety disorders according to DSM-5. This chapter provides an overview of research on sex and gender differences in anxiety disorders ranging from the well-established female preponderance in prevalence and severity to possible sex differences in the risk and protective factors associated with anxiety, sex differences in the clinical presentation of anxiety disorders, and potential sex differences in the effectiveness of different treatments. The chapter contains suggestions for future research, including important questions that remain to be answered.

Keywords: Sex differences, Gender differences, Anxiety disorders, OCD, PTSD, Acute stress disorder

1. Introduction

Anxiety disorders are the most prevalent group of psychiatric disorders [1]. It is well-documented that females are more likely than males to develop an anxiety disorder with lifetime and past-year rates of anxiety disorders being 1.5–2 times higher among females than males [2]. The increased prevalence of anxiety disorders in females has persisted independently of changes in the diagnostic criteria from DSM-III-R to DSM-IV [3, 4]. Sex differences in different anxiety disorders do not emerge at the same time, but sex differences in general anxiety levels emerge before the age of 4, and by age 6, anxiety levels in girls are about twice as high as in boys [5]. Once they have emerged, sex differences in DSM-IV anxiety disorders generally remain stable across age groups ranging from 18 years to 60+ years [6].

In spite of a few studies failing to find significant sex differences in the prevalence of anxiety disorders, clinical and community studies have generally reported higher rates of panic disorder (PD), agoraphobia (AG), specific phobias (SP), generalised anxiety disorder (GAD), separation anxiety (SA), and both acute and posttraumatic stress disorder (ASD and PTSD) in females compared to males [2, 3, 7, 8]. Sex differences are less pronounced for social anxiety disorder (SAD) and obsessive-compulsive disorder (OCD), and sex differences in the prevalence rates of these two disorders are not always significant [7, 9]. As can be seen in Table 1, lifetime prevalence rates of DSM-IV anxiety disorders range from 1.1% AG to 11.1% SAD in males and from 1.6% AG to 15.8% SP in females [3]. The three most prevalent anxiety disorders in males are SAD followed by SP and GAD [3]. In comparison, the three top-ranging anxiety disorders in females are SP, SAD, and PTSD. In spite of these widely reported sex differences in the prevalence and severity of anxiety disorders, sex differences in anxiety have been largely neglected compared to depression [10].

In the most recent edition of the diagnostic and statistical manual of mental disorders (DSM-5) [12], some of the anxiety disorders were re-arranged. As a consequence, ASD, PTSD, and OCD are no longer characterised as anxiety disorders. ASD and PTSD were moved to the new category trauma- and stressor-related disorders and OCD was relocated to the newly created category of obsessive-compulsive and related disorders. However, because these changes are still relatively recent, a limited amount of research has been published based on these categories of disorders. Furthermore, as a substantial amount of research has been conducted on these disorders in combination with other traditional anxiety disorders, it was considered expedient to include ASD, PTSD, and OCD in this chapter.

The inclusion of these three disorders further provides an opportunity to compare sex differences in ASD, PTSD, and OCD with sex differences in the disorders that have remained classified as anxiety disorders. Whereas ASD, PTSD, and OCD are no longer considered anxiety disorders, two new disorders have taken their place. In DSM-IV, selective mutism and SA were classified under the category of "Disorders usually first diagnosed in infancy, childhood, or adolescence" [13] but with the revisions carried out in the DSM-5, they were re-categorised as anxiety disorders [12]. Unfortunately, studies focusing specifically on sex differences in selective mutism are non-existing perhaps because the disorder is so rare that sex differences are rarely detected. Furthermore, this chapter will focus primarily on sex differences in adults, and research on selective mutism in adults is as hard to come by as research on sex differences. Thus, this chapter will examine the current status of research on sex differences in AG, ASD, GAD, OCD, PD, PTSD, SA, SAD, and SP.

Diagnosis	Males %[1]	Females %[1]	F:M ratio[2]	Classification[3]
AG	1.1	1.6	4:1	Substantial
ASD	-	-	-	-
GAD	4.2	7.1	3:1	Moderate
OCD	-	-	1:1	Moderate
PD	3.1	6.2	2:1 / 3:1[4]	Substantial
PTSD	3.6	9.7	2:1	Substantial
SA	-	-	OR = 1.4[5]	Substantial
SAD	11.1	13.0	1:1	Moderate
SP	8.9	15.8	2:1	Moderate
Any anxiety disorder	22.4	32.4	OR = 1.76[1]	-

Notes: GAD: generalised anxiety disorder; SAD: social anxiety disorder; PD: panic disorder; AG: agoraphobia; SP: specific phobia; PTSD: posttraumatic stress disorder; ASD: acute stress disorder; SA: separation anxiety; OR: Odds ratio for sex differences, OD >1 reflects higher prevalence in females.

[1]DSM-IV prevalence rates (and OR for any anxiety disorder) based on the NCS-R and published by Gum et al. [3].

[2]DSM-IV-TR female-to-male ratios published by Bekker et al. [7] (except for SA and any anxiety disorder).

[3]Classifications presented by Mackinaw-Koons & Vasey [11].

Substantial differences: females exceed males by at least 100%

Moderate differences: females exceed males by 33–99%

[4]PD with AG/PD without AG

[5]Prevalence for males and females combined is 6.6%. Prevalence and OR published by Shear et al. [8].

Table 1. Lifetime prevalence of DSM-IV anxiety disorders in adult males and females

1.1. Overview of relevant studies on sex differences in anxiety disorders since 2010

A search of studies on sex or gender differences in the different anxiety disorders published and indexed in PsycINFO and/or PubMed from 2010 until the end of 2014 was conducted. Search criteria can be seen in Table 2.

The literature search only included articles identified through the searches in PsycINFO and PubMed, even though articles published in the same period but not identified in these searches, may have been included in this chapter. The reasoning behind this is that the searches were intended to give an overview of the amount of sex/gender research published in relation to the different disorders over a period of 5 years. In addition, studies were excluded that did not focus primarily on anxiety disorders, focused on animals, focused primarily on children and younger adolescents, were not written in English, or were published as book chapters or dissertations. Articles were categorised as either relevant or not relevant based on whether their focus was on sex differences in the specific disorders. Furthermore, articles were classified as uniquely relevant to a specific anxiety disorder if that disorder was the sole focus of the article. Because many studies report sex differences in the prevalence or severity of anxiety without mentioning this in the abstract, only studies that examined sex differences beyond this level (i.e., tried to explain these differences – or absence thereof – or examined moderation effects or sex differences in specific symptoms etc.) were categorised as relevant. In addition, studies that did not focus on specific anxiety disorders and studies that examined specific subsamples of limited general relevance (e.g., sex differences in anxiety in patients undergoing treatment for substance dependence) were not categorised as relevant. Finally, articles that did not present original research or conduct thorough reviews or meta-analyses were not included.

An overview of articles identified in the searches can be seen in Table 3. Several of the studies were indexed in both of the databases. Such overlap was taken into account, which reduced the number of total articles identified somewhat. As can be seen in Table 3, more studies have been published on sex differences in PTSD than in any other anxiety disorder within the past 5 years.

	Keywords
Abstract	"General anxiety disorder" OR "generalised anxiety disorder" OR "generalized anxiety disorder" "Obsessive compulsive disorder" OR "obsessive-compulsive disorder" OR OCD "Specific phobia" "PTSD" OR "post-traumatic stress disorder" OR "posttraumatic stress disorder" "Acute stress disorder" "Panic disorder" "Agoraphobia" "Social phobia" OR "social anxiety disorder" "Separation anxiety"
Abstract	"Sex differences" OR "Gender differences"
Publication date	2010–2014

Note: At least one keyword from each row had to be present in the title/abstract for articles to be identified in the search

Table 2. Search criteria for sex/gender differences in anxiety studies published 2010–2015

Between 1 and 11 relevant studies were identified on sex differences in AG, GAD, OCD, PD, and SAD, whereas no relevant studies were identified on sex differences in ASD, SA, and PD. Quite a few of the studies published examined sex differences in several disorders, resulting in substantial overlap between the articles identified in the different searches. As a result of this, the number of unique articles identified in the searches of each disorder was substantially reduced for most of the disorders. The two exceptions to this were OCD where 5 of the 7 articles identified were unique and PTSD where a full 95.6% of the articles were unique. For the remaining diagnoses, between 0 and 5 articles were identified that were unique to each disorder. This overview of studies published within the past 5 years highlights the need for more research examining sex differences in anxiety. With the exception of PTSD, the number of published articles identified including sex or gender differences in the abstract is very low, and this number is reduced even further, when results are limited to those specifically focusing on sex or gender differences in relation to each disorder. The difference in numbers between the studies originally identified and the studies categorised as relevant suggests that future research on sex differences in anxiety should be much more focused. For this reason, the purpose of this chapter is to give an overview of what is presently known about sex differences in anxiety disorders and what still remains to be examined. Thus, this chapter may be read as a guide to research on sex and gender differences in anxiety disorders, summarising what is currently known and posing relevant questions for future research to answer.

Diagnosis	PubMed total	PsycINFO total	Total	Relevant	Uniquely relevant
AG	3	4	5	1	0
ASD	1	1	2	0	0
GAD	15	20	24	6	1
OCD	18	23	27	7	5
PD	23	21	27	9	4
PTSD	111	115	15	91	87
SA	6	6	9	0	0
SAD	23	28	21	11	5
SP	6	6	6	0	0

Note: AG: agoraphobia; ASD: acute stress disorder; GAD: generalised anxiety disorder; OCD: obsessive-compulsive disorder; PD: panic disorder; PTSD: posttraumatic stress disorder; SA: separation anxiety; SAD: social anxiety disorder; SP: specific phobia

Table 3. Results from literature search on sex/gender differences in the different anxiety disorders

2. Sex and gender differences in anxiety research

2.1. Sex differences in anxiety

A vast amount of research has documented sex differences in brain regions involved in cognition, memory, and affect [14]. In spite of important sex differences in the structure and function of the brain, most research on the brain's involvement in learning, memory, fear conditioning, and fear extinction has been conducted on male populations, as less than 2% of studies in these areas have focused on females [14]. However, what little research has been conducted has uncovered both structural and functional sex differences in brain regions relevant to anxiety, including the prefrontal cortex, hippocampus, and the extended amygdala complex. For example, significant genetic differences between males and females with OCD have been reported, although findings are sometimes contradictory and replication is needed [15, 16]. Furthermore, blood pressure and pulse have been reported to be more reactive to anxiety in females compared to males [17]. As a result of such sex differences, females appear to be more easily conditioned than males [7, 18], and males and females have also been found to differ in fear extinction [18]. One way through which biological sex differences can affect anxiety disorders is through gonadal hormones.

Important sex differences have been reported in several brain and bodily functions associated with anxiety [14]. Female gonadal hormones, such as oestrogen and progesterone appear to have substantial effects on the functions of anxiety-related neurotransmitter systems and affect fear extinction [14, 19]. Similarly, among the male gonadal hormones, testosterone has been found to have anxiolytic effects [20], possibly by reducing responsiveness to stress and suppressing activity of the hypothalamic pituitary adrenal (HPA) axis [20]. For this reason, gonadal hormones are likely to account for at least part of the increased prevalence and severity of anxiety disorders in females. Fluctuations in oestrogen and progesterone throughout the female menstrual cycle appear to affect HPA axis reactivity, glucocorticoid feedback sensitivity, and brain GABA connections, causing the homeostatic system to become less stable in females compared to males [17]. Such fluctuations may cause both short-term instability in females and be responsible for more long-term changes in the severity of anxiety symptoms occurring in relation to puberty, pregnancy, lactation, and menopause [17, 19, 20]. Support for the effects of monthly and major lifetime hormone fluctuations on anxiety in females comes from findings that self-reported changes in OCD and PD symptoms related to the female reproductive cycle and the occurrence of pregnancy and menopause have been found [10, 16, 17, 19]. The importance of gonadal hormones is further supported by findings that manipulating them can have consequences. For example, prolonged use of oral contraceptives appears to alter the reactivity of the HPA axis to psychological stress [21], thereby affecting the prevalence and severity of anxiety symptoms in females.

Altemus has made an interesting point in arguing that there may have been an evolutionary advantage in both the HPA axis and the catecholamine stress response system being suppressed during pregnancy and lactation, as it is a very recent development in evolutionary terms that females no longer spend the majority of the years between puberty and menopause being either pregnant or lactating [17]. Thus, the increased prevalence of depression and anxiety in females may be a recent development, as the primary female defence against these disorders is made ineffective in modern human society.

2.2. Gender differences in anxiety

It has been suggested, that sex differences in the development of internalising and externalising disorders may be partly attributable to differences in socialisation processes that are intensified during adolescence and activate concepts of masculinity and femininity [22]. Such gender-roles are likely to affect sex differences in anxiety. For example, there are some indications that sex differences in PTSD are smaller or even non-existing in male-dominated professions where females assume more masculine gender-roles [23]. Whereas femininity and masculinity were originally considered opposite ends of a continuum, they are now most commonly believed to exist independently of each other [24]. Masculinity/femininity measured on a single scale has been found to correlate negatively with manifest anxiety, indicating that males and females with high femininity scores report more anxiety [25]. However, when measured separately, femininity has been reported to be unassociated with AG and related measures, whereas masculinity is negatively associated with AG severity, trait anxiety, social anxiety, and avoidance behaviour in general [7, 24]. Furthermore, masculinity scores for both male and female patients with AG were found to be significantly lower than in community samples [26]. The protective function of masculinity is equally strong in males and females and has been found both in adults and in children suffering from various anxiety disorders [7, 24]. One study reported that sex was no longer associated with avoidance in patients with AG when masculinity was controlled for [26]. These findings suggest that the lower levels of masculinity in females compared to males may at least partly account for sex differences in anxiety. In contrast to masculinity, masculine gender-role stress, defined as stress resulting from rigid commitment to gender-roles in combination with dysfunctional coping, has been reported to be associated with certain characteristics of OCD as well as increased fears related to AG, blood, and social situations [7].

Gender-roles may affect sex differences in anxiety reports in at least two ways [27]. Identification with a masculine gender–role may cause a person to underreport anxiety symptoms [7, 27], resulting in a reporting bias. Some support for an underreporting of fear and anxiety in males has been found in a study that reported an increase in fear reports in males, but not in females, when their physiological fear reactions were being monitored and participants believed that lying would be detected [27]. However, other studies have found that sex differences in anxiety are not simply a result of sex differences in social desirability [10, 28]. In addition, it is possible for socialisation processes to result in actual sex differences in anxiety levels. From childhood, males are generally encouraged to confront feared objects, resulting in a greater exposure and extinction of fear responses in males compared to females, for whom avoidance and fearful behaviour is less likely to be dissuaded [9]. Furthermore, as females are more likely to ruminate than males [9], sex differences in recall bias may cause females to report more prior symptoms of anxiety. In accordance with this, depression research comparing baseline and follow-up reports of depressive episodes have found that females are more likely to recall new depressive episodes at follow-up, whereas males are more likely to forget previously reported episodes [22]. Finally, gender differences in the division of work status, socioeconomic status, and social roles may leave females more vulnerable to anxiety disorders than males [7], as males and females are exposed to different types of environmental stressors, which is likely to affect their susceptibility to anxiety disorders. For example, females are more at risk of being exposed to certain potentially traumatic events, such as sexual trauma and domestic abuse, as well as relationship stressors [9].

2.2.1. Summary and discussion of sex and gender influences in anxiety

Sex differences in anxiety have been reported universally and such consistencies in sex differences across cultures suggest a biological component. However, whereas sex differences in PTSD have been found to be culturally persistent, variations have been reported in the strength of these sex differences across cultures, suggesting that both biological sex and cultural gender play a role in differences between male and female PTSD severity [23]. Similarly, examining the lifetime prevalence of different DSM-III-R anxiety disorders, the National Comorbidity Survey (NCS) reported a significant interaction between sex and ethnic group on lifetime prevalence of anxiety disorders [29], suggesting that some inter-cultural variation in the extent of sex differences in anxiety disorders does occur. Also, in spite of their general presence, gender differences in anxiety symptoms are often non-significant in college students [28], suggesting that the strength of sex differences in anxiety may also differ between subcultures.

Unfortunately, potential interaction effects for specific anxiety disorders in the NCS were not examined, and thus it is unknown whether sex differences in the severity and prevalence of certain anxiety disorders are more stable than others across different ethnic groups and cultures. It has been suggested that PD may be more strongly related to physiological factors than the other anxiety disorders [30]. It is thus possible that differences between males and females with PD have more to do with sex and less to do with gender than what may be the case for the other anxiety disorders. Furthermore, the relative importance of sex and gender may differ for specific symptoms or groups of symptoms. There are some indications in PTSD research that sex differences in arousal are related primarily to biological sex differences, whereas sex differences in avoidance and re-experiencing are relatively more affected by social gender differences [23]. It is highly likely that similar variation can be found in other anxiety disorders, causing sex differences in certain symptoms, gender differences in others, and similarities between males and females in yet other symptoms.

Both sex and gender influences appear to contribute to the development of sex differences in anxiety, and telling them apart can be quite difficult. Whereas the changes in sex differences associated with the onset of puberty and menopause are often interpreted as support of the importance of gonadal hormones, such developments may equally well be explained by changes in gender-related variables, such as relationship and family status, social status, and gender-role identification [31]. Influences of sex and gender are likely to work together both at the societal and the individual level. Several gender differences in society are likely to build on pre-existing sex differences, such as those related to brain structure and functioning, physiological stress response, and influences of gonadal hormones. For example, features associated with femininity were probably originally based on sex differences and shaped by evolution. The increased prevalence of such traits in females is likely to have caused society to expect such traits in women, allowing socialisation processes to further strengthen the association between femininity and being female. Similarly, it is possible that if the same traits have been preferred in women by society for long enough for evolutionary processes to come into play, such traits may over time become biologically based, even if this was not originally the case. A similar process may take place at the individual level, where it has been argued that articulated traits are likely to reflect a complex, bidirectional process between inherent genetic vulnerabilities and socialisation experiences [2, 22].

Although sex differences in anxiety disorders are generally well-documented, the degree to which such differences can be accounted for by biological sex or cultural gender differences is unclear. More studies are needed to examine whether the impact of sex and gender influences are equal for different anxiety disorders. In spite of the fact that the female brain has been largely ignored in research on the brain processes behind fear and anxiety, sex differences have been reported in relevant areas of the brain, and gonadal hormones appear to be heavily involved in anxiety. These results are very promising and point strongly to the importance of more studies being conducted on the female brain. Such studies should include the impact of gonadal hormones, the female menstrual cycle, oral contraceptives, and HRT on anxiety symptoms as well as sex differences in fear networks and HPA axis reactivity. Also gender differences need to be more thoroughly studied in future research. Important gender-related concepts that invite further scrutiny include gender-roles, gender-role stress, and sexual identity. Another way to further examine the influences of gender on anxiety is to conduct more studies that examine cultural and subcultural influences on sex differences in anxiety. As previously mentioned, sex differences in trait anxiety were found to be more pronounced in Israeli compared to American college students [28]. However, although the American and Israeli college populations are likely to differ on a number of parameters, other cultures may differ even more, and these cultures will need to be included in future studies on cultural variations in sex differences in anxiety.

· Sex differences in anxiety are universally reported but their strength may vary across cultures, suggesting that both sex and gender influences are important.
· The relative importance of sex versus gender may vary for different disorders and specific symptoms or groups of symptoms.
· Biological sex can affect anxiety through differences in brain structuring and organisation and through gonadal hormones, and female hormonal fluctuations caused by the menstrual cycle and major lifetime hormonal influences (e.g., puberty, oral contraceptives, pregnancy, lactation, menopause).
· Sex differences in reactivity to stress associated with differences in HPA axis activation, increased fear conditioning in females, and a less stable female homeostatic system have been reported.
· Gender influences may be based on socialisation processes that activate gender-roles associated with masculinity and femininity.
· Masculinity is associated with decreased anxiety reports in both males and females, whereas femininity is unassociated with anxiety. Gender-role stress has been reported to increase anxiety.
· Socialisation processes may result in reporting bias, memory bias, and actual differences in anxiety levels.
· The latter may be affected by gender differences in work status, socioeconomic status, social roles, and exposure to different stressors (e.g., sexual assault, domestic abuse, relationship stressors).
· Future research should focus on gonadal hormones, the female menstrual cycle, oral contraceptives, HRT, HPA axis reactivity, fear networks, gender-roles, gender-role stress, sexual identity, and cultural/sub-cultural variations in sex differences in anxiety.

Table 4. Summary points for sex and gender influences in anxiety

2.3. Accounting for sex differences in anxiety severity

As both biological influences of sex and cultural influences of gender appear to be involved in the genesis of sex differences in anxiety, any model attempting to account for such differences must take both these types of influences into account. A thorough discussion of the different theories that have been used to explain different aspects of sex differences in anxiety is beyond the scope of this chapter. Furthermore, instead of simply explaining sex differences in the prevalence and severity of anxiety, a good theory should also be able to predict and explain differences between males and females once an anxiety disorder is present as well as sex differences between anxiety and associated variables and potential sex differences in the outcome of different approaches to treatment. As will be made clear later in this chapter, sex differences in these other areas of anxiety research are nowhere near as well-established as those in relation to the prevalence and severity of anxiety. Thus, rather than attempting to explain sex differences in anxiety, it is worth looking into how far research has come in its endeavours to account for sex differences in anxiety severity.

The mediation hypothesis suggests that sex differences in anxiety severity may be explained by the fact that several risk factors of anxiety are more prevalent in females than in males [10, 32]. Several such individual risk factors have been examined. In particular, prior sexual assault and abuse have been put forward as possible explanations for why females develop more anxiety, and specifically more PTSD, than males. However, sex differences in PTSD exist across all trauma types [33] and even prior sexual trauma has been found to account for only a small part of the association between sex and PTSD [32, 34]. In general, most studies have found that when examined individually, even the most promising potential mediators cannot fully account for sex differences in anxiety. Instead, several potential mediators are likely to work together.

A recent study found that a combination of 10 pre-, peri-, and posttraumatic risk factors could account for 83% of the association between sex and PTSD severity in bank employees exposed to robbery [32]. The strongest mediators in this mediation model were peritraumatic emotional responses and posttraumatic cognitions, although the authors argued that it was the combined effect of mediators, rather than the few uniquely significant variables, that were responsible for accounting for such a large proportion of sex differences in PTSD severity. Similarly, Leach and colleagues tested a multivariate mediation model consisting of 35 socio-demographic, psychological, and social mediators in three age groups [31]. Sex differences were most pronounced in the youngest age group (20–24 years) but were also significant in the other two (40–44 years and 60–64 years). Although several of these potential mediators contributed significantly to sex differences in anxiety, sex remained a significant predictor of anxiety in the youngest age group. In contrast, the combination of mediators fully accounted for sex differences in anxiety in the two older age groups. Adding rumination and neuroticism improved all three models, but sex still remained significant in the youngest age group [31]. The total and direct effects found in this study were obtained from the first author (Liana Leach, personal communication, January 2015). These were used to calculate how much of the association between sex and anxiety could be accounted for by the mediators. In the two older age groups, the mediators accounted for a similar amount of the association whether or not rumination and neuroticism were included (92–97%). Although this does look impressive, it is important to bear in mind that the total effects were very small in these two age groups (both c's <0.095), suggesting that the impact of sex on anxiety, though significant, was negligible. Thus, although mediation did occur in the two older age groups, this was not clinically relevant. However, in the younger population, sex had a much larger direct effect on anxiety ($c = 0.233$). In this population, the first mediation model accounted for 43.5% of the association between sex and anxiety. When rumination and neuroticism were included, the model accounted for 56.1% of the impact of sex on anxiety. Finally, Lewinsohn and colleagues used an ANOVA and logistic regression analysis to examine whether 10 psychosocial variables could account for sex differences in anxiety levels in high school students [10]. The impact of sex on diagnostic status remained largely unaltered after controlling for the impact of the 10 variables [10]. Together, results from these three studies suggest that several potential mediators are needed to fully account for sex differences in anxiety and particularly strong risk factors, such as neuroticism, emotional response, and subsequent negative cognitions and rumination, are necessary to include in such models. Interestingly, these variables appear to represent the presence of both biological and environmental influences on sex differences in anxiety. Whereas neuroticism appears to have a large hereditary component, emotional responses are more likely to be affected by socialisation processes [9]. Thus, it is most likely that any model attempting to account for sex differences in anxiety must include both sex-related and gender-related components.

One way in which gender and sex may work together to cause sex differences in anxiety is through a diathesis-stress model. Inspired by the arguments presented by Parker and Brotchie [22], the diathesis component of such a model may represent an inherent preparedness in females towards readily responding with anxiety when faced with a stressor. This inherent preparedness most likely consists of biologically grounded traits, such as neuroticism, anxiety sensitivity, and trait anxiety, along with HPA axis reactivity, limbic system hyperactivation, and similar biologically based systems. In accordance with this, it has been suggested that sex differences in anxiety may largely correspond with a larger genetic predisposition to anxiety and to general vulnerability traits in females compared to males [9]. Whereas biological sex differences result in an inherent vulnerability towards anxiety in females, cultural gender may further increase sex differences in the development of specific anxiety disorders through the stress component of the diathesis-stress model. The different roles that males and females hold in society are associated with exposure to different daily and traumatic stressors that can trigger the development of specific anxiety disorders and further increase sex differences in such disorders [20, 23]. Among the stressors that are most prevalent in females are sexual trauma, domestic abuse, and low socioeconomic status. In addition, it has been suggested that the social and environmental influences experienced by females may support the genetic predisposition, whereas experiences in males may be more likely to counteract such predispositions [9]. Some support has been offered for the possibility that the impact of genetic factors may be greater in females compared to males even in the absence of sex differences in the distribution of such genetic factors [9].

2.3.1. Summary and discussion of mediation studies

Mediation studies show great promise in helping researchers account for sex differences in the prevalence and severity of anxiety. However, very little is known about how different mediators may work together to account for sex differences. Furthermore, several potential mediators remain unstudied. For example, Bekker and Mens-Verhulst suggest that future studies examine sex/gender differences in the meanings being contributed to feared and avoided situations [7]. For example, although an interpersonal assault, such as a robbery, may not contain any element of sexual assault, it is still likely to be differently interpreted by a female compared to a male victim, as the whole experience is more likely to be shaped by fear of the assault becoming sexual in the female's case. The studies reviewed here suggest in accordance with the diathesis-stress model that both variables associated with biological sex and variables associated with cultural gender will need to be included as potential mediators for such mediation models to account for a substantial amount of sex differences in the prevalence and severity of anxiety. It is important that such future mediation studies are designed properly. In addition to being theoretically driven and including as many relevant potential mediators as possible, it is important that future studies build on prior research and include mediators that have previously been found to be among the strongest mediators of sex differences in anxiety. Neuroticism, rumination, emotional response, and negative cognitions have been found to be strong candidates to be included in future studies. Furthermore, potential mediators should represent both pre-existing risk and protective factors, stressor-related factors that appear to be involved in triggering the development of specific anxiety disorders, and maintaining factors involved in the continued presence or worsening of anxiety symptoms. Finally, future mediation studies should use statistical analyses designed specifically for testing multivariate mediation models [35].

· The mediation hypothesis suggests that the higher prevalence of anxiety symptoms in females can be accounted for by a higher female prevalence of related risk factors and a higher male prevalence of protective factors.
· Although several such variables have been proposed and examined, it appears that no single risk factor can sufficiently account for the increased anxiety in females. Instead, a combination of risk factors is needed.
· Multivariate mediation models show great promise helping researchers account for the preponderance of females in anxiety disorders.
· The diathesis-stress theory suggests that both an increased inherent vulnerability towards anxiety in females and different exposure to stressors contribute to sex differences in anxiety.
· The diathesis part of the model may manifest as a psychological (e.g., neuroticism, anxiety sensitivity, trait anxiety) and/or a physiological (HPA axis reactivity, limbic system hyperactivation) preparedness to respond to stressors with anxiety.
· The stress part of the model concerns different environmental factors that are associated with the development of anxiety (e.g., socioeconomic status, socialisation, minority status, everyday stressors, and traumatic exposure).
· The diathesis-stress theory is a great example of how influences of sex and gender can work together to affect the development of anxiety and increase prevalence rates in females compared to males.
· The diathesis-stress theory can be used to guide future mediation studies, as it suggests that both the diathesis and the stress component should be represented in multivariate mediation models.
· Future studies should include multiple mediators, including variables that have not previously been studied and variables found to be important in previous studies (e.g., neuroticism, rumination, emotional response, negative cognitions), as well as pre-existing, stressor-related, and maintaining factors.
· Future studies should use statistical methods developed specifically for testing multivariate mediation models.

Table 5. Summary points for accounting for sex differences in anxiety severity

The mediation hypothesis is neither a theory of sex differences in anxiety nor can it replace such theories. Rather, it may represent a way for sex differences in associated variables to affect sex differences in anxiety disorders. Which specific variables are relevant and why they affect anxiety levels are among the questions that we need good theories of sex differences in anxiety to answer. Furthermore, even if future mediation studies can fully account for sex differences in different anxiety disorders, this does not get us any closer to understanding these sex differences, if we still do not know why sex differences exist in the mediators [32]. In addition, sex differences in anxiety disorders appear to go beyond a higher prevalence and symptom severity in females. Even if a combination of different risk factors can fully account for why females report more anxiety symptoms than males, we still do not know whether these risk factors predict anxiety equally well in males and females. As has previously been suggested specifically for PTSD [23, 32], sex differences in anxiety are likely to involve both mediation and moderation effects. The association between anxiety symptoms and other variables, such as risk and protective factors, comorbidity, and treatment efficacy, may differ in males and females and may ultimately cause the two sexes to follow separate pathways to the different anxiety disorders.

2.4. Sex as a moderator in anxiety research

Doing a systematic review of moderation effects of sex in anxiety disorders is made extremely difficult by the fact that such moderation effects are rarely mentioned in the abstracts of the articles reporting them. Very often such moderation analyses appear to be conducted on little more than an afterthought and are rarely given much attention. For this reason, the results presented in this section do not represent a thorough or systematic discussion of how sex moderates important associations in anxiety research. Rather, the results presented here are meant as an appetizer, highlighting the importance of conducting such research – both within the field of anxiety and in relation to other mental disorders.

Some moderation effects may affect detection and self-reporting of anxiety in males and females. One study reported that primary care physicians detected ICD-10 GAD, panic disorder, and agoraphobia equally well in males and females, suggesting that sex differences in the prevalence rates of these disorders are not caused by detection bias [36]. However, the same study found that females were slightly more likely than males to be falsely diagnosed with an ICD-10 affective or anxiety disorder, suggesting that prevalence rates may be artificially inflated in females compared to males, although the impact of this on sex differences in prevalence rates are most likely negligible. Furthermore, whereas social desirability cannot account for sex differences in anxiety, males may be more likely than females to be biased by social desirability. One study reported that social desirability was only significantly correlated with state anxiety in males, and that the correlation between social desirability and trait anxiety, although significant in both males and females, was stronger in males [28]. However, the original study did not test whether these sex differences were significant. For the purpose of this chapter, the correlation coefficients and male and female population sizes reported in the original study were used to conduct a Z-test to examine the significance of the reported sex differences in the associations. This test revealed that sex did not significantly moderate the associations between social desirability and trait or state anxiety (both Z's < 1.75; two-tailed tests).

In addition to such moderation effects relevant to the prevalence and severity of anxiety disorders, moderation effects may be of tremendous theoretical and clinical importance when they affect associations between risk factors and the development of different anxiety disorders. The presence of such moderation effects may cause males and females to primarily follow different pathways to these disorders. For example, sex differences in the initial response to a traumatic event and subsequent moderation effects of sex on associations between PTSD and multiple correlates have been combined in a preliminary model suggesting sex-specific pathways to PTSD [23]. Although the existence of such sex-specific pathways have not been identified in adults, it is possible that they exist both in PTSD and other anxiety disorders where certain risk or protective factors are found to be predictive of symptoms only in males or females.

A study on SAD severity in graduate students found that the impact of independence and interdependence on social anxiety was moderated by sex. Whereas the association between social anxiety severity and independence was negative in males, it was positive in females [24]. The authors suggest that in accordance with self-discrepancy theory, social anxiety arises in individuals who perceive their social role and behaviour to be inconsistent with the expectations of others, causing social anxiety to arise in different situations for males and females. Similarly, another study found that there was a trend ($p = 0.07$) towards submissive behaviour being more strongly and positively associated with social anxiety in males compared to females [37]. These analyses were conducted in a relatively small sample, suggesting that submissive behaviour may prove in future studies to be more relevant to social anxiety, and possibly other types of anxiety, in males if examined in larger populations. Finally, more complicated analyses have found a significantly stronger association between submissive behaviours and shame in males compared to females with SAD [37]. This illustrates that sex is also an important variable to consider in future studies when examining the interactions between different variables and their impact on anxiety disorders.

Sex differences may also exist in the association between exposure to different stressors and the development of anxiety disorders. One study found that the occurrence of childhood trauma in patients with OCD differed between males and females, with sexual abuse being more common in females and emotional neglect being more common in males [16]. It is likely that such sex differences in prior traumatic events in clinical samples merely represent sex differences in the general exposure to such events. However, another possibility is that childhood trauma and severe stressors may play a stronger role in the development of OCD in males than in females. For example, it has been suggested that early brain trauma may be particularly involved in the early development of OCD in males [16, 38], whereas other stressful events are more likely to precipitate OCD in females [16]. It is further possible that sex differences exist in the associations between specific or general stressful and traumatic events and the development of different anxiety disorders. In addition to the possibility that different traumatic or stressful events may precipitate anxiety in males and females, it is possible that males and females may differ in the degree to which anxiety is associated with hereditary or environmental factors.

In general, the heritability of anxiety-related vulnerability factors, such as neuroticism, anxiety sensitivity, and trait anxiety have been found to be greater in females compared to males, and higher heritability estimates for fears and phobias have similarly been found in females in both child and adolescent samples [9]. In accordance with this, an Australian twin study found that 41% of SA in females was attributable to hereditary/genetic factors, whereas 58% was attributable to unique environmental factors, and only 2% to shared environmental factors [39]. In contrast, hereditary factors made no contribution to male SA, which could in turn be contributed to 73% unique environmental factors and 27% shared environmental factors. Two other studies have also reported sex differences in the influence of hereditary and environmental factors in SA. These studies found that the genetic contribution to SA was 50–75% in females but only 0–14% in males [11]. In accordance with a stronger environmental component to male SA, two studies have found that separation from fathers and overprotective parenting are associated with increased early separation anxiety symptoms in males only [39].

In contrast to the findings in SA, a study examining the heritability of OCD in children separately for males and females found that two out of three OCD dimensions were significantly inheritable in males with 60–65% of the variance in these two dimensions being attributable to genetic factors [28]. In contrast, none of the three dimensions were found to be inheritable in females. In addition, another study found a higher correlation between state and trait anxiety in males (0.456) compared to females (0.385). The authors deducted that situational factors may exert a greater impact on anxiety symptoms in females compared to males. However, they did not test whether this moderation effect was significant. For the purpose of this chapter, a Z-score was calculated using the information provided by the authors relating to the number of male and female participants and the two correlation coefficients [28]. This analysis provided a Z-score of 0.81, implying that although the correlation between state and trait anxiety appears to be stronger for males than females, this difference was not significant at the $p < 0.05$ level.

2.4.1. Summary and discussion of moderation effects

Research on moderation effects of sex on associations between anxiety and associated variables is very scarce. The few studies presented here are evidence that sex may have the potential to moderate important associations in anxiety research. In accordance with this, several researchers have called for more studies examining the impact of sex/gender on the epidemiology of anxiety disorders [2, 23]. Future research on moderation effects may involve any associations thought to be relevant in anxiety research. Whereas studies on mediation effects should focus on risk factors more prevalent in females and protective factors more prevalent in males, any variable thought to be associated with anxiety may be moderated by sex. Moderation effects are highly relevant to examine when studying risk and protective factors of anxiety disorders, as they may help researchers make sense of inconsistent findings. If a risk factor is only sometimes found to predict anxiety, this may be due to sex differences in its predictive value.

At this early stage, research may be guided by preliminary research hypotheses. For example, Christiansen and Elklit have presented a preliminary model of potential sex-specific pathways to PTSD based on sex differences in the physiological stress response [23]. This model suggests that variables such as dissociation, social support, and emotion-focused coping may be particularly involved in the development and maintenance of PTSD, and possibly other anxiety disorders, in females compared to males. In contrast, physiological arousal, anxiety, avoidant coping, and problem-focused coping may be more strongly associated with PTSD in males.

Another hypothesis used to guide moderation research could be based on the results regarding the apparently stronger genetic component in SA in females compared to males. It is possible that this moderation effect is specific to SA, perhaps because SA has represented an evolutionary advantage in females but not in males [39]. However, another possibility is that the increased hereditary effect in females is generalised to other anxiety disorders, with the likely exception of OCD. If that is the case, then biological risk and protective factors may prove more important in female compared to male anxiety disorders. Furthermore, this would suggest that personality traits with a high degree of heritability, such as neuroticism, trait anxiety, and similar variables are likely to be more strongly associated with SA in females compared to males. In contrast, variables associated with upbringing, personal experience, and environmental factors, such as employment status, socioeconomic status, and recent stressors, may be more important to male anxiety. In accordance with this, Silove and colleagues suggested that unless specifically challenged by distinctive environmental stressors, males are less likely to develop high levels of SA in childhood and adolescence [39]. If a similar hereditary component exists for females in other anxiety disorders, making females genetically more vulnerable to developing symptoms of anxiety, males may only develop such disorders if they are exposed to certain environmental stressors associated with each disorder.

Finally, the diathesis-stress model may be used to guide research on moderation effects of sex in anxiety. Because this model would suggest an inherent vulnerability to anxiety that is stronger in females compared to males, this would also result in hypotheses of physiological variables and hereditary traits being more important to anxiety in females compared to males. However, this model would not necessarily lead to hypotheses stating that environmental factors would be more strongly associated with anxiety in males. Rather, environmental factors could be expected to be equally important to anxiety in males and females, or certain variables could be particularly important in males and others in females. Regardless of the hypotheses used to guide moderation research, it is important that more such research is carried out. If sex differences exist in the ability of different risk and protective factors to predict anxiety disorders, this may point to the existence of sex-specific pathways to different anxiety disorders. Furthermore, if different risk factors dominate in males and females, this may result in sex differences once an anxiety disorder exists. Such sex differences may affect the age of onset, course, comorbidity, and general clinical presentation of different anxiety disorders in males and females.

There are different ways of examining moderation effects. One way is by examining interaction effects in ANOVA or regression analyses. These analyses make it easy to test for moderation effects while simultaneously controlling for other variables. However, the number of associations that can be examined in this way is limited. A different way of testing moderation is to conduct correlation or regression analyses separately in males and females. The benefit of this approach is that it presents an easy way of comparing multiple associations between males and females. An important limitation, however, is that the power of the analyses conducted is reduced, as the population sample is divided into two. Furthermore, there is a potential problem with these kinds of analyses. A number of studies have conducted correlation or regression analyses separately for males and females and have reported the results of such analyses without testing whether sex differences are significant. Even though the association between two variables is significant in males, but not in females, or is even positive in males and negative in females, such differences are not necessarily significant. Thus, in order to avoid reporting sex differences that are not significant, Z-tests should always be conducted to establish the significance levels of moderation effects in this type of analyses. There are several examples in the literature of authors who have based their conclusions on apparent moderation effects that are not actually significant. In addition, it is easy to overlook significant moderation effects if an association is significant in both males and females. In such cases, a Z-test can reveal that the association is significantly stronger in one sex, even though the main effect is significant in both. Thus, conducting Z-tests can reduce the risk of both type I and type II errors.

· Both mediation and moderation are likely to be involved in sex differences in anxiety.
· Whereas mediation effects can help account for sex differences in the severity and prevalence of anxiety, the presence of moderation effects would mean that the association between anxiety and certain variables are not equally strong in males and females.
· Moderation effects in the associations between anxiety and associated risk and protective factors may ultimately point to males and females primarily following different pathways to anxiety, which may result in sex differences in the expression and treatment of anxiety disorders.
· Moderation effects have been reported for both factors related to reporting and classification of anxiety (e.g., social desirability), genetic versus societal contributions to anxiety, and risk and protective factors (e.g., independence).
· Research is very scarce, non-significant moderation effects are likely to remain unreported, and all reported moderation effects should be replicated in other studies.
· Future studies could examine moderation effects for any associations in anxiety. However, associations that may be particularly relevant to examine in a moderation context include hereditary traits versus societal influences.
· There are different ways of examining moderation effects in anxiety research. Multivariate models can examine potential interaction effects or separate male and female correlation or regression analyses can be compared to each other. If the latter approach is used, the significance of potential moderation effects should always be examined in order to avoid both type I and type II errors.

Table 6. Summary points for sex as a moderator in anxiety research

2.5. Sex differences in clinical characteristics of anxiety disorders

Whereas it is well-established that females are more likely than males to develop most anxiety disorders, it is more uncertain whether sex differences exist once the disorder has developed. Several researchers have found that males and females do not differ in mean age of onset for anxiety disorders in general, nor for any specific anxiety disorder [2, 10]. However, other studies have reported a later onset of PD, GAD, and especially OCD in females compared to males [16, 30, 40, 41]. Only one disorder appears to have a later onset in males than in females. Although the vast majority of childhood cases of separation anxiety (SA) remit before adulthood, new as well as persisting cases of SA do exist in adults [8]. The odds ratio for females compared to males is 2.2 in childhood and 1.4 in adulthood [8]. Analyses have revealed that the higher female:male odds ratio in children compared to adults is caused by the fact that males are more likely than females to have a first onset of SA in adulthood [8].

In spite of a later onset for some of these disorders in females, PD and PTSD have both been found to be more chronic or recurrent in females compared to males [5, 9, 30, 11, 42, 43] although findings are inconsistent [30]. In contrast, OCD appears to take a more chronic course in males, as early onset OCD is often particularly severe [9]. Finally, studies have reported similar chronicity in males and females with SP, AG, SAD, and GAD [30]. Taking the high degree of comorbidity into account, one study found that females with a lifetime prevalence of any anxiety disorder were more likely than males to have met criteria for any anxiety disorder within the past year [2]. This suggests that females with anxiety disorders either have more re-occurrences or more onsets of different anxiety disorders than males.

Some sex differences have been reported in comorbidity. Overall, females who are diagnosed with one mental disorder are more likely than males to have three or more comorbid disorders [4]. Across different anxiety disorders, females appear to be more likely than males to report comorbid affective disorders, eating disorders, impulse control disorders, self-injurious behaviour, and other anxiety disorders [2, 10, 16, 38]. In contrast, males are more likely to report comorbid ADHD, intermittent explosive disorder, and substance use disorders [2, 16, 38]. Furthermore, males are more likely than females to have met criteria for hypersexual disorder and pyromania at an earlier time in their life [16], and specifically for OCD, comorbidity with Tourette syndrome and tics are much more pronounced in males compared to females [38, 44]. Finally, although the presence of any anxiety disorder is associated with high blood pressure and vascular disease in both males and females, the risk of suffering from vascular disease is more pronounced in males even after controlling for socio-demographic variables and risk factors for vascular disease [45].

The higher rates of comorbid disorders in females compared to males are likely to affect both symptom severity and clinical presentation. Some studies have reported comparable symptom levels in males and females suffering from GAD, PD (with or without agoraphobia), or SAD [24, 30, 37]. Similarly, in the NCS-R, no interaction effects were found between sex and disability on DSM-IV anxiety disorders when assessed together [3]. In contrast, other studies have found that females with PD, AG, GAD, SP, SAD, and PTSD report higher symptom levels than males with these disorders [7, 46]. Furthermore, sex differences in the clinical presentation of different anxiety disorders have been reported. For example, males and females with SP tend to differ in the specific content of their phobias [11]. Furthermore, whereas some studies have found that males and females with SAD report similar fears of social situations [24], others have found sex differences in regards to which specific social situations are most fear-provoking [37, 11]. Similar sex differences have been reported for OCD where obsessions and compulsions related to cleaning, contamination, and aggression are more prevalent in females, whereas those related to sexual content, exactness, ordering, repeating, hoarding, touching, and especially symmetry and checking, are more prevalent in males [9, 16, 38]. In PD, equal rates of panic attacks are generally reported by males and females, but physical panic symptoms, such as shortness of breath, faintness, and smothering sensations are more likely to be among the primary panic symptoms in females compared to males [9]. Furthermore, PD is more likely to be associated with AG in females than in males [42]. In AG, males are more likely than females to report fear of bodily illness and of the heart stopping, whereas females report more fears related to going into the street and into crowded shops and also appear to be more dependent on a companion when going out [26].

The generally higher symptom severity and more pronounced comorbidity in females may result a higher degree of functional impairment compared to males [41]. In contrast, it has been suggested that the earlier age of OCD onset in males may result in a higher impact on several areas of daily life in males, including both social adjustment and interpersonal relationships [38]. In accordance with this, sex differences have been reported specifically for OCD with several studies reporting better overall quality of life in females compared to males [47]. For anxiety disorders other than OCD, the degree of impairment tends to be similar for males and females. The clinical presentation of PD has been reported to be very similar in the two sexes [41], and males and females with an anxiety disorder are equally likely to miss work and to seek help for emotional and substance abuse issues [2]. In accordance with these findings, the symptom profiles of males and females with PTSD appear to be very similar [23].

2.5.1. Summary and discussion of sex differences in clinical characteristics

All in all, some sex differences occur in onset of anxiety with early onset of most disorders being more common in males. The one exception to this general rule appears to be SA, which may have a higher prevalence of adult onset in males compared to females. However, research on sex differences in adults with SA is practically non-existing, so this finding needs to be replicated. The most widely reported sex differences in the clinical presentation of anxiety disorders are those related to comorbidity. Females are more likely than males to report comorbid conditions, especially other anxiety disorders. In general, these findings regarding sex differences in comorbidity are hardly surprising, as they reflect the sex differences generally reported for these disorders, with males reporting higher degree of comorbidity with externalising disorders and females reporting higher degree of comorbidity with internalising disorders. In fact, a lack of sex differences in comorbid disorders would be a more interesting finding than the sex differences described here, as that would imply that males and females with anxiety disorders differ less on the prevalence of other disorders compared to the general population. That said, expected sex differences in comorbidity are not completely uninteresting, as the presence of comorbidity reduces the likelihood of remission and offers additional problems for the patient that are likely to affect everyday functioning and quality of life [5].

Males and females do appear to differ somewhat in the symptom profiles of different disorders. However, sex differences are generally not substantial and are mostly limited to the specific contents of phobias, social fears, obsessions, and compulsions. Furthermore, the general impairment related to the different disorders appears to be mostly comparable between males and females, although females generally report higher symptom levels. All in all, these results suggest that in spite of the substantial impact of sex on the prevalence and severity of anxiety in the general population, there appear to be more similarities than differences once an anxiety disorder has developed.

The biggest exception to this rule is OCD. Early onset OCD is significantly more prevalent in males compared with females. Furthermore, OCD in males is more likely to be associated with tics, and possibly also with early brain injury, compared to females. OCD is also the only disorder that is sometimes found to be associated with a higher degree of impairment in males. In fact, the differences between male and female OCD are so substantial that researchers have suggested they are etiologically different from one another [15]. This hypothesis is supported by findings that male OCD patients show distinct patterns of neuropsychological dysfunction [15]. Perhaps it is not surprising that sex differences in OCD appear to be more substantial compared to sex differences in the other anxiety disorders, as OCD is no longer considered an anxiety disorder. In contrast, sex differences in PTSD appear to be more similar to those found in other anxiety disorders. Although sex differences in ASD have been less extensively studied, the influence of sex in ASD is likely to be comparable to that in PTSD because of the general similarities and partial symptom overlap between the two disorders. However, whereas sex differences in PTSD, and presumably also ASD, are similar to those found in conditions still categorised as anxiety disorders, the unique requirement of traumatic exposure in ASD and PTSD sets them aside from the other disorders discussed in this chapter.

· Whereas it is clear that females have a higher risk of developing anxiety disorders than males, it is less clear whether differences exist once the disorders have developed.
· Whereas findings are inconsistent, there is some support for sex differences related to age of onset, chronicity, comorbidity, severity, and clinical presentation.
· Females may have later onset of PD, GAD, and OCD but earlier onset of SA compared to males.
· OCD may be more chronic in males, but females appear to have more chronic and/or more recurrent anxiety disorders in general.
· Males and females appear to differ in their patterns of comorbid disorders. These sex differences generally follow the common clinical pattern of more external disorders in males and more internal disorders in females.
· Females with anxiety disorders tend to have higher symptom levels than their male counterparts.
· Sex differences in the clinical presentation of anxiety disorders are generally not substantial and have mostly been reported in relation to the specific content of phobias, social fears, obsessions, and compulsions.
· The degree of impairment and reduced quality of life associated with having an anxiety disorder is generally similar for males and females. The exception is OCD, as male OCD patients tend to be more negatively affected than their female counterparts.
· In general, there appear at present to be more similarities than differences between males and females diagnosed with an anxiety disorder.
· Only for OCD do sex differences appear to be so substantial that it has been suggested that male and female OCD are etiologically distinct disorders.
· More research is needed to further examine sex differences and similarities in patients suffering from different anxiety disorders.
· Future research should among other things examine the temporal association between anxiety and comorbid disorders along with the potential impact of sex on such associations.
· Even minor sex differences once an anxiety disorder has developed can potentially affect impairment, quality of life, and treatment response.

Table 7. Summary points for sex differences in clinical characteristics of anxiety disorders

McLean and colleagues have suggested that future research move beyond documenting sex differences in the differential patterns of comorbidity to examine how sex affects the sequential association between anxiety diagnoses and comorbidity [2]. As suggested by Christiansen and Elklit, gonadal hormones are likely to affect male and female stress responses over long periods of time [23]. Thus, it is possible that such stress response patterns may affect both the development of a first anxiety disorder and the development of comorbidity over time. If more is learned about how one anxiety disorder affects the development of other anxiety disorders along with depression and other types of comorbidity, we may be able to do more to prevent the generalisation of fears and anxiety. Such research should account for sex as a potential moderator from the very beginning to increase our understanding of interaction effects and to better help males and females suffering from anxiety and other disorders. In addition, more research should examine how sex affects other aspects of anxiety disorders once they have developed. Although such research is unlikely to find anxiety disorders, other than OCD, to be etiologically different in males and females, even minor sex differences are relevant to identify, as they may have the potential to affect both impairment and quality of life. Finally, such differences may affect how males and females respond to both pharmacotherapy and psychotherapy.

2.6. Sex differences in treatments of anxiety disorders

Males are generally significantly less likely to seek and receive mental health services compared to females [48], and females suffering from anxiety disorders have a significantly higher health care usage compared to their male counterparts [2]. This general tendency has been confirmed in a study of GAD [49] but disconfirmed in a study of SAD [24]. In the latter study, males were more likely than females to seek treatment, which may explain why sex differences are not always found in clinical populations of SAD [9]. Finally, one study examined help-seeking behaviour across the life span separately in males and females with different anxiety and mood disorders. They found that females were more likely than males to seek help for all the anxiety disorders that were examined [48]. According to this study, 25–32% of males suffering from GAD, PTSD, PD, SAD, or SP sought treatment, whereas the numbers for females were 68–75%. However, it is possible that a large proportion of the increased help-seeking behaviour in females is due to the higher prevalence of comorbid disorders in females.

In addition to sex differences in treatment-seeking behaviour, sex differences in anxiety have the potential to greatly influence treatment outcomes. Variables that are found to be moderated by sex in their effects on anxiety are particularly relevant to sex differences in treatment outcome, as they may be targeted in therapy aimed specifically at male or female patients. In addition, sex differences have been reported in the physiological stress response involving both the HPA axis and the serotonergic system [23, 50]. Such sex differences are likely to affect treatment outcomes and possibly cause sex differences in response to psychotropic medication. Several researchers have suggested that knowledge about sex and gender should be implemented in research on treatment of anxiety disorders [7, 23]. Furthermore, both sex and gender influences may affect how males and females respond to different treatments, including how well they tolerate them and how different aspects of treatment affect different symptoms.

Unfortunately, sex and gender differences are very rarely examined in studies of treatment effects on different anxiety disorders. Bekker and Mens-Verhulst conducted a literature search for empirical studies of the influence of sex on outcomes in treatment studies [7]. Although this search initially resulted in the identification of 33 studies, only four reported the results of sex-specific analyses, two studies on pharmacotherapy and two studies on psychotherapy. For the remaining studies, it was unclear whether no such results were reported because no significant interaction effects were found or because sex-specific analyses were not conducted. Finally, the authors identified a meta-analysis that had divided 33 treatment studies into studies based primarily on male or female populations and found no significant differences in treatment efficacy between the two groups [7]. A review of sex differences specifically in PTSD treatment efficacy published in 2010 identified only nine randomised controlled trials that had analysed sex differences in PTSD treatment [51].

2.6.1. *Pharmacotherapy*

There are several reasons to expect that sex differences in the impact of different psychopharmacological treatments on different anxiety symptoms may exist. Although research in this area is very scarce, the existence of some sex differences have been reported for the metabolism, and side-effects of benzodiazepines, tricyclic antidepressants (TCAs), and selective serotonin reuptake inhibitors (SSRIs) [5, 19]. Sex differences may further depend on age as well as reproductive status, use of oral contraceptives, and HRT in females. For example, lower concentrations of benzodiazepines may be expected in premenopausal females, but not postmenopausal females, compared to males [19]. Furthermore, use of oral contraceptives and HRT appear to affect the impact of benzodiazepines, TCAs, and SSRIs [19, 41], and probably also other types of anxiolytic and psychotropic medication. However, whereas significant sex differences have been identified in both the pharmacokinetics and pharmacodynamics of antidepressants [52], the clinical implications of these sex differences have not been properly examined [19]. In spite of the fact that such sex differences may result in more adverse effects occurring in females compared to males when receiving the same dose of anxiolytic medications [19], such clinically relevant sex differences are rarely examined in research on pharmacotherapy in patients with different anxiety disorders.

Whereas several studies have found an increased effect of SSRIs on depression in females compared to males [52, 53], only few studies have examined the effects of SSRIs on anxiety separately in males and females. One study found that there were no sex differences in the efficacy of sertraline over placebo in the treatment of GAD [49]. In contrast, another study found that female patients with PD benefitted more from sertraline treatment than males on some of the outcome measures [41]. It is possible that the lack of significant sex differences in the former study is related to the finding that a significantly greater proportion of females had prior experience with psychotropic medication, thereby suggesting that a greater proportion of female compared to male patients may have been particularly difficult to treat. Furthermore, although males and females had similar scores on most pre-treatment measures, females did score significantly higher on a few, including overall clinical severity. Thus, any potentially stronger effect of sertraline in female patients may have been cancelled out by a higher severity level and more treatment-resistant symptoms in females. Finally, in spite of a very small sample size, one study found that females with GAD had a significantly worse response to 6 weeks of treatment with the SSRI fluoxetine compared to males [53]. In this study, patients with current comorbid anxious or affective disorders were not excluded from the study, whereas patients with alcohol or substance abuse/dependence were. However, this is unlikely to explain the differences in treatment outcome, as there were no significant sex differences in comorbid mood or anxiety disorders, and comorbidity did not predict treatment outcome.

In contrast to the apparently greater effect of SSRIs in females, results from research on depression suggest that both TCAs and tetracyclic antidepressants (TeCAs) may result in better outcomes in males [52]. A study of OCD patients found that females responded better to treatment with either the TCA clomipramine or the SSRI flovixamine than males [54]. However, due to an already small sample size and high drop-out rates, it is unclear whether these differences were equal for the two drugs and whether interactions between treatment and response to a prior symptom-provoking agent differed for males and females. In addition to these studies of antidepressives, a pilot study examining the effects of propranolol found promising results that this beta-blocker decreases PTSD severity in males, but may actually increase symptom levels in females [55].

Finally, one of the treatment studies examined sex differences in tolerance levels for males and females undergoing sertraline treatment for GAD. It was reported that sertraline was generally tolerated equally well by males and females with comparable reports of side-effects and similar dropout rates [49]. The exceptions were nausea for which a larger placebo versus treatment effect was found in males and increased sweating which was more commonly reported by females in the sertraline group. In accordance with these minor sex differences, other studies have reported that males and females differ in the specific side effects associated with different antidepressives [52]. This may cause sex differences in the attrition rates associated with different drugs used for treating anxiety. In accordance with this, there is some support that females are more likely to drop out from TCA treatment, whereas males are more likely to drop out from SSRI treatment [52]. One study treating male and female OCD patients with either a TCA or an SSRI found no significant sex differences in drop-out rates [54]. However, as 46% of males compared to 29% of females failed to complete the treatment, it is possible that the lack of significant sex differences were due to low power. Furthermore, because of the low power, a sex by treatment interaction effect could not be examined for attrition rates.

2.6.2. Psychotherapy

Males and females may also differ in how they respond to psychotherapy. Possibly because of oestrogen effects, sex differences have been reported in both fear conditioning and extinction [18]. As exposure therapy is commonly used to treat anxiety disorders, it is very likely that sex differences may exist in the effectiveness of such therapies. A review of sex differences in PTSD treatment identified a few studies that in spite of low sample sizes reported that females responded significantly better to trauma-focused therapy than males [51]. In contrast, a more recent study comparing the effects of exposure therapy given alone to exposure therapy combined with cognitive restructuring reported similar outcomes for males and females with

PTSD [56]. However, although the combined treatment was superior to exposure given alone for both sexes, females maintained their gains from exposure therapy significantly better than males, suggesting that the difference between the two treatments was greater for males than for females.

Studies examining the impact of behavioural therapy for other anxiety disorders have reported inconsistent findings. One study on cognitive behavioural therapy (CBT) combined with acceptance and commitment therapy (ACT) reported that the treatment was equally effective in males and females with different anxiety disorders [57]. Another study examined the effects of intensive behavioural therapy in severely affected treatment-resistant OCD patients and reported greater symptom decrease in females than in males [58]. Sex differences in treatment outcome remained even after controlling for initial OCD severity and psychosocial functioning. Finally, a study on cognitive processing therapy in patients with PTSD found that males and females did not differ significantly on the primary outcomes of PTSD and depression [59]. This was found both following the last session and at 3 months follow-up in spite of medium effect sizes favouring females. In contrast, females did score significantly higher than males on the secondary outcomes of guilt, anger, and dissociation with medium-to-large effect sizes. Furthermore, the improvement on these measures occurred at a significantly higher rate in females compared to males.

Finally, there are some indications that males and females may differ in their tolerance of different aspects of psychotherapy, although results are inconsistent. One study reported comparable attrition rates and treatment length for males and females undergoing cognitive processing therapy for PTSD [59]. Other studies have found that males are more likely than females to drop out of treatments including aspects of exposure [26, 51, 57]. Similarly, females appear to be more compliant in CBT compared to males [58]. It is possible that these differences in compliance and attrition are at least partly responsible for the superior response rates in females that have sometimes been reported.

2.6.3. Summary and discussion of sex differences in treatment

In general, very little research exists that has examined sex differences in the effectiveness of anxiety treatment. Most such research is designed to have adequate statistical power for detecting treatment differences, rather than gender by treatment interactions, and is often limited by small sample sizes, resulting in higher risk of type II errors. Sex differences are rarely a primary focus in treatment research, and even when significant moderation effects are found, this may not even be mentioned in the abstract. In addition, studies that do examine the impact of sex on treatment outcomes are often characterised by a failure to examine other potential moderators, such as comorbidity. In fact, patients with comorbid disorders are often excluded from treatment studies, which is likely to result in the exclusion of the worst-functioning females who are likely to benefit less from treatment. Whereas such studies may better reflect the direct impact of sex, they may prevent the identification of actual sex differences likely to be present in clinical populations. Whereas it is indeed relevant to examine whether potential sex differences in treatment effects are caused by a higher degree of comorbidity in females, such associations should be examined in mediation and moderation analyses, rather than by

http://dx.doi.org/10.5772/60662

individuals with comorbidity being excluded from the study. Furthermore, most studies examining sex differences in the effects of pharmacological treatment are of relatively short duration (8–12 weeks) and do not assess whether the presence or absence of sex differences remain over time. Finally, sex-specific analyses are often limited to the primary outcome measures. Sex differences in treatment effects may be more likely to be found for secondary outcomes, as these may be related to differences in comorbidity.

· Overall, females are more likely than males to seek and receive mental health services.
· Although knowledge of sex and gender ought to be routinely implicated in research on treatment outcomes, this is very rarely done.
· Sex differences in gonadal hormones, metabolism, fear conditioning, and extinction are likely to cause males and females to respond differently to both pharmacotherapy and psychotherapy.
· Although evidence stems mainly from research on depression, there is some support that females respond better to SSRIs than males, whereas males respond better to TCAs and TeCAs.
· Results from research on psychotherapy are even more inconsistent, but may suggest that females benefit more from CBT (particularly exposure) than males.
· Sex differences in secondary outcomes (e.g., guilt, anger, dissociation) may be found even in the absence of sex differences in primary outcome.
· Although results are inconsistent, sex differences may exist in treatment tolerance, side effects, compliance, and drop-out rates. However, the impact of such sex differences on treatment outcome remains unexplored.
· Research on sex differences in treatment response is often limited by small populations, inadequate statistical power, failure to take potential moderators and mediators into account, and short follow-up range. Furthermore, sex differences are rarely a primary focus, non-significant sex differences often go unreported, and even significant sex differences may not be mentioned in the abstracts of the studies reporting them.
· In addition to avoiding these limitations, future studies should examine whether the effects of specific elements of psychotherapy are moderated by sex and whether female use of oral contraceptives, HRT, reproductive status, and menstrual cycle affect the outcomes of pharmacotherapy and psychotherapy.

Table 8. Summary points for sex differences in treatments of anxiety disorders

In addition to more research examining sex differences in the general efficacy of different treatments, future studies should also begin to examine the unique role of different treatment elements in male and female treatment outcomes. For example, even if CBT is found to work equally well in males and females, it is possible that certain features (e.g., exposure) are particularly beneficial for males, if they can tolerate it, whereas others (e.g., cognitive elements) are particularly beneficial for females. Identifying sex differences in the effects of different treatment elements may help improve interventions offered to males and females. It is possible that future research will teach us that males and females benefit from the same pharmacotherapeutic and psychotherapeutic interventions, in which case they can continue to be offered the same treatments. However, another possibility is that future research may identify specific interventions and specific elements of psychotherapy or anxiolytic medications that are substantially more beneficial to one sex compared to the other, and that this will call for sex-specific interventions tailored specifically to males or to females with general or specific symptom profiles. Whatever the answer may be, it is highly important that we begin to ask the necessary questions.

Future studies on sex differences in treatment outcomes should make an effort to include more variables that may contribute to sex differences. This is especially true for psychotropic treatment trials where a great gap exists in knowledge on hormonal influences on treatment outcomes, particularly in females. Despite the fact that data from the United States suggest that one in four females between the ages of 15 and 44 years receive oral contraceptives, and one in three females between the ages of 50 and 65 years receive some kind of HRT [19], the effects of oral contraceptives and HRT on anxiety levels remain largely unexamined. Future research should also examine whether it is beneficial, when prescribing psychotropic therapy to females, to adjust for phase of the menstrual cycle [50]. Future studies should examine the impact of gonadal hormones on the effectiveness of both pharmacotherapy and psychotherapy, as both appear to be affected by oestrogen.

3. Conclusion

The chapter examined the current status of research on sex differences in agoraphobia, general anxiety disorder, panic disorder, separation anxiety, social anxiety disorder, acute stress disorder, posttraumatic stress disorder, and obsessive-compulsive disorder. Although the extent of sex differences across the different anxiety disorders varies, a higher symptom severity in females compared to males has been reported for all these disorders. Studies using multivariate mediation models to examine whether the influence of sex on the severity and prevalence of anxiety can be accounted for by sex differences in associated variables show some promise, especially if a combination of several variables are taken into account and if these represent both biological and environmental risk and protective factors. However, mediation analyses can only account for a small part of the contribution of sex to anxiety, as sex differences in anxiety appear to go beyond sex differences in the prevalence and severity of the different anxiety disorders. Although studies on sex as a moderator in anxiety research are few and far between certain risk factors have been reported to be significantly more strongly associated with anxiety in one sex compared to the other. Thus, much more research is needed to examine the extent of such moderation effects. Future studies should strive to conduct proper moderation analyses, making sure to report not just sex differences in relevant associations, but also report whether such sex differences are significant. Furthermore, moderation effects of sex should be confirmed in more than one study, and it should be examined whether the same moderation effects exist across different anxiety disorders. At the present time, so little research has been conducted on moderation effects in anxiety disorders, that a lack of significant sex differences in such associations will be as interesting a finding as the identification of significant differences. As has been suggested for PTSD [23], even small sex differences in associations between anxiety and related variables may point to the involvement of different mechanisms in the development of anxiety disorders in males and females. Sex differences in the association between anxiety and important risk and protective factors have the potential to affect the clinical expression of such anxiety disorders. However, although some sex differences have been reported in relation to age of onset, specific symptoms, and comorbidity, more similarities than differences appear to exist between the clinical profiles of males and females with anxiety disorders. Finally, very little research has examined whether different approaches to treat anxiety are equally effective in males and females. Although findings are inconsistent, there are some indications that SSRIs may be more effective in females, TCAs may be more effective in males, and males may be more likely to drop out of exposure-based psychotherapy than females. The fact that no studies were published during the past 5 years examining sex differences specifically in AG, ASD, SA, and SP suggests that research on sex differences in these disorders is particularly warranted. However, the generally low numbers found for all anxiety disorders, except for PTSD, highlight the importance for much more research focusing on sex differences in anxiety disorders in general.

The present review of sex differences in diagnoses previously or currently classified as anxiety disorders has generally found many similarities across the different disorders. Thus, although ASD and PTSD are no longer categorised as anxiety disorders, it remains defensible to compare findings to those reported in relation to anxiety disorders. As much more research has been conducted on sex differences in PTSD compared to any of the other disorders, there may be some benefit to letting the design of future studies on other anxiety disorders be inspired by research on sex differences in PTSD. For example, moderation effects reported in PTSD research are likely to also be found in relation to other anxiety disorders. Whereas more similarities than differences exist in the clinical profiles of males and females with most anxiety disorders, once the disorder has developed, this does not appear to be the case with OCD. OCD in males have been found to be more genetically based, have an earlier onset, be associated with tics and Tourette syndrome, and be associated with a lower quality of life compared to OCD in females. All these findings support the possibility of OCD in males being etiologically distinct from OCD in females, which is further consistent with the removal of OCD from the anxiety disorder category. When it comes to sex differences, at least, OCD does not appear to have much in common with other traditional anxiety disorders.

Nomenclature

Diagnoses:

- AG: agoraphobia
- ASD: acute stress disorder
- GAD: generalised anxiety disorder
- OCD: obsessive-compulsive disorder
- PD: panic disorder
- PTSD: posttraumatic stress disorder
- SA: separation anxiety

- SAD: social anxiety disorder
- SP: specific phobia

Other abbreviations:

- ACT: acceptance and commitment therapy
- DSM-III-R: diagnostic and statistical manual of mental disorders 3rd edition revised
- DSM-IV: diagnostic and statistical manual of mental disorders 4th edition
- DSM-IV-TR: diagnostic and statistical manual of mental disorders 4th edition – text revision
- DSM-5: diagnostic and statistical manual of mental disorders 5th edition
- HPA axis: hypothalamic-pituitary-adrenal axis
- NCS: national comorbidity survey
- NCS-R: national comorbidity survey-replication
- SSRI: selective serotonin re-uptake inhibitors
- TCA: tricyclic antidepressives
- TeCA: tetracyclic antidepressives

Author details

Dorte M. Christiansen[1,2]

Address all correspondence to: dochristiansen@health.sdu.dk

1 Institute of Psychology, Aarhus University, Denmark

2 National Center for Psychotraumatology, University of Southern Denmark, Denmark

References

[1] Kessler RC, Chiu WT, Demler O, Walters EE. Prevalence, severity, and comorbidity of 12-month DSM-IV disorders in the National Comorbidity Survey Replication. Archives of General Psychiatry 2005;62(6) 617–627.

[2] McLean CP, Asnaani A, Litz BT, Hofmann SG. Gender differences in anxiety disorders: Prevalence, course of illness, comorbidity and burden of illness. Journal of Psychiatric Research 2011;45(8) 1027–1035.

[3] Gum AM, King-Kallimanis B, Kohn R. Prevalence of mood, anxiety, and substance-abuse disorders for older Americans in the national comorbidity survey-replication. The American Journal of Geriatric Psychiatry 2009;17(9) 769–781.

[4] Kessler RC, McGonagle KA, Zhao S, Nelson CB, Hughes M, Eshleman S, et al. Lifetime and 12-month prevalence of DSM-III-R psychiatric disorders in the United States: Results from the National Comorbidity Survey. Archives of General Psychiatry 1994;51(1) 8–19.

[5] Howell HB, Brawman-Mintzer O, Monnier J, Yonkers KA. Generalized anxiety disorder in women. Psychiatric Clinics of North America 2001;24(1) 165–178.

[6] Kessler RC, Berglund P, Demler O, Jin R, Merikangas KR, Walters EE. Lifetime prevalence and age-of-onset distributions of DSM-IV disorders in the National Comorbidity Survey Replication. Archives of General Psychiatry 2005;62(6) 593–602.

[7] Bekker MH, van Mens-Verhulst J. Anxiety disorders: Sex differences in prevalence, degree, and background, but gender-neutral treatment. Gender Medicin 2007;4(Suppl. B) S178–S193.

[8] Shear K, Jin R, Ruscio AM, Walters EE, Kessler RC. Prevalence and correlates of estimated DSM-IV child and adult separation anxiety disorder in the National Comorbidity Survey Replication. The American Journal of Psychiatry 2006;163(6) 1074–1083.

[9] McLean CP, Anderson ER. Brave men and timid women? A review of the gender differences in fear and anxiety. Clinical Psychology Review 2009;29(6) 496–505.

[10] Lewinsohn PM, Gotlib IH, Lewinsohn M, Seeley JR, Allen NB. Gender differences in anxiety disorders and anxiety symptoms in adolescents. Journal of Abnormal Psychology 1998;107(1) 109–117.

[11] Mackinaw-Koons B, Vasey MW. Considering sex differences in anxiety and its disorders across the life span: A construct-validation approach. Applied & Preventive Psychology 2000;9(3) 191–209.

[12] American Psychiatric Association. Diagnostic and statistical manual of mental disorders: DSM-5. Washington, DC: Author; 2013.

[13] American Psychiatric Association. Diagnostic and statistical manual of mental disorders: DSM-IV-TR. Washington, DC: Author; 2000.

[14] Lebron-Milad K, Milad MR. Sex differences, gonadal hormones and the fear extinction network: Implications for anxiety disorders. Biology of Mood & Anxiety Disorders 2012;2(1). doi:10.1186/2045-5380-2-3

[15] Segalàs C, Alonso P, Labad J, Real E, Pertusa A, Jaurrieta N, et al. A case-control study of sex differences in strategic processing and episodic memory in obsessive-compulsive disorder. Comprehensive Psychiatry 2010;51(3) 303–311.

[16] Lochner C, Hemmings SMJ, Kinnear CJ, Moolman-Smook JC, Corfield VA, Knowles JA, et al. Gender in obsessive–compulsive disorder clinical and genetic findings. European Neuropsychopharmacology 2004;14(2) 105–113.

[17] Altemus M. Sex differences in depression and anxiety disorders: Potential biological determinants. Hormones and Behavior 2006;50(4) 534–538.

[18] Farrell MR, Sengelaub DR, Wellman CL. Sex differences and chronic stress effects on the neural circuitry underlying fear conditioning and extinction. Physiology & Behavior 2013;122 208–215. doi:10.1016/j.physbeh.2013.04.002

[19] Pigott TA. Gender differences in the epidemiology and treatment of anxiety disorders. Journal of Clinical Psychiatry 1999;60(Suppl. 18) 4–15.

[20] McHenry J, Carrier N, Hull E, Kabbaj M. Gender differences in anxiety and depression: Role of testosterone. Frontiers in Neuroendocrinology 2014;35(1) 42–57.

[21] Biondi M, Picardi A. Psychological stress and neuroendocrine function in humans: The last two decades of research. Psychotherapy and Psychosomatics 1999;68(3) 114–150.

[22] Parker GB, Brotchie HL. From diathesis to dimorphism: The biology of gender differences in depression. The Journal of Nervous and Mental Disease 2004;192(3) 210–216.

[23] Christiansen D, Elklit A. Sex differences in PTSD. In: Ovuga E (ed.) Post Traumatic Stress Disorder in a Global Context. Rijeka: InTech; 2012. p113–142.

[24] Moscovitch DA, Hofmann SG, Litz BT. The impact of self-construals on social anxiety: A gender-specific interaction. Personality and Individual Differences 2005;38(3) 659–672.

[25] Gall MD. The relationship between masculinity-femininity and manifest anxiety. Journal of Clinical Psychology 1969;25(3) 194–195.

[26] Chambless DL, Mason J. Sex, sex-role stereotyping and agoraphobia. Behaviour Research and Therapy 1986;24(2) 231–235.

[27] Pierce KA, Kirkpatrick DR. Do men lie on fear surveys? Behaviour Research and Therapy 1992;30(4) 415–418.

[28] Ben-Zur H, Zeidner M. Sex differences in anxiety, curiosity, and anger: A cross-cultural study. Sex Roles 1988;19(5/6) 335–347.

[29] Breslau J, Kendler KS, Su M, Gaxiola-Aguilar S, Kessler RC. Lifetime risk and persistence of psychiatric disorders across ethnic groups in the United States. Psychological Medicine 2005;35(3) 317–327.

[30] Yonkers KA, Bruce SE, Dyck IR, Keller MB. Chronicity, relapse, and illness – course of panic disorder, social phobia, and generalized anxiety disorder: Findings in men and women from 8 years of follow-up. Depression and Anxiety 2003;17(3) 173–179.

[31] Leach LS, Christensen H, Mackinnon AJ, Windsor TD, Butterworth P. Gender differences in depression and anxiety across the adult lifespan: The role of psychosocial mediators. Social Psychiatry and Psychiatric Epidemiology 2008;43(12) 983–998.

[32] Christiansen DM, Hansen M. Accounting for sex differences in PTSD: A multivariable mediation model. European Journal of Psychotraumatology 2015;6(26068). doi: 10.3402/ejpt.v6.26068

[33] Tolin DF, Foa EB. Sex differences in trauma and posttraumatic stress disorder: A quantitative review of 25 years of research. Psychological Trauma: Theory, Research, Practice, and Policy 2008;S(1) 37–85.

[34] Stein MB, Walker JR, Forde DR. Gender differences in susceptibility to posttraumatic stress disorder. Behaviour Research and Therapy 2000;38(6) 619–628.

[35] Preacher KJ, Hayes AF. Asymptotic and resampling strategies for assessing and comparing indirect effects in multiple mediator models. Behavior Research Methods 2008;40(3) 879–891.

[36] Gater R, Tansella M, Korten A, Tiemens BG, Mavreas VG, Olatawura MO. Sex differences in the prevalence and detection of depressive and anxiety disorders in general health care settings: Report from the World Health Organization collaborative study on psychological problems in general health care. Archives of General Psychiatry 1998;55(5) 405–413.

[37] Zimmerman J, Morrison AS, Heimberg RG. Social anxiety, submissiveness, and shame in men and women: A moderated mediation analysis. British Journal of Clinical Psychology 2015;54(1) 1–15.

[38] de Mathis MA, de Alvarenga P, Funaro G, Torresan RC, Moraes I, Torres AR, et al. Gender differences in obsessive-compulsive disorder: A literature review. The Revista Brasileira de Psiquiatria 2011;33(4) 390–399.

[39] Silove D, Manicavasagar V, O'Connell D, Morris-Yates A. Genetic factors in early separation anxiety: Implications for the genesis of adult anxiety disorders. Acta Psychiatrica Scandinavica 1995;92(1) 17–24.

[40] Ruscio AM, Stein DJ, Chiu WT, Kessler RC. The epidemiology of obsessive-compulsive disorder in the National Comorbidity Survey Replication. Molecular Psychiatry 2010;15(1) 53–63.

[41] Clayton AH, Stewart RS, Fayyad R, Clary CM. Sex differences in clinical presentation and response in panic disorder: Pooled data from sertraline treatment studies. Archives of Women's Mental Health 2006;9(3) 151–157.

[42] Nillni YI, Berenz EC, Rohan KJ, Zvolensky MJ. Sex differences in panic-relevant responding to a 10% carbon dioxide-enriched air biological challenge. Journal of Anxiety Disorders 2012;26(1) 165–172.

[43] Breslau N, Kessler RC, Chilcoat HD, Schultz LR, Davis GC, Andreski P. Trauma and posttraumatic stress disorder in the community: The Detroit area survey of trauma. Archives of General Psychiatry 1998;55(7) 626–632.

[44] Moore J, Smith GW, Shevlin M, O'Neill FA. Alternative factor models and heritability of the Short Leyton Obsessional Inventory-Children's Version. Journal of Abnormal Child Psychology 2010;38(7) 921–934.

[45] Fiedorowicz JG, He J, Merikangas KR. The association between mood and anxiety disorders with vascular diseases and risk factors in a nationally representative sample. Journal of Psychosomatic Research 2011;70(2) 145–154.

[46] Kessler RC, Sonnega A, Bromet E, Hughes M, Nelson CB. Posttraumatic stress disorder in the National Comorbidity Survey. Archives of General Psychiatry 1995;52(12) 1048–1060.

[47] Farooqi YN, Rasul F. Gender differences in perceived quality of life of patients suffering from obsessive-compulsive disorder. Pakistan Journal of Psychological Research 2011;26(1) 61–71.

[48] Mackenzie CS, Reynolds K, Cairney J, Streiner DL, Sareen J. Disorder-specific mental health service use for mood and anxiety disorders: Associations with age, sex, and psychiatric comorbidity. Depression and Anxiety 2012;29(3) 234–242.

[49] Steiner M, Allgulander C, Ravindran A, Kosar H, Burt T, Austin C. Gender differences in clinical presentation and response to sertraline treatment of generalized anxiety disorder. Human Psychopharmacology 2005;20(1) 3–13.

[50] Steiner M, Lepage P, Dunn EJ. Serotonin and gender-specific psychiatric disorders. International Journal of Psychiatry in Clinical Practice 1997;1(1) 3–13.

[51] Blain LM, Galovski TE, Robinson T. Gender differences in recovery from posttraumatic stress disorder: A critical review. Aggression and Violent Behavior 2010;15(6) 463–474.

[52] Keers R, Aitchison KJ. Gender differences in antidepressant drug response. International Review of Psychiatry 2010;22(5) 485–500.

[53] Simon NM, Zalt AK, Worthington III JJ, Hoge EA, Christian KM, Stevens JC, et al. Preliminary support for gender differences in response to fluoxetine for generalized anxiety disorder. Depression and Anxiety 2006;23(6) 373–376.

[54] Mundo E, Bareggi SR, Pirola R, Bellodi L. Effect of acute intravenous clomipramine and antiobsessional response to proserotonergic drugs: Is gender a predictive variable? Biological Psychiatry 1999;45(3) 290–294.

[55] Nugent NR, Christopher NC, Crow JP, Browne L, Ostrowski S, Delahanty DL. The efficacy of early propranolol administration at reducing PTSD symptoms in pediatric injury patients: A pilot study. Journal of Traumatic Stress 2010;23(2) 282–287.

[56] Felmingham KL, Bryant RA. Gender differences in the maintenance of response to cognitive behavior therapy for posttraumatic stress disorder. Journal of Consulting and Clinical Psychology 2012;80(2) 196–200.

[57] Wolitsky-Taylor KB, Arch JJ, Rosenfield D, Craske MG. Moderators and non-specific predictors of treatment outcome for anxiety disorders: A comparison of cognitive behavioral therapy to acceptance and commitment therapy. Journal of Consulting and Clinical Psychology 2012;80(5) 786–799.

[58] Stewart SE, Yen C-H, Stack DE, Jenike MA. Outcome predictors for severe obsessive-compulsive patients in intensive residential treatment. Journal of Psychiatric Research 2006;40(6) 511–519.

[59] Galovski TE, Blain LM, Chappuis C, Fletcher T. Sex differences in recovery from PTSD in male and female interpersonal assault survivors. Behaviour Research and Therapy 2013;51(6) 247–255.

Chapter 3

Psychobiological Aspects of Panic Disorder

Daniel C. Mograbi, Vitor Castro-Gomes,
Elie Cheniaux and J. Landeira-Fernandez

Additional information is available at the end of the chapter

http://dx.doi.org/10.5772/60663

Abstract

Anxiety is a useful warning sign that helps an individual face potential or real danger. At appropriate levels, it serves as a warning for the presence of internal or external threats, causing a person to be alert and prepare to deal appropriately with such situations. Moreover, moderate levels of anxiety can lead to improved performance in several activities. However, anxiety becomes pathological when its duration is excessively long or its intensity is extremely high and leads to significant suffering and distress. In such cases, anxiety is appropriately described as part of a pathological response, characterizing an anxiety disorder. The historical concept of a unitary anxiety disorder has been replaced by a heterogeneous group of psychopathologies with different etiologies. Panic disorder is a complex anxiety disorder that involves both recurrent, unexpected panic attacks, and persistent concern about having additional attacks. The present chapter reviews current psychobiological perspectives in the etiology and treatment of panic disorder. The first section describes the current classification of this anxiety disorder. We then explore possible neural circuitry associated with panic disorder. Finally, the chapter addresses current treatment approaches, considering the efficacy of different forms of psychotherapy and pharmacological treatments.

Keywords: Anxiety, Panic Disorder, Neural Circuitry, Behavioral Therapy, Pharmacological Therapy

1. Introduction

Anxiety is a useful warning sign that helps an individual face potential or real danger. At appropriate levels, it serves as a warning for the presence of internal or external threats, causing a person to be alert and prepare to deal appropriately with such situations. Moreover, moderate levels of anxiety can lead to improved performance in several activities [1]. This notion was originally suggested by Yerkes and Dodson [2], who described the relationship between anxiety and performance as an inverted U-shaped curve. According to the Yerkes-Dodson Law, arousal and anxiety have optimal levels for the execution of different tasks, and anxiety that is above or below this level is detrimental to performance. As shown in Figure 1, the level of task difficulty influences this optimal anxiety level to maximize performance. More difficult tasks demand lower levels of anxiety compared with simpler tasks. Regardless of the difficulty of the task, however, very high levels of anxiety are always detrimental to performance. Clearly, anxiety becomes pathological when its duration or intensity is such that it prevents the normal range of daily activities, leading to social isolation and difficulties at work. In such cases, anxiety is appropriately described as part of a pathological response, characterizing an anxiety disorder.

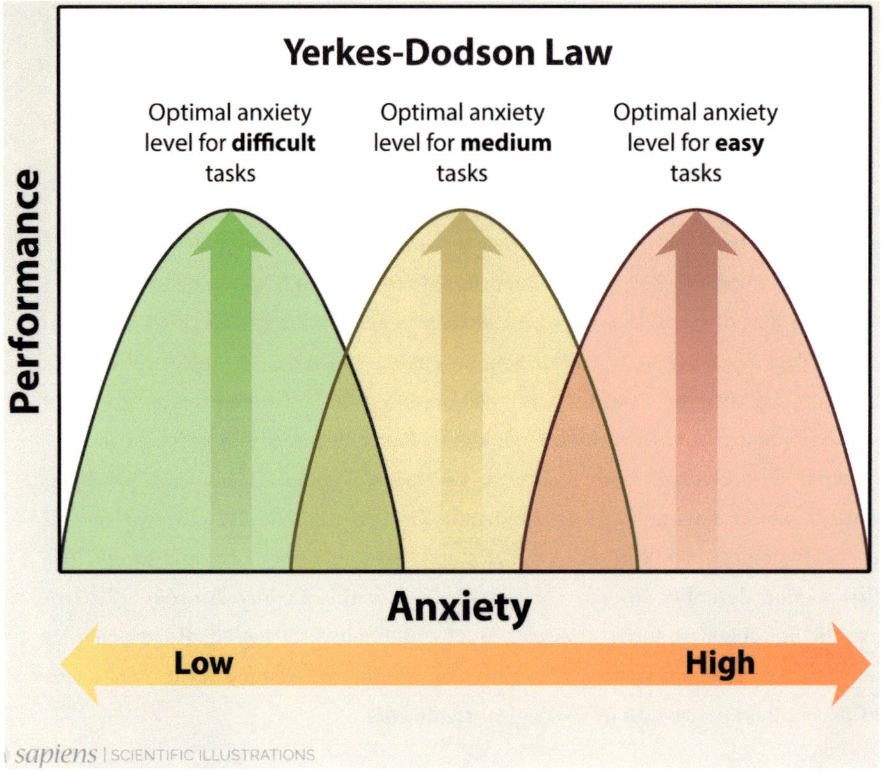

Figure 1. Yerkes-Dodson Law that illustrates a possible relationship between anxiety level and task performance according to task difficulty.

Several indications can characterize an anxiety reaction. They can be typically divided into physiological reactions (e.g., autonomic activation that leads to sweating, palpitations, nausea, dizziness, and feeling an empty stomach, among others), behavioral responses (e.g., constant movement of the hands and feet, trembling, and facial expressions), and conscious feelings (e.g., the subjective experience of tension or apprehension and hypervigilance). Figure 2 illustrates these three elements associated with anxiety reactions. Although several attempts have been made to understand and classify these anxiety reactions, it was only with Sigmund Freud that anxiety disorders acquired a large clinical emphasis, and different pathological conditions that involve anxiety began to be systematically studied. Freud [3] described several clearly related disorders, among them anxiety attacks and anxiety neurosis, that are now called panic attacks and panic disorder, respectively [4].

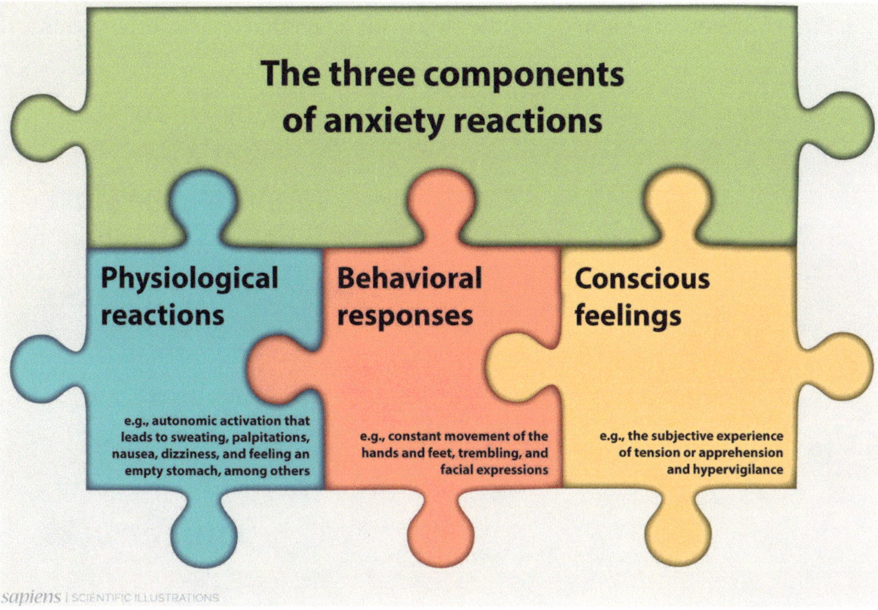

Figure 2. Three components of anxiety reactions.

The present understanding of anxiety disorders made a departure from an earlier view of a single unitary construct that ranged in intensity from normal to pathological or neurotic levels. Anxiolytic agents were the main prescription drugs to treat this unitary disorder. The main shift toward the current view of anxiety disorder occurred with the discovery that imipramine had a selective effect in the treatment of panic attacks [5]. Additionally, anxiety disorders differ from each other in the primary object or specificity of threat. Fear of a circumscribed and well-defined object or situation is a characteristic of specific phobias, whereas diffuse and chronic sustained anxiety is the main feature of generalized anxiety disorder. Therefore, anxiety disorders appear to represent a heterogeneous group of psychopathologies with different etiologies.

The present chapter reviews current psychobiological perspectives in the etiology and treatment of panic disorder. The first section below describes the current classification of this anxiety disorder. We then explore possible neural circuitry associated with panic disorder. Finally, the chapter addresses current treatment approaches, considering the efficacy of different forms of psychotherapy and pharmacological treatments.

2. Panic disorder diagnosis

The diagnosis of panic disorder involves two main components. The first component comprises unexpected and recurrent panic attacks. The second component includes constant worrying over the possibility of new attacks and behavioral changes in response to panic attacks [6]. Figure 3 presents a scheme of the two symptoms that characterize a panic disorder diagnosis.

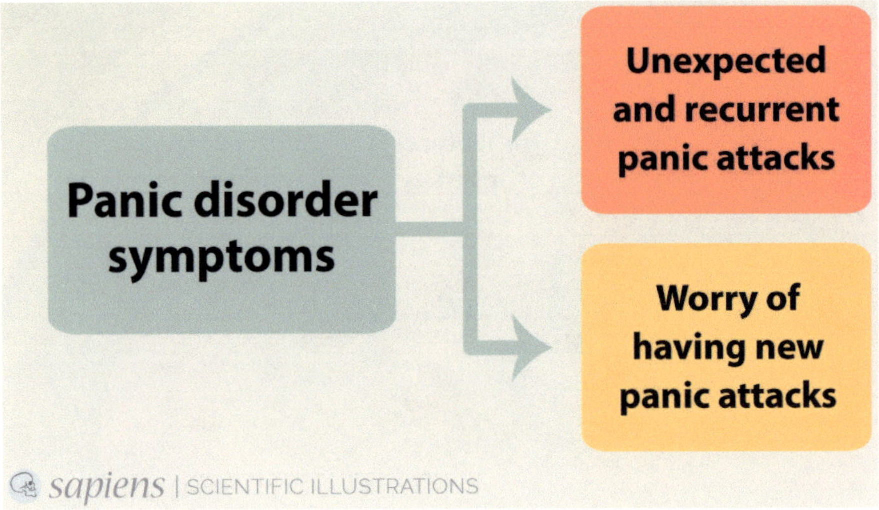

Figure 3. Two main symptoms related to panic disorder diagnosis.

A panic attack is a severe crisis that involves anxiety of great intensity, with an abrupt onset and short duration. Symptoms include shortness of breath (dyspnea), dizziness, fainting, palpitations, tremor, sweating, nausea, tingling (paresthesia), hot flashes or chills, and chest pain. These alterations express a state of autonomic discharge, involving both the sympathetic and parasympathetic nervous systems. These physiological changes can be accompanied by depersonalization (feelings of detachment from oneself), de-realization (feelings of unreality), fear of losing control or going insane, and a sense of impending death. Panic attacks typically peak quickly and last between 5 and 20 minutes. Because of its signs and symptoms, a panic attack is often mistaken as a heart attack, which reinforces the sensation of impending death.

Importantly, panic attacks are not exclusive to panic disorder; they are also present in other anxiety disorders, such as specific phobias, social phobia, and posttraumatic stress disorder. In this case, the panic attack is evoked by an object, event, or specific situation. Panic attacks that characterize panic disorders occur unexpectedly or in an unjustified manner (i.e., they appear "out of nowhere"). Panic attacks can occur even in situations of high relaxation, such as during sleep.

Although the recurrence of these panic attacks is a hallmark of panic disorder, the chronic condition of this anxiety disorder is defined by the constant and persistent fear of experiencing further attacks or worry about the possible consequences of a panic attack. This chronic form of anxiety, which is less intense but causes considerable damage to the person because of its constancy and duration, is quite different from a panic attack.

Patients who suffer from panic disorder may live in a nearly constant state of apprehension. The frightening prospect of experiencing another panic attack might be so extreme that the patient develops agoraphobia. This term originally referred to the fear of open spaces or crowds (from the Greek *Ágora*). The current concept of agoraphobia is more extensive and includes avoidance behavior that is caused by places or situations where escape would be difficult or embarrassing or situations in which help may not be available. The patient avoids going through tunnels or bridges, riding on a train, subway, or airplane, or being in a crowd or queue. In more severe cases, the patient refuses to be alone or never leaves home. When the person is in one of these situations, he might present feelings of intense helplessness. Moreover, the presence of a trusted companion can change the behavior of these patients. For example, a person who suffers from agoraphobia can leave the house, make long trips, and perform virtually almost all daily activities as long as the patient is accompanied by a close relative or friend.

The recent revision of the *Diagnostic and Statistical Manual of Mental Disorders*, 5th edition [6] introduced only minor changes to the classification of panic disorder. The description of panic attacks was simplified to include expected and unexpected attacks, differentiating between contextually bound/cued attacks and un-cued attacks. Additionally, panic disorder and agoraphobia are now considered two different conditions, which can, in some cases, be comorbid [6].

With regard to epidemiology, the prevalence of panic disorder varies between 1% and 3% in community samples and between 3% and 8% in clinical samples [7]. The first panic attacks typically appear during adolescence or early adulthood, and women are up to twice more likely to develop the disorder than men [7]. The prevalence of panic disorder varies very little across different regions of the world [8], suggesting an important biological component of the disorder.

3. Neural circuitry associated with panic disorder

The complex nature of the symptoms that are involved in panic disorders suggests that several brain regions may be implicated in this pathology. Some of these neural structures and their possible connections are presented in Figure 4. One of the main regions involved in panic attack is the dorsal portion of the periaqueductal gray (dPAG), a phylogenetically older brain structure that is located in the mesencephalon. Electrical stimulation of the dPAG in humans can produce symptoms that are very similar to panic attacks, such as feelings of terror and imminent death, accompanied by increased heart rate and diffuse pain in the face and chest [9].

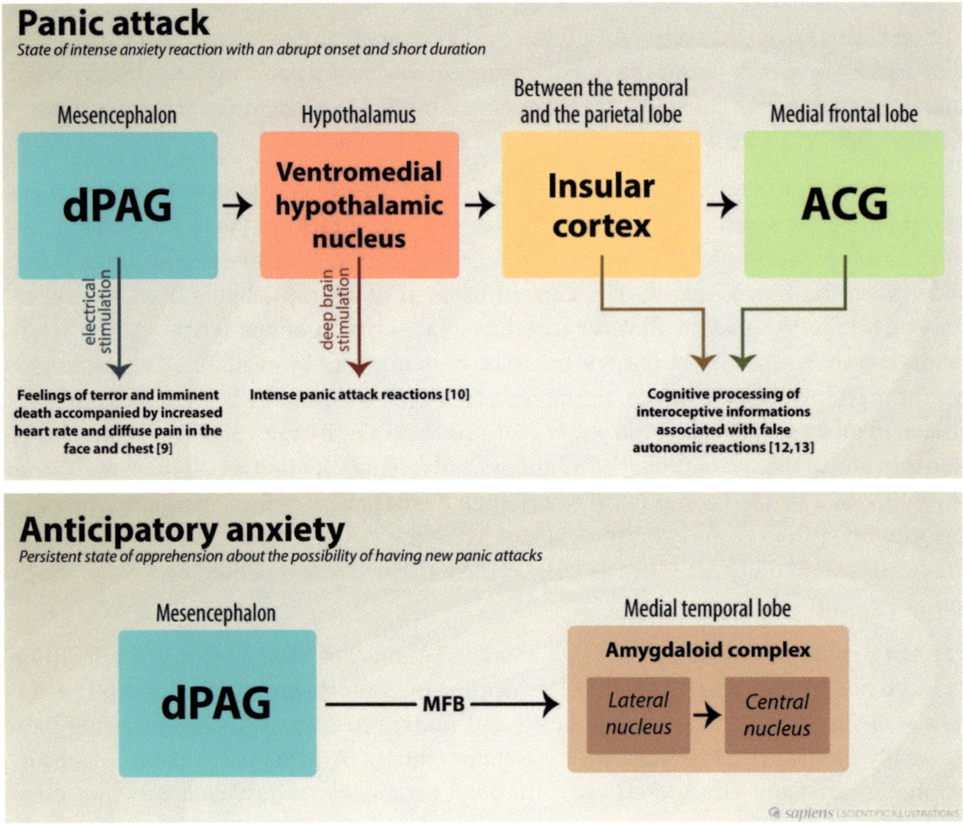

Figure 4. Flow diagram of the neural circuitry associated with the two main symptoms of panic disorder: panic attack (top) and anticipatory anxiety (bottom). dPAG, dorsal periaqueductal gray; ACG, anterior cingulate gyrus; MFB, medial forebrain bundle.

The physiological reactions that are present during a panic attack are likely mediated though neural circuitries that involve ascending projections from the dPAG to hypothalamic areas. Results from an awake patient who received bilateral implantation of deep brain stimulation electrodes in the ventromedial hypothalamic nucleus indicated that stimulation of either hemisphere of the central area of this hypothalamic nucleus evoked intense panic attack reactions [10].

One of the main functions of the hypothalamic region is autonomic regulation. The awareness of these autonomic responses is an extremely important aspect of panic attack. Patients who suffer from panic disorder are extremely sensitive to autonomic responses and thus overreactive to somatic signs [11]. This high sensitivity generates a belief that the autonomic reactions can have disastrous consequences. For example, a person with high sensitivity to autonomic reactions might have a greater propensity to interpret such somatic signs as palpitations, dizziness, nausea, and sweating as signs of a high anxiety reaction, as opposed to someone else who is less sensitive to these symptoms of anxiety.

This misinterpretation of false autonomic reactions might be attributable to dysfunction in brain structures that are responsible for interoceptive integration, such as the insular cortex and the anterior cingulate gyrus [12]. Both of these brain structures are associated with the cognitive processing of interoceptive information, and problems in the representation of internal body information might be one of the causes of panic disorder. Indeed, brain imaging studies indicated that anxiety reactions in patients who suffer from panic disorder recruit several forebrain areas, such as the insular cortex and anterior cingulate gyrus [13].

Acute autonomic reactions and physiological responses that are triggered by the hypothalamic area are processed by the insular cortex, which in turn sends projections to the anterior cingulate gyrus where subjective experiences of these autonomic reactions are generated. The conscious processing of these intense physiological responses in the absence of a potential or real external stimulus of danger is a critical issue in the etiology of panic disorder. Considering the neural circuitry, the symptoms associated with a panic attack are a consequence rather than the cause of physiological changes in the body. The concept of becoming conscious of an emotion as a consequence of autonomic changes is consistent with a classic theory that was independently proposed by William James [14] and Carl Lange [15].

The occurrence of several panic attacks can lead to the development of panic disorder, whose main characteristic, in addition to the presence of panic attacks, is apprehension and persistent concern about the possibility of having new panic attacks. This aspect of panic disorder is likely mediated by ascending projections from the dPAG to amygdaloid complex through the medial forebrain bundle. The amygdaloid complex is located in the medial temporal lobe of both hemispheres and can be subdivided into at least 12 nuclei, each associated with different aspects of an emotional experience. Two of these nuclei are particularly important. The lateral nucleus is the input pathway and responsible for processing external environmental stimuli. The central nucleus is the main output of this complex neural circuitry.

As mentioned above, agoraphobia is one of the main conditions that can develop together with panic disorder. This association between agoraphobia and panic disorder is likely attributable to the fact that the amygdaloid complex is intimately involved in associative aversive leaning. The convergence of environmental neutral stimuli with aversive information, triggered by ascending projections from the dPAG to the lateral nucleus of the amygdala, might result in a constant state of anticipatory anxiety.

Increasing the sensitivity of the lateral nucleus of the amygdala can make the patient more reactive to environmental stimuli, causing him to react defensively to situations that other people simply ignore. In this case, the central nucleus of the amygdala responds adequately to overactivity of the lateral nucleus of the amygdala. Another possibility might be that the lateral nucleus of the amygdala is functioning properly, but the central nucleus of the amygdala, in the absence of any real danger, has excessively high activity. Understanding this neuronal circuitry that involves both internal and external stimulus processing and interpretation is extremely useful for psychotherapeutic interventions to treat panic disorder.

4. Psychological and pharmacological interventions

There are basically two mains strategies to manage the symptoms of panic disorder: psychotherapeutic and pharmacological interventions. Figure 5 illustrates these two types of interventions. Most of the psychotherapeutic techniques that are used for the treatment of panic disorder involve a process of reflection by the patient regarding his emotional dysfunction. Cognitive behavioral therapy, for example, seeks to change the thought patterns and beliefs that these patients have while experiencing symptoms of anxiety. An important issue concerning psychotherapeutic interventions for panic disorder is to change patterns of thinking to appropriately deal with the physiological reactions that the patient has during the panic attack. This technique consists of producing, under controlled conditions, some of the physiological symptoms associated with panic attack so that immediate thinking reactions, such as "I will die, " can be replaced by more appropriate interpretations, such as "I am experiencing great physiological arousal, but it will pass" [16]. The purpose of this technique is to make the patient reinterpret these physiological reactions by changing their patterns of catastrophic thinking (or "catastrophizing") so the patient can adequately deal with these autonomic reactions [17].

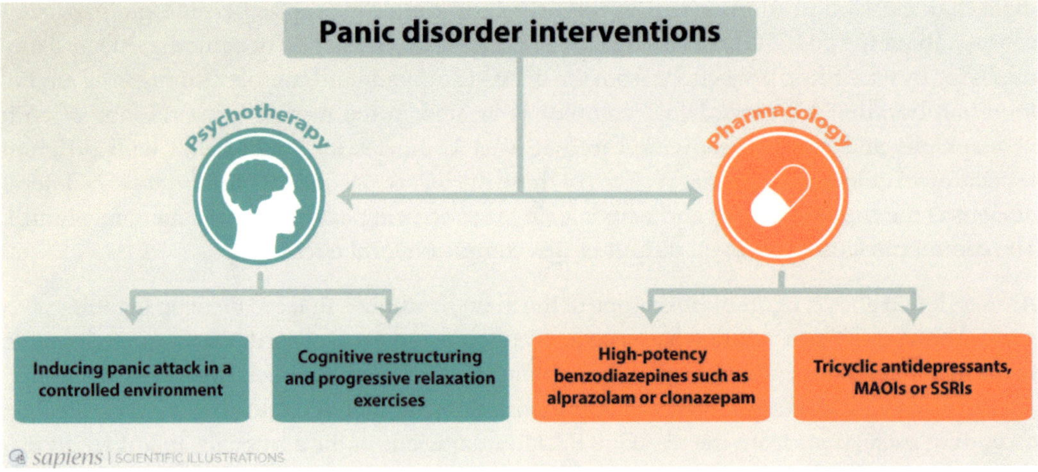

Figure 5. Psychotherapeutic and pharmacological interventions for the treatment of panic disorder. SSRIs, selective serotonin reuptake inhibitors; MAOIs, monoamine oxidase inhibitors.

Panic attacks hardly manifest exclusively by themselves. Panic attacks are often comorbid with symptoms of constant worry and anxiety reactions, especially with agoraphobia. Therefore, in addition to specific techniques that are related to the treatment of panic attacks, the use of relaxation training is common for the treatment of the phobic reactions and constant eager expectation that these patients display.

The effects of psychotherapeutic interventions on the symptoms of panic disorder appear to be related to cortical structures. These phylogenetically newer structures have the ability to inhibit the activity of older structures that are related to exacerbated defense reactions that characterize panic disorder. Indeed, experiments that used animal models of anxiety indicated that rats require the amygdaloid complex but not cortical areas to acquire a fear response to an auditory stimulus that was previously associated with an electric shock. However, cortical regions were necessary for the extinction of fear in response to the auditory stimulus [18]. Recent studies that used two breeding lines of rats that were selected for high and low anxiety-like behavior [19, 20] indicated that long extinction training was able to extinguish phenotypic differences between the two lines, but the divergence was restored after just one fear reacquisition training session [21].

These results allow us to infer that the psychotherapeutic treatment of anxiety disorders does not change the neural structures that are responsible for the etiology of the disorder but rather strengthens other structures that are responsible for its inhibition. Supporting this view is the finding that patients with intense feelings of panic attack exhibited low activity in the prefrontal cortex, thereby causing a lack of inhibition of the amygdaloid complex [22]. Indeed, patients who were diagnosed with panic disorder and received cognitive behavioral therapy exhibited a strong association between clinical improvement and a bilateral increase in the activity of the medial prefrontal cortex [23]. Therefore, a particular anxiety disorder may remain latent after a good response to psychotherapy but might reappear when this inhibitory system loses strength, such as in situations where a patient faces new situations of stress.

Anxiolytic drugs have also been used to manage anxiety symptoms in panic disorder. The first anxiolytic agents that were used to control anxiety were barbiturates, such as phenobarbital, amobarbital, pentobarbital, and secobarbital, which began to be used to control anxiety in the early 20th century. Side effects such as drowsiness, sedation, and high dependence potential prompted the search for other, more effective anxiolytics. In the early 1960s, benzodiazepines were introduced, such as chlordiazepoxide, diazepam, bromazepam, clobazam, clorazepam, estazolam, flunitrazepam, flurazepam, lorazepam, and nitrazepam, whose high efficacy combined with lower toxicity and ability to produce dependence allowed these compounds to be adopted as the drugs of choice for the treatment of anxiety symptoms.

Recently, drugs with actions on serotonin (5-hydroxytryptamine [5-HT]) neurotransmission have been used to treat anxiety symptoms. Among these drugs is buspirone, a 5-HT_{1A} autoreceptor agonist. The stimulation of these receptors leads to a reduction of serotonin transmission. The therapeutic effect of buspirone takes approximately 2–3 weeks to become apparent. This period appears to be related to a reduction of serotonergic activity that is caused by continuous 5-HT_{1A} autoreceptor stimulation. Thus, the therapeutic effects of buspirone appear to be related to a reduction of serotonergic activity.

A main issue when dealing with panic disorder is the fact that the occurrence of panic attacks appears to be resistant to the action of traditional anxiolytic agents. Only high-potency benzodiazepines, such as alprazolam or clonazepam, when used at high doses, can be extremely useful for managing anxious features of the acute phase of panic disorder. In such cases, however, high doses can produce undesirable side effects, such as sleepiness, memory impairment, and ataxia.

As discussed earlier, the pharmacological treatment of panic disorder has relied on the pioneering work of Donald Klein, who in the early 1960s showed that imipramine, a tricyclic antidepressant that inhibits the reuptake of norepinephrine and serotonin, alleviated the occurrence of panic attacks [5]. Tricyclic antidepressants, such as amitriptyline, clomipramine, and nortriptyline, were the first drugs that were used in the treatment of panic disorder. Subsequently, older antidepressants that inhibit monoamine oxidase (MAOIs), such as phenelzine nialamide, tranylcypromine, and isocarboxazid, were also effective in the treatment of panic disorder [24]. Currently, selective serotonin reuptake inhibitors (SSRIs), such as fluoxetine, paroxetine, and sertraline, are employed in the treatment of panic disorder. SSRIs have the common ability to inhibit the protein that is responsible for transporting serotonin back into the presynaptic neuron, thereby increasing the activity of this neurotransmitter in the synaptic cleft.

Notably, the use of SSRIs in the treatment of panic attack paradoxically increases symptoms of anxiety mainly during the beginning of the treatment. This paradox has been clarified through a theory developed by the Brazilian neuroscientist Frederick Graeff and British psychiatrist William Deakin. According to this theory [25], the stimulation of serotonergic receptors in the amygdala enhances the sensitivity of individuals to dangerous stimuli, thereby producing an anxiogenic effect. Thus, serotonergic antagonists, such as buspirone, tend to reduce anxiety. The stimulation of serotonergic systems in the dPAG reduces the occurrence of panic attacks. In this case, serotonergic agonists have the ability to reduce the occurrence of panic attacks but with a side effect of increasing the incidence of anxiety reactions through the action of these compounds in more rostral structures, such as the amygdaloid complex. Neuroimaging studies have indicated that the anxiety-induced activation of forebrain structures inhibits the activation of brainstem structures that is caused by panic attacks, and *vice versa* [26]. Patients with bilateral amygdala damage were shown to be more prone to panic attacks than healthy volunteers [27].

Clinical evidence also supports this theory. For example, relaxation therapy that is used for the treatment of anxiety symptoms can precipitate panic attacks [28]. Furthermore, the frequency of panic attacks is higher during the initial course of panic disorder, when anticipatory anxiety levels are relatively low, than in the late phases of panic disorder, when anticipatory anxiety is extremely high [29]. Other clinical studies indicated that patients who suffer from panic disorder and are acutely treated with serotonin releaser and uptake blocker D-fenfluramine presented a decrease in the occurrence of panic attacks but displayed an increase in anxiety symptoms [30]. Conversely, clinical trials with the 5-$HT_{2A/2C}$ receptor antagonist ritanserin reduced symptoms of anticipatory anxiety [31] but exacerbated the incidence of panic attacks [32]. Finally, experimental studies that used animal models of anxiety supported the view that the activation of neural circuitry that is involved in anxiety might, in fact, inhibit the incidence of panic attacks [33, 34, 35].

5. Concluding remarks

Although anxiety is important in our everyday lives, it becomes a pathological phenomenon when its duration or intensity is extremely high and leads to significant suffering and distress. The historical concept of a unitary anxiety disorder has been replaced by a heterogeneous group of psychopathologies with different etiologies. Panic disorder is a complex anxiety disorder that involves both recurrent, unexpected panic attacks and persistent concern about having additional attacks. Several brain structures participate in different components of panic disorder. The dPAG is a core structure remove involved in the genesis of panic attacks. Projections to the hypothalamus and then to the insular cortex and anterior cingulate gyrus through the nucleus of the solitary tract might be responsive for misinterpreting interoceptive information that is associated with false autonomic reactions. Projections to the amygdaloid complex might be associated with anticipatory anxiety as a consequence of recurrent panic attacks. Psychological interventions combine *in vivo* exposure to interoceptive and autonomic symptoms that are present during a panic attack with relaxation training to manage the anxiety associated with having another panic attack. Pharmacological treatment combines high-potency benzodiazepines and substances with antidepressant properties, suggesting relative independence between the mechanisms that modulate panic attack and the constant anticipatory anxiety associated with new panic attacks. Indeed, clinical and experimental results with animal models of anxiety suggest that anticipatory anxiety might have an inhibitory effect on panic attacks.

Author details

Daniel C. Mograbi[1,2], Vitor Castro-Gomes[3], Elie Cheniaux[4,5] and J. Landeira-Fernandez[1*]

*Address all correspondence to: landeira@puc-rio.br

1 Pontifícia Universidade Católica – Rio, Department of Psychology, Brasil

2 King's College London, Institute of Psychiatry, Department of Psychology, UK

3 Universidade Federal de São João Del-Rei, Department of Biossystems Engineering, Brasil

4 Universidade Federal do Rio de Janeiro, Institute of Psychiatry, Brasil

5 Universidade do Estado do Rio de Janeiro, Department of Medical Sciences, Brasil

References

[1] Lupien, S.J., Maheu, F., Tu, M., Fiocco, A., & Schramek, T.E.: The effects of stress and stress hormones on human cognition: implications for the field of brain and cognition. Brain and Cognition. 2007; 65, 209-237.

[2] Yerkes, R.M. & Dodson, J.D.: The relation of strength of stimulus to rapidity of habit-formation. Journal of Comparative Neurology and Psychology. 1908; 18, 459-482.

[3] Freud, S: On the grounds for detaching a particular syndrome from neurasthenia under the description "anxiety neurosis." In: *The standard edition of the complete psychological works of Sigmund Freud.* 1978 [1895]; (III, pp. 87-115). London: Hogarth Press.

[4] Glas, G. (2003). A conceptual history of anxiety and depression. In: S. Kasper & J.A. den Boer (Eds.), *Handbook of Anxiety and Depression* (2nd edition, pp. 1-48). New York: Marcel Dekker.

[5] Klein, D.F. & Fink, M.: Psychiatric reaction patterns to imipramine. American Journal of Psychiatry. 1962; 119, 432-438.

[6] American Psychiatric Association (2013). *Diagnostic and statistical manual of mental disorders* (5th edition, pp. 5-25). Washington, DC: American Psychiatric Publishing.

[7] Katon, W.J.: Panic disorder. New England Journal of Medicine. 2006; 354, 2360-2367.

[8] Ayuso-Mateos, J.L.: Global burden of panic disorder in the year 2000. Geneva: World Health Organization. [http://www.who.int/healthinfo/statistics/bod_posttraumatic-stressdisorder.pdf; Retrieved February 17, 2015]

[9] Nashold, B.S. Jr., Wilson, W.P., & Slaughter, D.G.: Sensations evoked by stimulation in the midbrain of man. Journal of Neurosurgery. 1969; 30, 14-24.

[10] Wilent, W.B, Oh, M.Y., Buetefisch, C.M., Bailes, J.E., Cantella, D., Angle, C., & Whiting, D.M.: Induction of panic attack by stimulation on the ventromedial hypothalamus. Journal of Neurosurgery. 2010; 112, 1295-1298.

[11] Reiss, S. & McNally, R.J. (1985). Expectancy model of fear. In: S. Reiss & R.R. Bootzin (Eds.), *Theoretical issues in behavior therapy* (pp. 107-121). Orlando: Academic Press.

[12] Uchida, R.R., Del-Bem, C.M., Busatto, G.F., Duran, F.L., Guimarães, F.S., Crippa, J.A., Araújo, D., Santos, A.C., & Graeff, F.G.: Regional gray matter abnormalities in panic disorder: a voxel-based morphometry study. Psychiatry Research. 2008; 163, 21-29.

[13] De Carvalho, M.R., Dias, G.P., Cosci, F., De Melo-Neto, V.L., Bevilaqua, M.C., Gardino, P.F., & Nardi, A.E.: Current findings of fMRI in panic disorder: contributions for the fear neurocircuitry and CBT effects. Expert Review of Neurotherapeutics. 2010; 10, 291-303.

[14] James, W.: What is an emotion? Mind. 1884; 9, 188-205.

[15] Lange, C. G.: Om sindsbevaegelser: et psychkofysiologisk studie. (1885 [1967])[The mechanism of the emotions: a psychophysiological study; originally pub. by Jacob Lunds, Copenhagen].

[16] Sanchez-Meca, J., Rosa-Alcazar, A., Marin-Martinez, F., & Gomez-Conesa, A.: Psychological treatment of panic disorder with or without agoraphobia: a meta-analysis. Clinical Psychology Review. 2010; 30, 37-50.

[17] Ito, L.M., de Araujo, L.A., Tess, V.L., de Barros-Neto, T.P., Asbahr, F.R., & Marks, I.: Self-exposure therapy for panic disorder with agoraphobia: randomised controlled study of external v. interoceptive self-exposure. British Journal of Psychiatry. 2001; 178, 331-336.

[18] Morgan, M.A. & LeDoux, J.E.: Differential contribution of dorsal and ventral medial prefrontal cortex to the acquisition and extinction of conditioned fear in rats. Behavioral Neuroscience. 1995; 109, 681-688.

[19] Castro-Gomes, V.C and Landeira-Fernandez, J.: Amygdaloid lesions produced similar contextual fear conditioning disruption in the Carioca high- and low-conditioned freezing rats. Brain Research. 2008; 1233, 137-145.

[20] Castro-Gomes, V.C., Silva, C.E.B., & Landeira-Fernandez, J. (2011). The Carioca high- and low-conditioned freezing lines: a new animal model of generalized anxiety disorder. In: V. Kalinin (Ed.), *Anxiety disorder* (pp. 121-134). Rijeka: Intech.

[21] Castro-Gomes, V.C., León, L., Mograbi, D., Cardenas, L.F., Landeira-Fernandez, J.: Contextual fear extinction and re-extinction in Carioca high- and low-conditioned freezing rats. World Journal of Neuroscience. 2014; 4, 247-252.

[22] Berkowitz, R.L., Coplan, J.D., Reddy, D.P., Gorman, J.M.: The human dimension: how the prefrontal cortex modulates the subcortical fear response. Reviews in the Neurosciences. 2007; 18, 191-207.

[23] Sakai, Y., Kumano, H., Nishikawa, M., Sakano, Y., Kaiya, H., Imabayashi, E., Ohnishi, T., Matsuda, H., Yasuda, A., Sato, A., Diksic, M., & Kuboki, T. (2006). Changes in cerebral glucose utilization in patients with panic disorder treated with cognitive-behavioral therapy. Neuroimage. 2006; 33, 218-226.

[24] Sheehan, D.V., Ballenger, J., & Jacobsen, G.: Treatment of endogenous anxiety with phobic, hysterical, and hypochondriacal symptoms. Archives of General Psychiatry. 1980; 37, 51-59.

[25] Deakin, J.W.F. & Graeff, F.G. 5-HT and mechanisms of defense. Journal of Psychopharmacology. 1991; 5, 305-315.

[26] Mobbs, D., Marchant, J.L., Hassabis, D., Seymour, B., Tan, G., Gray, M., Petrovic, P., Dolan, R.J., & Frith, C.D.: From threat to fear: the neural organization of defensive fear systems in humans. Journal of Neuroscience. 2009; 29, 12236-12243.

[27] Feinstein, J.S., Buzza, C., Hurlemann, R., Follmer, R.L., Dahdaleh, N.S., Coryell, W.H., Welsh, M.J., Tranel, D., & Wemmie, J.A.: Fear and panic in humans with bilateral amygdala damage. Nature Neuroscience. 2013; 16, 270-272.

[28] Adler, C.M., Craske, M.G., & Barlow, D.H.: Relaxation-induced panic (RIP): when resting isn't peaceful. Integrative Psychiatry. 1987; 5(2), 94-112.

[29] Klein, D.F. & Klein, H.M. (1989). The definition and psychopharmacology of spontaneous panic and phobia. In: P.J. Tyrer (Ed.), *Psychopharmacology of anxiety* (pp. 135-162). Oxford: Oxford University Press.

[30] Targum, S.D. & Marshall, L.E.: Fenfluramine provocation of anxiety in patients with panic disorder. Psychiatry Research. 1989; 28, 295-306.

[31] Ceulemans, D.L., Hoppenbrouwers, M.L., Gelders, Y.G., & Reyntjens, A.J.: The influence of ritanserin, a serotonin antagonist, in anxiety disorders: a double-blind placebo-controlled study versus lorazepam. Pharmacopsychiatry. 1985; 18, 303-305.

[32] Deakin, J.F.W., Wang, M., & Guimarães, F.S. (1990). Early clinical experience with ritanserin in neurotic patients. In: *Clinical profile of ritanserin* (series title: *Proceedings of the World Federation of Societies of Biological Psychiatry Symposium*, pp. 16-33). Chester: Adis International.

[33] Magierek, V., Ramos, P.L., da Silveira-Filho, N.G., Nogueira, R.L., Landeira-Fernandez, J.: Context fear conditioning inhibits panic-like behavior elicited by electrical stimulation of dorsal periaqueductal gray. Neuroreport. 2003; 14, 1641-1644.

[34] Galvão, B., Larrubia, B., Hommes, W.J., Cardenas, F.P., Cruz, A.P.M., & Landeira-Fernandez, J.: Effects of contextual fear conditioning and pentylenetetrazol on panic-like reactions induced by dorsal periaqueductal gray stimulation with N-methyl-D-aspartate. Psychology & Neuroscience. 2010; 3, 67-72.

[35] Galvão, B.O., Castro-Gomes, V.C., Maisonnette, S., Landeira-Fernandez, J.: Panic-like behaviors in Carioca high-and low-conditioned freezing rats. Psychology & Neuroscience. 2011; 4, 205-210.

Chapter 4

Genetics of Posttraumatic Stress Disorder — Candidate Genes and Their Implication in the Disease-Associated Molecular Pathomechanisms

Boyajyan Anna, Avetyan Diana, Hovhannisyan Lilit and Mkrtchyan Gohar

Additional information is available at the end of the chapter

http://dx.doi.org/10.5772/60443

Abstract

Posttraumatic stress disorder (PTSD) is a complex psychiatric disorder (DSM-V code: 309.81; ICD-10 codes: F43.1). PTSD is an anxiety disorder developed in a person experiencing, witnessing, or learning about an extreme physically or/and psychologically distressing event. Its incidence and the number of this disease-affected people are threateningly increasing in contemporary society. Therefore, the development of prognostic strategies and novel efficient methods on early diagnostics and treatment of PTSD is currently considered as one of the most important healthcare problems worldwide.

Results of epidemiologic, clinical, and experimental studies suggest implication of both environmental and genetic factors in pathomechanisms of PTSD and that, most probably, PTSD belongs to complex disorders with polygenic inheritance. Whereas the environmental factors triggering PTSD are well defined, less is known about PTSD-associated genetic variations and molecular etiopathomechanisms.

Several studies, including our own reports, suggest the involvement of neuro-immune alterations in the pathophysiology of PTSD. These include changes in neuronal plasticity, synaptic connectivity, humoral and cellular immune-mediated responses, and apoptosis rate leading to cognitive deficit and behavioral changes in patients with PTSD accompanied with development of low-grade inflammatory reactions. Currently, many research groups working on elucidation of molecular mechanisms of PTSD are exploring whether these changes have genetic background or are induced by other external or internal environmental factors.

In the present chapter, we provide overview and discussion of the existing data, including our own results, on variations in genes encoding neuro-immune and apoptotic mediators and regulators and related transcription factors in PTSD patients. Potential role of these genetic variations in generation and development of PTSD is considered and the implication of relevant candidate genes in mechanisms responsible for disease progression is proposed.

Keywords: Apoptosis, candidate genes, complement system, posttraumatic stress disorder, synaptic plasticity

---

1. Introduction

Posttraumatic stress disorder (PTSD; DSM-V code: 309.81; ICD-10 codes: F43.1) is a complex, severe, and chronic psychiatric illness [1–2]. PTSD is an anxiety disorder developed in a person experiencing, witnessing, or learning about an extreme physically and/or psychologically distressing event [3–7]. Its incidence and the number of disease-affected people are threateningly increasing in contemporary society. They usually remain out of society, become drug addicted, alcoholic, and often commit suicide [8–10]. Therefore, development of prognostic strategies, novel efficient methods on early diagnostics and treatment of PTSD is currently considered as one of the most important health care problems worldwide.

Results of epidemiologic, clinical, and experimental studies suggest implication of both environmental and genetic factors in pathomechanisms of PTSD, and that, most probably, PTSD belongs to the complex disorders with polygenic inheritance. PTSD is also unique in its exposure to an environmental (traumatic) event as the first criterion for diagnosis. Whereas the environmental factors triggering PTSD are well defined, less is known about PTSD-associated genetic variations and molecular etiopathomechanisms [11–17]. Although it is beyond the scope of many studies to comprehensively discuss the genetics of PTSD, it should be noted that there is an emerging literature on genetic variations in those neurobiological systems which drive responses to trauma and, consequently, are risk factors to develop PTSD. Many studies on detection of candidate genes association with PTSD are being carried up to date [18–26].

In the present chapter, we provide overview and discussion of the existing data, including genetic variants of serotonergic and dopaminergic systems, hypothalamic–pituitary–adrenal (HPA) axis, and other genes related to neurotransmission, neuromodulation, and stress physiology. Here, we have also included our own results on variations in genes encoding neuro, immune, and apoptotic mediators and regulators, and related transcription factors in PTSD patients. Potential role of these genetic variations in generation and development of PTSD is considered and the implication of relevant candidate genes in mechanisms responsible for disease progression is proposed.

2. Genetic Studies of PTSD

2.1. Neuroendocrine system candidate genes

Many studies indicate association between PTSD and polymorphisms of number of genes, suggesting a polygenic nature of PTSD. Several studies indicate that functional abnormalities in neuroendocrine system detected in PTSD patients are conditioned with hereditary factor [21–26]. Thus, as it follows from Table 1, PTSD is associated with the genetic mutations in a number of genes encoding neurotransmitters, hormones and their enzymes, hormone receptors and transporters.

Candidate genes	Cytogenetic location	Studied SNPs	Source
Dopaminergic system			
Dopamine D2 receptor *(DRD2)*	11q23	rs1800497	[24-30]
Dopamine D3 receptor *(DRD3)*	3q13.3	rs2134655, rs201252087, rs4646996, rs9868039	[31]
Dopamine D4 receptor *(DRD4)*	11p15.5	VNTR	[32]
Dopamine transporter type 1 *(SLC6A3, DAT1)*	5p15.3	VNTR	[33]
Dopamine beta-hydroxylase *(DBH)*	9q34	rs1611115	[37, 38]
Catechol-O-methyltransferase *(COMT)*	22q11	rs4680 rs4633C	[39-41]
Serotonergic system			
Serotonin transporter *(SLC6A4, SERT)*	17q11	rs4795541, rs25531	[42-45]
Serotonin type-2A receptor *(HTR2A)*	13q14.2	rs6311	[46, 47]
Tryptophan hydroxylase 1 *(TPH1)*	11p15.1	rs2108977	[48]
Tryptophan hydroxylase 2 *(TPH2)*	12q21.1	rs11178997	[41, 48]
GABAergic system			
Gamma-aminobutyric acid receptor alpha-2 *(GABRA2)*	4p12	rs279836, rs279826	[49]
Hypothalamic-pituitary-adrenal axis			
Cannabinoid receptor 1 *(CNR1)*	6q15		[50]

Candidate genes	Cytogenetic location	Studied SNPs	Source
Glucocorticoid receptor GCCR *(NR3C1)*	5q31.3	rs41423247 rs258747	[51, 52]
Corticotropin-releasing hormone receptor-1 *(CRHR1)*	17q21.31	rs12944712	[53]
Pituitary adenylate cyclase 1 receptor *(ADCYAP1R1, PAC1)*	7p14.3	rs2267735	[54, 55]
FK506 binding protein 5 *(FKBP5)*	6p21	rs9296158, rs3800373, 1360780, rs9470080	[56-62]
Neurotrophic factor			
Brain-derived neurotrophic factor *(BDNF)*	11p14.1	rs6265	[30, 63-66]
Other genes			
Apolipoprotein E *(ApoE)*	19q13	rs429358, rs7412	[67]
Monoamine oxidase B *(MAOB)*	Xp11.3	rs1799836	[70]
Neuropeptide Y *(NPY)*	7p15.3	rs16139	[71]
Phosphoribosyl transferase domain-containing protein 1 *(PRTFDC1)*	10p12.1	rs6482463	[73]
Regulator of G-protein signalling 2 *(RGS2)*	1q31.2	rs4606	[74]

Table 1. Neuroendocrine system candidate genes in PTSD

2.1.1. Dopaminergic system

Dopaminergic system dysregulation has long been implicated in the pathophysiology of PTSD. A positive association between the risk for development of PTSD and Taq1A (rs1800497) polymorphism of the dopamine D2 receptor gene was found [24–30]. The dopamine D3 receptor (*DRD3*) gene's 4 SNPs (rs2134655, rs201252087, rs4646996, and rs9868039) showed evidence of association with PTSD [31]. Also, positive association was revealed between tandem repeat polymorphism of dopamine transporter gene and PTSD, as well as between dopamine D4 transporter gene long allele and severity of PTSD symptoms [32]. Recent publications reported that carriers of the 9R of allele of the gene, encoding the dopamine transporter (*SLC6A3, DAT, or DAT1*), had increased the risk of PTSD [33–36]. This finding suggests that genetically determined features of *DAT* may contribute to the development of PTSD among trauma survivors. Genetic variants in dopamine beta-hydroxylase (*DBH*) gene represent a likely candidate for examining genetic contributions to PTSD because of the role this enzyme plays in converting dopamine to norepinephrine as a part of catecholamine synthesis [37, 38]. A significant association between one or more copies of the rs4680 allele of

COMT and PTSD has been reported. Thus, regulation of COMT and subsequent catecholamine neurotransmitter cascades may be an important factor in fear processing for those with PTSD and similar psychiatric disorders [39, 40]. Moreover, a recent study has shown a significant association of the *COMT* allele rs4633C with total PTSD, and severity scores of D category (negative alterations in cognitions and mood) of DSM-V categories [41].

2.1.2. Serotonergic system candidate genes

Dysregulation of brain serotonergic systems has been implicated in the pathophysiology of PTSD; indeed, this pathway represents the most studied candidate in PTSD. The most studied polymorphism in this system is located in the promoter region of the serotonin transporter encoding gene (*SLC6A4, 5-HTTLPR*). Several studies indicated that this risk was associated with rs4795541, rs25531 genotypes, and PTSD [35, 42–45]. Serotonin receptor 2A rs6311 polymorphism has also been found to be associated with PTSD [46–47].

Goenjian and colleagues' studies have suggested association of *TPH1, TPH2,* and *5HTTLPR* with PTSD and depressive symptoms [48]. It was shown that the *TPH-2* allele rs11178997T and *COMT* allele rs4633C together accounted for 7% of the variance in severity scores of PTSD. Carriers of these *COMT* and *TPH-2* alleles may be at increased risk for PTSD. These findings provided biological support for dividing DSM-IV category C symptoms into DSM-V categories C and D [41].

2.1.3. GABAergic system

Inhibitory neurotransmitter, gamma-aminobutyric acid receptor gene (*GABAA*) has been studied in relation to PTSD. Three polymorphisms in the *GABAA* receptor subunit alpha 2 (*GABRA2*) had significant interactions with childhood trauma to predict PTSD [49].

2.1.4. HPA axis candidate genes

PTSD is also characterized by dysfunction of the stress response system, such that activity of the HPA axis is altered. Recent studies reported associations between PTSD and cannabinoid receptor (*CNR1*) gene variants NM_016083 and NM_033181; [50], glucocorticoid receptor (*NR3C1,* rs41423247, and rs258747) gene [51, 52], and between SNP in corticotropin-releasing hormone receptor-1 (*CRHR1,* rs12944712) and PTSD [53]. Also neuropeptide pituitary adenylate cyclase-activating polypeptide is regulating the stress response. Recently, a genetic variant in the PAC1 receptor (*ADCYAP1R1;* rs2267735) was found to be associated with PTSD [54, 55]. Of particular interest were the findings that a genetic variation of the glucocorticoid receptor cochaperone protein, FKBP5, moderates risk of developing PTSD in childhood abuse cases [56–61]. Binder and colleagues found that 4 SNPs in *FKBP5* (rs9296158, rs3800373, 1360780, rs9470080) interacted with child abuse severity to predict adult PTSD symptoms [62].

2.1.5. Neurotrophic factor candidate genes

Brain derived neurotrophic factor (BDNF) is involved in the neural plasticity underlying the extinction of fear and recovery from stress, both disrupted in PTSD. Based on its role in hippocampal-dependent learning and the neurobiology of anxiety and depression, the *BDNF* gene has been studied in relation to PTSD. A significant interaction between *DRD2* Taq1A (rs1800497) and Val66Met (rs6265) predicts PTSD severity [30]. Interestingly, a recent study in humans and rats suggested that *BDNF* overexpression may be a critical stress response underlying PTSD by showing that the Val66Met allele confers vulnerability to PTSD via startle data and plasma BDNF levels [63–66].

2.1.6. Other candidate genes

Apolipoprotein E (ApoE) is involved in stress dysregulation. A significant association between the ApoE2 allele and impaired memory and greater re-experiencing symptoms has been found in combat-exposed PTSD patients [67–69]. The monoamine oxidase B gene (*MAOB*) rs1799836 polymorphism has been studied in relation with PTSD because *MAOB* expression in platelets has been implicated in several psychopathologies and may represent a biomarker for vulnerability to psychiatric illness [70]. Recent studies of the link between neuropeptide Y (NPY) and PTSD were published [71]. However, another study did not find any association between polymorphism in *NPY* (Leu7Pro; rs16139) and PTSD in a population of Caucasian combat veterans [72]. Nievergelt and colleagues found evidence for phosphoribosyl transferase domain-containing protein 1 (*PRTFDC1*) as a potential novel PTSD gene, but this finding needs further replication [73]. Finally, it was reported that the regulator of G-protein signaling 2 (RGS2) belongs to a protein family that has been widely involved in neural plasticity, particularly associated with learning and memory, and may play a critical role in PTSD-associated cognitive dysfunction. In PTSD patients experiencing high stress and low social support, an association with *RGS2* (rs4606) was found [74].

2.2. Complement system candidate genes

The complement system is major effector of the immune response, which acts on the interface of innate and adaptive immunity, and is a key component and trigger of many immunoregulatory mechanisms. Changes in the functional activity of the complement cascade contribute to the pathology of many human diseases [75–77], including mental disorders [78–83], and are also detected during physiological stress [84, 85]. It has already been demonstrated that complement system alterations are involved in PTSD pathogeneses, particularly hypoactivation state of the complement alternative pathway in PTSD patients, which positively and significantly correlates ($p < 0.05$) with total (frequency and intensity) PTSD symptom cluster of re-experiencing, avoidance, and hyperarousal, and with PTSD total symptom score [13]. Now, our interest is focused on studying the genetic basis of complement system regulators, particularly the role and genetic variants of complement factors B, H, and I (*CFB, CFH,* and *CFI,* accordingly) in PTSD. The distributions of genotypes for *CFB, CFH,* and *CFI* SNPs in both patients and control groups were in compliance with Hardy–Weinberg equilibrium ($p > 0.05$). The allele and phenotype frequencies of *CFB, CFH,* and *CFI* genetic variants in the groups of PTSD patients and controls are shown in Table 2.

Gene (SNP)	Genotypes			Alleles		Carriage
***CFB* rs12614**	CC	CT	TT	C	T	T
PTSD	87 (0.58)	59 (0.4)	3 (0.02)	233 (0.78)	65 (0.22)	62 (0.42)
Controls	125 (0.55)	89 (0.4)	12 (0.05)	339 (0.75)	113 (0.25)	101 (0.45)
p				0.32		0.56
OR				0.84		1.13
95% CI:				0.59-1.19		0.75-1.72
***CFB* rs1048709**	GG	GA	AA	G	A	A
PTSD	134 (0.918)	11 (0.075)	1 (0.007)	279 (0.955)	13 (0.045)	12 (0.08)
Controls	167 (0.92)	14 (0.08)	0 (0)	348 (0.96)	14 (0.04)	14 (0.08)
p				0.7		0.87
OR				1.16		0.94
95% CI:				0.54-2.50		0.42-2.09
***CFH* rs424535**	TT	TA	AA	T	A	A
PTSD	56 (0.38)	47 (0.32)	44 (0.3)	159 (0.54)	135 (0.46)	91 (0.62)
Controls	74 (0.344)	108 (0.502)	33 (0.154)	256 (0.6)	174 (0.4)	141 (0.6)
p				0.145		0.47
OR				1.25		1.17
95% CI:				0.93-1.69		0.76-1.81
***CFH*rs1061170**	CC	CT	TT	C	T	T
PTSD	30 (0.21)	53 (0.36)	63 (0.43)	113 (0.39)	179 (0.61)	83 (0.47)
Controls	24 (0.11)	104 (0.46)	97 (0.43)	152 (0.34)	298 (0.66)	128 (0.57)
p				0.17		1.0
OR				0.81		1.92
95% CI:				0.60-1.10		1.05-3.52
***CFH* rs800292**	CC	CT	TT	C	T	T
PTSD	117 (0.8)	25 (0.17)	4 (0.03)	259 (0.89)	33 (0.11)	29 (0.2)
Controls	166 (0.74)	55 (0.24)	4 (0.02)	387 (0.86)	63 (0.14)	59 (0.26)
p				0.29		0.16
OR				0.78		1.43
95% CI:				0.50-1.23		0.87- 2.37
***CFI* rs10033900**	TT	TC	CC	T	C	C
PTSD	38 (0.3)	62 (0.4)	49 (0.3)	138 (0.46)	160 (0.54)	111 (0.75)
Controls	69 (0.31)	99 (0.44)	57 (0.25)	237 (0.53)	213 (0.47)	156 (0.69)

Gene (SNP)	Genotypes			Alleles		Carriage
P				0.089		0.279
OR				1.29		0.77
95% CI:				0.962-1.73		0.486-1.23
***CFI*rs1000954**	GG	GA	AA	G	A	A
PTSD	98 (0.66)	40 (0.27)	10 (0.07)	236 (0.8)	60 (0.2)	50 (0.34)
Controls	84 (0.488)	75 (0.436)	12 (0.076)	243 (0.71)	101 (0.29)	87 (0.51)
P				**0.02**[a]		**0.006**[b]
OR				0.61		2.03
95% CI:				0.42-0.88		1.29-3.2
***CFI* rs4469075**	CC	CG	GG	C	G	G
PTSD	19 (0.13)	60 (0.42)	65 (0.45)	98 (0.34)	190 (0.66)	79 (0.55)
Controls	17 (0.1)	76 (0.5)	71 (0.4)	110 (0.3)	218 (0.7)	93 (0.57)
P				1.0		0.75
OR				0.98		1.32
95% CI:				0.7-1.37		0.64– 2.70

[a]$p_{corrected}$ values for comparison of mutant allele frequency between PTSD patients and controls.

[b]$p_{corrected}$ values for comparison of mutant allele carriage between PTSD patients and controls.

Table 2. Distribution of genotypes, alleles and carriage of minor alleles of CFB, CFH and CFI polymorphisms in patients with PTSD and controls.

According to the results obtained, the *CFI* rs1000954*A allele was more frequent in controls than in patients (0.29 vs. 0.20, $p_{nominal} = 0.008$, OR = 0.61, 95 %CI: 0.42-0.88). Also, the carriers of this allele were overrepresented in the group of controls compared to patients (0.51 vs. 0.34, $p_{nominal}$ = 0.002, OR = 2.03, 95% CI: 1.29–3.2). In case of other selected polymorphisms, no significant association with PTSD was found ($p > 0.05$).

2.3. Candidate genes of apoptosis

Apoptosis is a genetically programmed, morphologically distinct form of cell death that can be triggered by a variety of physiological and pathological stimuli [86]. According to various apoptotic stimuli, apoptosis can be induced by two major pathways: the intrinsic pathway (mitochondria-dependent pathway) and the extrinsic pathway (death receptor-dependent pathway) [87]. Recent studies reported that neuronal apoptosis of amygdala, hippocampus, and medial prefrontal cortex (mPFC) have a certain relationship with the pathogenesis of PTSD [88]. However, the role of apoptosis in the pathogenesis of PTSD is not yet entirely clear.

Apoptosis is the process of strict control multigene, known in the process of apoptosis with a series of apoptosis-related genes, such as Bcl-2 family, caspase family, C-myc oncogenes, and tumor suppressor gene P53, etc. The Bcl-2 family proteins play a crucial role in the process of apoptosis and are considered to be the final passage of apoptosis. Bcl-2 family proteins regulate mitochondrial structure and functional stability with the help of other apoptosis protein synergy. According to the recent study, the increase of the Bcl-2 and Bax expression and the imbalance in the Bcl-2/Bax ratio were few of the mechanisms causing mPFC neuronal apoptosis, which may be one of the reasons of PTSD development in rat [88].

According to our study, the rs956572*A minor allele of the *BCL2* gene was overrepresented in patients with PTSD compared to healthy subjects (0.64 vs. 0.41, $p_{nominal}$ = 6.02E-11, OR = 2.59, 95% CI: 1.94–3.44). In addition, the carriers of this allele were more in the group of patients compared to controls (0.87 vs. 0.65, $p_{nominal}$ = 4.11E-7, OR = 3.53, 95% CI: 2.14–5.81). Further, we found that the rs1801018*G minor allele of the *BCL2* gene was more frequent among controls compared to patients (0.5 vs. 0.4, $p_{nominal}$ = 0.0036, OR = 0.66, 95% CI: 0.50–0.87). Also, the carriers of the rs1801018*G minor allele were more frequent in controls than in patients (0.79 vs. 0.61, $p_{nominal}$ = 8.6E-5, OR = 2.41, 95% CI: 1.54–3.75). After Bonferroni correction, difference in allele frequency between the patient and the control groups minor alleles remained significant (Table 3).

Gene (SNP)	**Genotypes**			**Alleles**		**Carriage**
***ANXA5* rs11575945**	CC	CT	TT	C	T	T
PTSD	63 (0.79)	14 (0.17)	3 (0.04)	140 (0.875)	20 (0.125)	17 (0.21)
Controls	53 (0.71)	21 (0.28)	1 (0.01)	127 (0.85)	23 (0.15)	22 (0.29)
p				1.4[a]		0.75[b]
OR				0.79		0.65
95% CI:				0.41 - 1.5		0.31 - 1.35
***ANXA11* rs1049550**	GG	GA	AA	G	A	A
PTSD	83 (0.415)	101 (0.505)	16 (0.08)	267 (0.67)	133 (0.33)	117 (0.59)
Controls	68 (0.34)	97 (0.485)	35 (0.175)	233 (0.58)	167 (0.42)	132 (0.66)
p				**0.013**[a]		0.12[b]
OR				0.695		1.38
95% CI:				0.52 - 0.93		0.92 - 2.07
***BCL2* rs956572**	GG	GA	AA	G	A	A
PTSD	27 (0.135)	89 (0.445)	84 (0.42)	143 (0.36)	257 (0.64)	173 (0.87)
Controls	71 (0.355)	94 (0.47)	35 (0.175)	236 (0.59)	164 (0.41)	129 (0.65)
p				**1.20E-10**[a]		**8.22E-07**[b]
OR				2.59		3.53
95% CI:				1.94 - 3.44		2.14 - 5.81
***BCL2* rs1801018**	AA	AG	GG	A	G	G

Gene (SNP)	Genotypes			Alleles		Carriage
PTSD	78 (0.39)	83 (0.415)	39 (0.195)	239 (0.6)	161 (0.4)	122 (0.61)
Controls	42 (0.21)	114 (0.57)	44 (0.22)	198 (0.5)	202 (0.5)	158 (0.79)
p				**0.0072[a]**		**0.00017[b]**
OR				0.66		2.41
95% CI:				0.5 - 0.87		1.54 - 3.75

[a]$p_{corrected}$ values for comparison of mutant allele frequency between PTSD patients and controls.

[b]$p_{corrected}$ values for comparison of mutant allele carriage between PTSD patients and controls.

Table 3. Distribution of genotypes, alleles and carriage of minor alleles of *ANXA5, ANXA11* and *BCL2* polymorphisms in patients with PTSD and controls.

The externalization of phosphatidylserine is one of the leading indicators of apoptosis. The annexins are multigene family of Ca^{2+}-regulated phospholipid-dependent and membrane-binding annexin proteins [89]. One member of the annexin gene family, annexin A5, is known as a Ca^{2+}-dependent, phospholipid-binding protein that inhibits protein kinase C (PKC) signaling. Although annexin A5 has been used for the detection of apoptosis, it shows high affinity for surface-exposed phosphatidylserine during apoptosis and may directly involve in apoptotic pathway [90]. Another member of annexins family is annexin A11, which is involved in calcium signaling, apoptosis, vesicle trafficking, cell growth, and the terminal phase of cell division [91].

According to the results obtained, the blood level of annexin-A5 was significantly lower in PTSD and which may also be one of the factors responsible for development of PTSD-associated low-grade inflammation [92, 93]. The results of annexin family proteins encoding genes association with PTSD are shown in Table 3. The *ANXA11* gene rs1049550*A allele was more frequent among controls than in patients (0.42 vs. 0.33, $p_{nominal} = 0.013$, OR = 0.695, 95% CI: 0.52–0.93). There were no significant differences of carriers of rs1049550*A minor allele in the group of patients compared to controls.

2.4. Candidate genes of synaptic plasticity

Synaptic plasticity change, which is a fundamental characteristic of the nervous system, underlies numerous aspects of cognition. Plasticity is essential for the recovery of the nervous system after injury, stroke, and other pathological processes and can permit remarkable functional recovery even after devastating damage, especially in a young and otherwise healthy brain. However, the very mechanisms of plasticity that permit development, learning, resilience, memory, and recovery can also contribute to behavioral dysfunction and to psychopathology [94].

Complexins are small, cytosolic proteins that bind to the soluble N-ethylmaleimide-sensitive factor attachment protein receptor (SNARE) complex to regulate synaptic vesicle exocytosis. Complexin 1 and 2 are the two major isoforms in the brain [95, 96]. Significant alterations of complexins 2 expression levels are seen in a number of neurological and psychiatric disorders, including bipolar disorder [97–99], major depression [98, 100], Huntington's disease (HD) [101, 102], schizophrenia [97, 100, 103–107], Parkinson's disease [108], Alzheimer's disease [109], and PTSD [93].

Neurotrophin family are traditionally recognized for their nerve growth promoting function and are recently identified as crucial factors in regulating neuronal activity in the central and peripheral nervous systems. The family members including brain-derived neurotrophic factor (*BDNF*), nerve growth factor (*NGF*), and its receptor (*NGFR*) are the essential mediators of synaptic and morphological plasticity, neuronal growth, survival, and differentiation; especially in the developing brain, thought may play an important role in pathogenesis of PTSD. [110]

We have reviewed data related neurotransmitter/neuroendocrine systems that are known to be involved in the pathophysiology of PTSD and that may contribute to the symptoms and cognitive dysfunctions in these patients. In Table 4, we have collected our data concerning candidate genes of the proteins involved in synaptic plasticity which may contribute to PTSD.

Gene (SNP)	**Genotypes**			**Alleles**		**Carriage**
***BDNF* rs6265**	GG	GA	AA	G	A	A
PTSD	150 (0.75)	48 (0.24)	2 (0.01)	348 (0.87)	52 (0.13)	50 (0.25)
Controls	129 (0.645)	67 (0.335)	4 (0.02)	325 (0.81)	75 (0.19)	71 (0.36)
p				**0.03**[a]		**0.02**[b]
OR				0.65		1.65
95% CI:				0.44 - 0.95		1.07 - 2.54
***CPLX2* rs1366116**	CC	CT	TT	C	T	T
PTSD	34 (0.39)	36 (0.41)	17 (0.2)	104 (0.6)	70 (0.4)	53 (0.61)
Controls	45 (0.6)	24 (0.32)	6 (0.08)	114 (0.76)	36 (0.24)	30 (0.4)
p				**0.006**[a]		**0.02**[b]
OR				2.2		0.43
95% CI:				1.4 – 3.6		0.2 - 0.8
***CPLX2* rs3892909**	CC	CT	TT	C	T	T
PTSD	16 (0.18)	45 (0.52)	26 (0.3)	77 (0.44)	97 (0.56)	71 (0.82)
Controls	15 (0.2)	41 (0.55)	19 (0.25)	71 (0.47)	79 (0.53)	60 (0.8)
p				1.7[a]		2.4[b]
OR				1.13		0.9
95% CI:				0.73 – 1.76		0.4 – 1.97
***NTNG1* rs628117**	AA	AG	GG	A	G	G
PTSD	47 (0.36)	66 (0.5)	19 (0.14)	160 (0.6)	104 (0.4)	85 (0.64)

Gene (SNP)	Genotypes			Alleles		Carriage
Controls	36 (0.34)	43 (0.41)	26 (0.25)	115 (0.55)	95 (0.45)	69 (0.66)
p				0.2[a]		0.8[b]
OR				0.79		1.06
95% CI:				0.55 – 1.14		0.62 - 1.82
***NGF* rs6330**	CC	CT	TT	C	T	T
PTSD	66 (0.33)	106 (0.53)	28 (0.14)	238 (0.6)	162 (0.4)	134 (0.67)
Controls	130 (0.65)	58 (0.29)	12 (0.06)	318 (0.8)	82 (0.2)	70 (0.35)
p				**2.04E-09**[a]		**4.20E-10**[b]
OR				2.64		3.77
95% CI:				1.9 - 3.6		2.5 - 5.7
***NGF* rs4839435**	GG	GA	AA	G	A	A
PTSD	130 (0.65)	66 (0.33)	4 (0.02)	326 (0.8)	74 (0.2)	70 (0.35)
Controls	85 (0.425)	97 (0.485)	18 (0.09)	267 (0.67)	133 (0.33)	115 (0.58)
p				**4.00E-06**[a]		**1.20E-05**[b]
OR				0.46		0.4
95% CI:				0.33 - 0.63		0.27 - 0.6
***NGFR* rs11466155**	CC	CT	TT	C	T	T
PTSD	109 (0.545)	82 (0.41)	9 (0.045)	300 (0.75)	100 (0.25)	91 (0.46)
Controls	110 (0.55)	75 (0.375)	15 (0.075)	295 (0.74)	105 (0.26)	90 (0.45)
p				1.37[a]		2[b]
OR				0.94		0.98
95% CI:				0.68 - 1.29		0.66 - 1.45
***NGFR* rs734194**	CC	CT	TT	C	T	T
PTSD	164 (0.82)	34 (0.17)	2 (0.01)	362 (0.9)	38 (0.1)	36 (0.18)
Controls	109 (0.545)	74 (0.37)	17 (0.085)	292 (0.73)	108 (0.27)	91 (0.46)
p				**2.74E-10**[a]		**8.82E-09**[b]
OR				0.284		0.263
95% CI:				0.19 - 0.42		0.17 - 0.42
***CHN1* rs14228**	CC	CT	TT	C	T	T
PTSD	79 (0.395)	86 (0.43)	35 (0.175)	244 (0.61)	156 (0.39)	121 (0.6)
Controls	82 (0.41)	62 (0.31)	56 (0.28)	226 (0.565)	174 (0.435)	118 (0.59)
p				0.39[a]		1.52[b]
OR				0.83		0.94
95% CI:				0.63 - 1.1		0.63 - 1.4

Gene (SNP)	Genotypes			Alleles		Carriage
***CHN1* rs2646153**	AA	AG	GG	A	G	G
PTSD	50 (0.25)	86 (0.43)	64 (0.32)	186 (0.465)	214 (0.535)	150 (0.75)
Controls	57 (0.285)	90 (0.45)	53 (0.265)	204 (0.51)	196 (0.49)	143 (0.72)
p				0.4[a]		0.86[b]
OR				1.2		0.84
95% CI:				0.9 - 1.6		0.54 – 1.3
***FOS* rs7101**	CC	CT	TT	C	T	T
PTSD	12 (0.06)	71 (0.355)	117 (0.585)	95 (0.24)	305 (0.76)	188 (0.94)
Controls	94 (0.47)	85 (0.43)	21 (0.1)	273 (0.68)	127 (0.31)	106 (0.53)
p				**4.04E-37**[a]		**1.31E-21**[b]
OR				6.9		13.9
95% CI:				5.1 - 9.4		7.3 - 26.5
***FOS* rs1063169**	GG	GT	TT	G	T	T
PTSD	161 (0.8)	36 (0.18)	3 (0.02)	358 (0.9)	42 (0.1)	39 (0.2)
Controls	92 (0.46)	80 (0.4)	28 (0.14)	264 (0.66)	136 (0.34)	108 (0.54)
p				**1.50E-15**[a]		**1.70E-12**[b]
OR				0.23		0.21
95% CI:				0.16 - 0.33		0.13 - 0.32
***JUN* rs11688**	GG	GA	AA	G	A	A
PTSD	34 (0.17)	113 (0.565)	53 (0.265)	181 (0.45)	219 (0.55)	166 (0.83)
Controls	47 (0.24)	111 (0.56)	42 (0.2)	205 (0.51)	195 (0.49)	153 (0.77)
p				0.09[a]		0.11[b]
OR				1.27		0.67
95% CI:				0.96 - 1.68		0.4 - 1.1
***IER5* rs6425663**	GG	GT	TT	G	T	T
PTSD	29 (0.145)	78 (0.39)	93 (0.465)	136 (0.34)	264 (0.66)	171 (0.86)
Controls	20 (0.1)	74 (0.37)	106 (0.53)	114 (0.285)	286 (0.715)	180 (0.9)
p				0.09[a]		0.17[b]
OR				0.77		1.53
95% CI:				0.57 - 1.04		0.83 - 2.8

[a] $p_{corrected}$ values for comparison of mutant allele frequency between PTSD patients and controls.

[b] $p_{corrected}$ values for comparison of mutant allele carriage between PTSD patients and controls.

Table 4. Distribution of genotypes, alleles and carriage of minor alleles of *BDNF, CPLX2, NTNG1, NGF, NGFR, CHN1, FOS, JUN*and *IER5* polymorphisms in patients with PTSD and controls.

According to the data obtained, the rs6265*A allele of the*BDNF* gene was more frequent in controls than in patients (0.19 vs. 0.13, $p_{nominal}$ = 0.03, OR = 0.65, 95% CI: 0.44–0.95). Also, the carriers of rs6265*A minor allele were overrepresented in the group of controls compared to patients (0.36 vs. 0.25, $p_{nominal}$ = 0.02, OR = 1.65, 95% CI: 1.07–2.54). In contrast, the rs1366116*T minor allele of the *CPLX2* gene was more frequent among patients compared to controls (0.4 vs. 0.24, $p_{nominal}$ = 0.002, OR = 2.2, 95% CI: 1.4–3.6). Also, the carriers of this allele were more in the group of patients compared to controls (0.61 vs. 0.4, $p_{nominal}$ = 0.008, OR = 0.43, 95% CI: 0.2–0.8). Further, we found that the rs6330*T allele of the *NGF* gene was overrepresented in patients with PTSD compared to healthy subjects (0.4 vs. 0.2, $p_{nominal}$ = 1.02E-9, OR = 2.64, 95% CI: 1.93–3.61). Also, the carriers of the rs6330*T minor allele (CT + TT) were more frequent in patients than in controls (0.67 vs. 0.35, $p_{nominal}$ = 2.1E-10, OR = 3.77, 95% CI: 2.49–5.70). On the contrary, the frequency (0.33 vs. 0.2, $p_{nominal}$ = 2.0E-6, OR = 0.46, 95% CI: 0.33–0.63) and carriers (0.58 vs. 0.35, $p_{nominal}$ = 6.0E-6, OR = 0.40, 95% CI: 0.27–0.60) of the rs4839435*A minor allele of the *NGF* gene were higher in controls than in PTSD patients. The *NGFR* rs734194*T minor allele frequency again was higher in controls than in patients (0.27 vs. 0.1, $p_{nominal}$ = 1.37E-10, OR = 0.28, 95% CI: 0.19–0.42). The same applies to the carriers of the *NGFR* rs734194*T allele (0.46 vs. 0.18, $p_{nominal}$ = 4.41E-9, OR = 0.26, 95% CI: 0.17–0.42). Also, rs7101*T allele of the *FOS* gene was more frequent in patients than in controls (0.76 vs. 0.31, $p_{nominal}$ = 2.02E-37, OR = 6.90, 95% CI: 5.05–9.43). The carriers of rs7101*T minor allele were overrepresented in the group of patients compared to controls (0.94 vs. 0.53, $p_{nominal}$ = 6.57E-22, OR = 13.89, 95% CI: 7.28–26.51). In contrast, the rs1063169*T minor allele of the *FOS* gene was more frequent among controls compared to patients (0.34 vs. 0.1, $p_{nominal}$ = 7.48E-16, OR = 0.23, 95% CI: 0.16–0.33). Also, the carriers of this allele were more in the group of controls compared to patients (0.54 vs. 0.2, $p_{nominal}$ = 8.51E-13, OR = 0.21, 95% CI: 0.13–0.32). After Bonferroni correction, difference in allele frequency between the patient and the control groups for these minor alleles remained significant.

3. Conclusion

As found in several mental disorders, the risk for PTSD following traumatic event has limited genetic heritability. The genetic understanding of PTSD through candidate gene studies is premature at this point, although several genes hold promise as potential biomarkers. Identifying and understanding the genetics of PTSD will enrich our ability of diagnosis of PTSD. In Figure 1, we summarized the candidate genes responsible for generation and development of PTSD.

Several studies indicated the association between PTSD and polymorphisms of number of genes of dopaminergic, serotonergic, and GABAergic systems, HPA axis, and other genes related to neurotransmission, neuromodulation, etc. We also compiled a list of genes that have been reported in the literature to be significantly associated with PTSD, also adding our own results on variations in genes encoding neuro-, immune and apoptotic mediators and regulators, and related transcription factors. Profound understanding of risks in PTSD is possible through classic and convergent genomic approaches and this will lead to development of

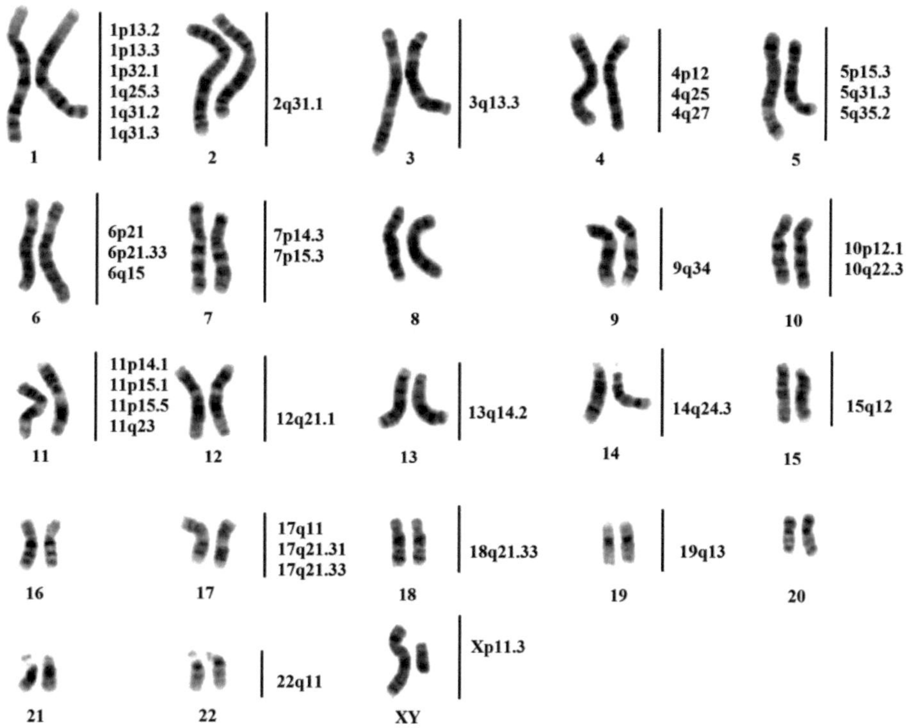

Figure 1. Candidate genes responsible for development of PTSD.

targeted treatment and prevention approaches. Overall, such researches highlight the potential usefulness of the assessment of target genes' alteration in diagnosis of PTSD.

Author details

Boyajyan Anna, Avetyan Diana, Hovhannisyan Lilit and Mkrtchyan Gohar*

*Address all correspondence to: g_mkrtchyan@mb.sci.am

Institute of Molecular Biology, National Academy of Sciences, Yerevan, Republic of Armenia

References

[1] ICD-10. International Statistical Classification of Diseases and Related Health Problems (Edition: 10). Geneva: World Health Organization; 1992.

[2] Diagnostic and Statistical Manual of Mental Disorders by American Psychiatric Association (edition 5). Washington, DC; 2013.

[3] Dietrich AM. As the pendulum swings: the etiology of PTSD, complex PTSD, and revictimization. Traumatology 2000;6:41–59.

[4] Yehuda R, Giller EL, Levengood RA, Southwick SM, Siever LJ. Hypotalamic-pituitary-adrenal functioning in post-traumatic stress disorder: expanding the concept of the stress response spectrum. Neurobiologial and clinical consequences of stress: from normal adaptation to post-traumatic stress disorder. Hagerstown. MD: Lippincott-Raven; 1991. p. 351–66.

[5] Yehuda R. Biology of posttraumatic stress disorder. J Clin Psychiatry 2001;62(17):41–6.

[6] Connor MD, Butterfield MI. Post-traumatic stress disorder. FOCUS 2003;1(3):247–62.

[7] Kinchin D. Post traumatic stress disorder: the invisible injury. UK: Success Unlimited; 2005.

[8] Amir M, Kaplan Z, Efroni R, Kotler M. Suicide risk and coping styles in post-traumatic stress disorder patients. Psychother Psychosom 1999;68(2):76–81.

[9] Young RM, Lawford BR, Noble EP, Kann B, Wilkie A, Ritchie T, Arnold L, Shadforth S. Harmful drinking in military veterans with post-traumatic stress disorder: association with the D2 dopamine receptor A1 allele. Alcohol 2002;37(5):451–6.

[10] Ben-Ya'acov Y, Amir M. Posttraumatic symptoms and suicide risk. Person Indiv Diff 2004;36:1257–64.

[11] Helzer JE, Robins LN, McEvoy L. Post-traumatic stress disorder in the general population. Findings of the epidemiologic catchment area survey. N Engl J Med 1987;317(26):1630–34.

[12] Breslau N. The epidemiology of posttraumatic stress disorder: what is the extent of the problem? J Clin Psychiatry 2001;62(17):16–22.

[13] Breslau N. Epidemiologic studies of trauma, posttraumatic stress disorder, and other psychiatric disorders. Can J Psychiatry 2002;47(10):923–29.

[14] Eley TC, Sugden K, Corsico A, Gregory AM, Sham P. Gene-environment interaction analysis of serotonin system markers with adolescent depression. Mol Psychiatry 2004;9(10):908–15.

[15] Afifi TO, Asmundson GJ, Taylor S, Jang KL. The role of genes and environment on trauma exposure and post-traumatic stress disorder symptoms: a review of twin studies. Clin Psychol Rev 2010;30:101–12.

[16] Cornelis MC, Nugent NR, Amstadter AB, Koenen KC. Genetics of post-traumatic stress disorder: review and recommendations for genome-wide association studies. Curr Psychiatry Rep 2010;12:313–26.

[17] Mehta D, Binder EB. Gene × environment vulnerability factors for PTSD: the HPA-axis. Neuropharmacology 2012;62:654–62.

[18] Segman RH, Shalev AY. Genetics of posttraumatic stress disorder. CNS Spectr 2003;8(9):693–8.

[19] Grabe HJ, Lange M, Wolff B, Völzke H, Lucht M. Mental and physical distress is modulated by a polymorphism in the 5-HT transporter gene interacting with social stressors and chronic disease burden. Mol Psychiatry 2005;10(2):220–4.

[20] Koenen KC. Genetics of posttraumatic stress disorder: review and recommendations for future studies. J Trauma Stress 2007;20:737–50.

[21] Broekman BF, Olff M, Boer F. The genetic background to PTSD. Neurosci Biobehav Rev 2007;31:348–62.

[22] Amstadter AB, Nugent NR, Koenen KC. Genetics of PTSD: fear conditioning as a model for future research. Psych Ann 2009;39:358–67.

[23] Koenen KC, Aiello AE, Bakshis E, Amstadter AB, Ruggiero KJ, Acierno R, Kilpatrick DG, Gelernter J, Galea S. Modification of the association between serotonin transporter genotype and risk of posttraumatic stress disorder in adults by county-level social environment. Am J Epidemiol 2009;169:704–11.

[24] Skelton K, Ressler KJ, Norrholm SD, Jovanovic T, Bradley-Davino B. PTSD and gene variants: new pathways and new thinking. Neuropharmacology 2012;62:628–37.

[25] Digangi J, Guffanti G, McLaughlin KA, Koenen KC. Considering trauma exposure in the context of genetics studies of post-traumatic stress disorder: a systematic review. Biol Mood Anxiety Disord 2013;3:2.

[26] Almli LM, Fani N, Smith AK, Ressler KJ. Genetic approaches to understanding post-traumatic stress disorder. Int J Neuropsychopharmacol. 2014; 7(2):355–70.

[27] Young RM, Lawford BR, Noble EP, Kann B, Wilkie A, Ritchie T, Arnold L, Shadforth S. Harmful drinking in military veterans with post-traumatic stress disorder: association with the D2 dopamine receptor A1 allele. Alcohol 2002;37(5):451–6.

[28] Comings DE, Muhleman D, Gysin R. Dopamine D2 receptor (DRD2) gene and susceptibility to posttraumatic stress disorder: a study and replication. Biol Psychiatry 1996;40:368–72.

[29] Voisey J, Swagell CD, Hughes IP, Morris CP, Van Daal A, Noble EP, Kann B, Heslop KA, Young RM, Lawford BR. The DRD2 gene 957C > T polymorphism is associated with posttraumatic stress disorder in war veterans. Depress Anxiety 2009;6(1):28–33.

[30] Hemmings SM, Martin LI, Klopper M, van der Merwe L, Aitken L, de Wit E, Black GF, Hoal EG, Walzl G, Seedat S. BDNF Val66Met and DRD2 Taq1A polymorphisms interact to influence PTSD symptom severity: a preliminary investigation in a South African population. Prog Neuropsychopharmacol Biol Psychiatry 2013;40:273–80.

[31] Wolf EJ, Mitchell KS, Logue MW, Baldwin CT, Reardon AF, Aiello A, Galea S, Koenen KC, Uddin M, Wildman D, Miller MW. The dopamine D3 receptor gene and posttraumatic stress disorder. J Trauma Stress 2014;27(4):379–87.

[32] Dragan WL, Oniszczenko W. The association between dopamine D4 receptor exon III polymorphism and intensity of PTSD symptoms among flood survivors. Anxiety Stress Coping 2009;22:483–95.

[33] Segman RH, Cooper-Kazaz R, Macciardi F, Goltser T, Halfon Y, Dobroborski T, Shalev AY. Association between the dopamine transporter gene and posttraumatic stress disorder. Mol Psychiatry 2002;7:903–7.

[34] Drury SS, Theall KP, Keats BJ, Scheeringa M. The role of the dopamine transporter (DAT) in the development of PTSD in preschool children. J Trauma Stress 2009;22:534–9.

[35] Valente NL, Vallada H, Cordeiro Q, Miguita K, Bressan RA, Andreoli SB, Mari JJ, Mello MF. Candidate-gene approach in post-traumatic stress disorder after urban violence: association analysis of the genes encoding serotonin transporter, dopamine transporter, and BDNF. J Mol Neurosci 2011;44:59–67.

[36] Chang SC, Koenen KC, Galea S, Aiello AE, Soliven R, Wildman DE, Uddin M. Molecular variation at the SLC6A3 locus predicts lifetime risk of PTSD in the Detroit Neighborhood Health Study. PLoS ONE 2012;7:e39184.

[37] Mustapic M, Pivac N, Kozaric-Kovacic D, Dezeljin M, Cubells JF, Mück-Seler D. Dopamine beta-hydroxylase (DBH) activity and -1021C/T polymorphism of DBH gene in combat-related post-traumatic stress disorder. Am J Med Genet Neuropsychiatr Genet 2007;144B(8):1087–9.

[38] Tang YL, Li W, Mercer K, Bradley B, Gillespie CF, Bonsall R, Ressler KJ, Cubells JF. Genotype-controlled analysis of serum dopamine beta-hydroxylase activity in civilian post-traumatic stress disorder. Prog Neuropsychopharmacol Biol Psychiatry 2010;34:1396–401.

[39] Kolassa IT, Kolassa S, Ertl V, Papassotiropoulos A, De Quervain DJ. The risk of post-traumatic stress disorder after trauma depends on traumatic load and the catechol-o-methyltransferaseVal(158)Met polymorphism. Biol Psychiatry 2010;67:304–8.

[40] Valente NL, Vallada H, Cordeiro Q, Bressan RA, Andreoli SB, Mari JJ, Mello MF. Catechol-O-methyltransferase (COMT) val158met polymorphism as a risk factor for PTSD after urban violence. J MolNeurosci 2011;43:516–23.

[41] Goenjian AK, Noble EP, Steinberg AM, Walling DP, Stepanyan ST, Dandekar S, Bailey JN. Association of COMT and TPH-2 genes with DSM-5 based PTSD symptoms. J Affect Disord 2014;22(172C):472–8.

[42] Kilpatrick DG, Koenen KC, Ruggiero KJ, Acierno R, Galea S, Resnick HS, Roitzsch J, Boyle J, Gelernter J. The serotonin transporter genotype and social support and moderation of posttraumatic stress disorder and depression in hurricane exposed adults. Am J Psychiatry 2007;164:1693–9.

[43] Thakur GA, Joober R, Brunet A. Development and persistence of posttraumatic stress disorder and the 5-HTTLPR polymorphism. J Trauma Stress 2009;22:240–3.

[44] Xie P, Kranzler HR, Poling J, Stein MB, Anton RF, Brady K, Weiss RD, Farrer L, Gelernter J. Interactive effect of stressful life events and the serotonin transporter 5-HTTLPR genotype on posttraumatic stress disorder diagnosis in 2 independent populations. Arch Gen Psychiatry 2009;66:1201–9.

[45] Grabe HJ1, Spitzer C, Schwahn C, Marcinek A, Frahnow A, Barnow S, Lucht M, Freyberger HJ, John U, Wallaschofski H, Völzke H, Rosskopf D., Serotonin transporter gene (SLC6A4) promoter polymorphisms and the susceptibility to posttraumatic stress disorder in the general population. Am J Psychiatry 2009;166:926–33.

[46] Lee H, Kwak S, Paik J, Kang R, Lee M. Association between serotonin 2A receptor gene polymorphism and posttraumatic stress disorder. Psychiatry Investig 2007;4:104–8.

[47] Mellman TA, Alim T, Brown DD, Gorodetsky E, Buzas B, Lawson WB, Goldman D, Charney DS. Serotonin polymorphisms and post-traumatic stress disorder in a Trauma exposed African American population. Depress Anxiety 2009;26:993–7.

[48] Goenjian AK, Bailey JN, Walling DP, Steinberg AM, Schmidt D, Dandekar U, Noble EP. Association of TPH1, TPH2, and 5HTTLPR with PTSD and depressive symptoms. J Affect Disord 2012;140(3):244–452.

[49] Nelson EC, Agrawal A, Pergadia ML, Lynskey MT, Todorov AA, Wang JC, Todd RD, Martin NG, Heath AC, Goate AM, Montgomery GW, Madden PA. Association of childhood trauma exposure and GABRA2 polymorphisms with risk of posttraumatic stress disorder in adults. Mol Psychiatry 2009;14:234–5.

[50] Lu AT, Ogdie MN, Jarvelin MR, Moilanen IK, Loo SK, McCracken JT, McGough JJ, Yang MH, Peltonen L, Nelson SF, Cantor RM, Smalley SL. Association of the cannabinoid receptor gene (CNR1) with ADHD and posttraumatic stress disorder. Am J Med Gene Neuropsychiatr Genet 2008;147B:1488–94.

[51] Hauer D, Weis F, Papassotiropoulos A, Schmoeckel M, Beiras-Fernandez A, Lieke J, Kaufmann I, Kirchhoff F, Vogeser M, Roozendaal B, Briegel J, de Quervain D, Schelling G. Relationship of a common polymorphism of the glucocorticoid receptor gene

to traumatic memories and posttraumatic stress disorder in patients after intensive care therapy. Crit Care Med 2011;39(4):643–50.

[52] Lian Y, Xiao J, Wang Q, Ning L, Guan S, Ge H, Li F, Liu J. The relationship between glucocorticoid receptor polymorphisms, stressful life events, social support, and post-traumatic stress disorder. BMC Psychiatry 2014;12(14):232.

[53] Amstadter AB, Nugent NR, Yang BZ, Miller A, Siburian R, Moorjani P, Haddad S, Basu A, Fagerness J, Saxe G, Smoller JW, Koenen KC. Corticotrophin-releasing hormone type 1 receptor gene (CRHR1) variants predict posttraumatic stress disorder onset and course in pediatric injury patients. Dis Markers 2011;30(2–3):89–99. DOI: 10.3233/DMA-2011-0761.

[54] Ressler KJ, Mercer KB, Bradley B, Jovanovic T, Mahan A, Kerley K, Norrholm SD, Kilaru V, Smith AK, Myers AJ, Ramirez M, Engel A, Hammack SE, Toufexis D, Braas KM, Binder EB, May V. Post-traumatic stress disorder is associated with PACAP and the PAC1 receptor. Nature 2011;470(7335):492–7.

[55] Uddin M, Chang SC, Zhang C, Ressler K, Mercer KB, Galea S, Keyes KM, McLaughlin KA, Wildman DE, Aiello AE, Koenen KC. Adcyap1r1 genotype, posttraumatic stress disorder, and depression among women exposed to childhood maltreatment. Depress Anxiety 2013;30(3):251–8.

[56] Xie P, Kranzler HR, Poling J, Stein MB, Anton RF, Farrer LA, Gelernter J. Interaction of FKBP5 with childhood adversity on risk for post-traumatic stress disorder. Neuropsychopharmacology 2010;35(8):1684–92.

[57] Rothbaum BO, Kearns MC, Reiser E, Davis JS, Kerley KA, Rothbaum AO, Mercer KB, Price M, Houry D, Ressler KJ. Early intervention following trauma may mitigate genetic risk for PTSD in civilians: a pilot prospective emergency department study. J Clin Psychiatry 2014;75(12):1380–7.

[58] Sabbagh JJ, O'Leary JC 3rd, Blair LJ, Klengel T, Nordhues BA, Fontaine SN, Binder EB, Dickey CA. Age-associated epigenetic upregulation of the FKBP5 gene selectively impairs stress resiliency. PLoS One 2014;9(9):e107241.

[59] Wilker S, Pfeiffer A, Kolassa S, Elbert T, Lingenfelder B, Ovuga E, Papassotiropoulos A, de Quervain D, Kolassa IT. The role of FKBP5 genotype in moderating long-term effectiveness of exposure-based psychotherapy for posttraumatic stress disorder. Transl Psychiatry 2014;4:e403.

[60] Szabó C, Kelemen O, Kéri S. Changes in FKBP5 expression and memory functions during cognitive-behavioral therapy in posttraumatic stress disorder: a preliminary study. Neurosci Lett 2014;569:116–20.

[61] Zhang H, Ozbay F, Lappalainen J, Kranzler HR, van Dyck CH, Charney DS, Price LH, Southwick S, Yang BZ, Rasmussen A, Gelernter J. Brain derived neurotrophic factor (BDNF) gene variants and Alzheimer's disease, affective disorders, posttrau-

matic stress disorder, schizophrenia, and substance dependence. Am J Med Genet B Neuropsychiatr Genet 2006;141:387–93.

[62] Binder EB, Bradley RG, Liu W, Epstein MP, Deveau TC, Mercer KB, Tang Y, Gillespie CF, Heim CM, Nemeroff CB, Schwartz AC, Cubells JF, Ressler KJ. Association of FKBP5 polymorphisms and childhood abuse with risk of posttraumatic stress disorder symptoms in adults. JAMA 2008; 299(11):1291–305.

[63] Pivac N, Kozaric-Kovacic D, Grubisic-Ilic M, Nedic G, Rakos I, Nikolac M, Blazev M, Muck-Seler D. The association between brain-derived neurotrophic factor Val66Met variants and psychotic symptoms in posttraumatic stress disorder. World J Biol Psychiatry 2012;13(4):306–11.

[64] Felmingham KL, Dobson-Stone C, Schofield PR, Quirk GJ, Bryant RA. The brain-derived neurotrophic factor Val66Met polymorphism predicts response to exposure therapy in posttraumatic stress disorder. Biol Psychiatry 2013;73(11):1059–63.

[65] Miller JK, Wiener JM. PTSD recovery, spatial processing, and the val66met polymorphism. Front Hum Neurosci 2014;8:100.

[66] Zhang L, Benedek DM, Fullerton CS, Forsten RD, Naifeh JA, Li XX, Hu XZ, Li H, Jia M, Xing GQ, Benevides KN, Ursano RJ. PTSD risk is associated with BDNF Val66Met and BDNF overexpression. Mol Psychiatry 2014;19(1):8–10.

[67] Freeman T, Roca V, Guggenheim F, Kimbrell T, Griffin WS. Neuropsychiatric associations of apolipoprotein E alleles in subjects with combat-related posttraumatic stress disorder. J Neuropsychiatry Clin Neurosci 2005;17(4):541–3.

[68] Lyons MJ, Genderson M, Grant MD, Logue M, Zink T, McKenzie R, Franz CE, Panizzon M, Lohr JB, Jerskey B, Kremen WS. Gene-environment interaction of ApoE genotype and combat exposure on PTSD. Am J Med Genet B Neuropsychiatr Genet 2013;162B(7):762–9.

[69] Kim TY, Chung HG, Shin HS, Kim SJ, Choi JH, Chung MY, An SK, Choi TK, So HS, Cho HS. Apolipoprotein E gene polymorphism, alcohol use, and their interactions in combat-related posttraumatic stress disorder. Depress Anxiety 2013;30(12):1194–201.

[70] Pivac N, Knezevic J, Kozaric-Kovacic D, Dezeljin M, Mustapic M, Rak D, Matijevic T, Pavelic J, Muck-Seler D. Monoamine oxidase (MAO) intron 13 polymorphism and platelet MAO-B activity in combat-related posttraumatic stress disorder. J Affect Disord 2007;103(1–3):131–8.

[71] Sah R, Geracioti TD. Neuropeptide Y and posttraumatic stress disorder. Mol Psychiatry 2013;18(6):646–55.

[72] Lappalainen J, Kranzler HR, Malison R, Price LH, Van Dyck C, Rosenheck RA, Cramer J, Southwick S, Charney D, Krystal J, Gelernter J. A functional neuropeptide Y Leu7Pro polymorphism associated with alcohol dependence in a large population sample from the United States. Arch Gen Psychiatry 2002;59:825–31.

[73] Nievergelt CM, Maihofer AX, Mustapic M, Yurgil KA, Schork NJ, Miller MW, Logue MW, Geyer MA, Risbrough VB, O'Connor DT, Baker DG. Genomic predictors of combat stress vulnerability and resilience in U.S. Marines: a genome-wide association study across multiple ancestries implicates PRTFDC1 as a potential PTSD gene. Psychoneuroendocrinology 2015;51:459–71.

[74] Amstadter AB, Koenen KC, Ruggiero KJ, Acierno R, Galea S, Kilpatrick DG, Gelernter J. Variant in RGS2 moderates post-traumatic stress symptoms following potentially traumatic event exposure. J Anxiety Disord 2009;23:369–73.

[75] Sakamoto M, Fujisawa Y, Nishioka K. Physiologic role of the complement system in host defense, disease, and malnutrition. Nutrition 1998;14(4):391–8.

[76] Volankis JE, Frank MM: The human complement system in health and disease. New York: Mircel Dekker Inc; 1998.

[77] Mollnes TE, Song W-C, Lambris JD. Complement in inflammatory tissue damage and disease. Trends Immunol Today 2002;23(2):61–6.

[78] Morgan BP, Gasque P, Singhrao SK, Piddlesden SJ. The role of complement in disorders of the nervous system. Immunopharmacology 1997;38(1–2):43–50.

[79] Yasojima K, Schwab C, McGeer EG, McGeer PL. Up-regulated production and activation of the complement system in Alzheimer's disease brain. Amer J Pathol 1999;154(3):927–36.

[80] Gasque P, Neal JW, Singhrao SK, McGreal EP, Dean YD, Van BJ, Morgan BP. Roles of the complement system in human neurodegenerative disorders: pro-inflammatory and tissue remodeling activities. MolNeurobiol 2002;25(1):1–17.

[81] Francis K, Van Beek J, Canova C, Neal JW, Gasque P: Innate immunity and brain inflammation: the key role of complement. Expert Rev Mol Med 2003;5(15):1–19.

[82] Van Beek J, Elward K, Gasque P. Activation of complement in the central nervous system: roles in neurodegeneration and neuroprotection. Ann N Y AcadSci 2003;992:56–71.

[83] Boyajyan A, Zakharyan R, Khoyetsyan A. Chapter XI. Molecular and genetic indicators of aberrant immunity and apoptosis in schizophrenia In: Sumiyoshi T editor. Schizophrenia Research: Recent Advances: Nova Science Publishers; 2012, pp.183–240.

[84] Maes M, Hendriks D, Van Gastel A, Demedts P, Wauters A, Neels H, Janca A, Scharpé S. Effects of psychological stress on serum immunoglobulin, complement, and acute phase protein concentrations in normal volunteers. Psychoneuroendocrinology 1997;22:397–409.

[85] Burns V, Edwards K, Ring C, Drayson M, Carroll D: Complement cascade activation after an acute psychological stress task. Psychosomatic Medicine 2008;70:387–396.

[86] Liu D, Xiao B, Han F, Wang E, Shi Y. Single-prolonged stress induces apoptosis in dorsal raphe nucleus in the rat model of posttraumatic stress disorder. BMC Psychiatry 2012;12:211.

[87] Han F, Yan S, Shi Y. Single-prolonged stress induces endoplasmic reticulum-dependent apoptosis in the hippocampus in a rat model of post-traumatic stress disorder. PLoS One 2013;8(7):e69340.

[88] Li Y, Han F, Shi Y. Increased neuronal apoptosis in medial prefrontal cortex is accompanied with changes of Bcl-2 and Bax in a rat model of post-traumatic stress disorder. J Mol Neurosci 2013;51(1):127–37.

[89] Wang J, Guo C, Liu S, Qi H, Yin Y, Liang R, Sun MZ, Greenaway FT. Annexin A11 in disease. Clin Chim Acta 2014;431:164–8.

[90] Hong M, Park N, Chun YJ. Role of annexin a5 on mitochondria-dependent apoptosis induced by tetramethoxystilbene in human breast cancer cells. Biomol Ther 2014;22(6):519–24.

[91] Shibata H, Kanadome T, Sugiura H, Yokoyama T, Yamamuro M, Moss SE, Maki M2. Anew role for annexin A11 in the early secretory pathway via stabilizing Sec31A at the endoplasmic reticulum exit sites (ERES). J Biol Chem 2014;pii:jbc.M114.592089. [Epub ahead of print].

[92] Mkrtchyan GM, Boyadzhyan AS, Avetyan DG, Sukiasyan SG. Involvement of anomalous apoptosis in impairments to synaptic plasticity in post-traumatic stress disorder. Neurosci Behav Physiol 2014;44(4):442–6.

[93] Boyajyan A, Mkrtchyan G, Hovhannisyan L, Avetyan D. Chapter 5 Alterations in the immune response, apoptosis and synaptic plasticity in posttraumatic stress disorder: molecular indicators and relation to clinical symptoms. In: Durbano F ed. New Insights Into Anxiety Disorders: In Tech 2013;p.105–33.

[94] Glynn D, Gibson HE, Harte MK, Reim K, Jones S, Reynolds GP, Morton AJ. Clorgyline-mediated reversal of neurological deficits in a Complexin 2 knockout mouse. Hum Mol Genet 2010;19(17):3402–12.

[95] McMahon HT, Missler M, Li C, Sudhof TC. Complexins: cytosolic proteins that regulate SNAP receptor function. Cell 1995;83:111–9.

[96] Reim K, Wegmeyer H, Brandstatter JH, Xue M, Rosenmund C, Dresbach T, Hofmann K, Brose N. Structurally and functionally unique complexins at retinal ribbon synapses. J. Cell Biol 2005;169:669–80.

[97] Eastwood SL, Harrison PJ. Hippocampal synaptic pathology in schizophrenia, bipolar disorder and major depression: a study of complexin mRNAs. Mol Psychiatry 2000;5:425–32.

[98] Eastwood SL, Harrison PJ. Synaptic pathology in the anterior cingulate cortex in schizophrenia and mood disorders. A review and a Western blot study of synaptophysin, GAP-43 and the complexins. Brain Res Bull 2001;55:569–78.

[99] Knable MB, Barci BM, Webster, MJ, Meador-Woodruff J, Torrey EF. Stanley Neuropathology Consortium Molecular abnormalities of the hippocampus in severe psychiatric illness: postmortem findings from the Stanley Neuropathology Consortium. Mol Psychiatry 2004;9:609–20.

[100] Sawada K, Young CE, Barr AM, Longworth K, Takahash S, Arango V, Mann JJ, Dwork AJ, Falkai P, Phillips AG, Honer WG. Altered immunoreactivity of complexin protein in prefrontal cortex in severe mental illness. Mol Psychiatry 2002;7:484–92.

[101] Morton AJ, Faull RL, Edwardson JM. Abnormalities in the synaptic vesicle fusion machinery in Huntington's disease. Brain Res Bull 2001;56:111–7.

[102] DiProspero NA, Chen EY, Charles V, Plomann M, Kordower JH, Tagle DA. Early changes in Huntington's disease patient brains involve alterations in cytoskeletal and synaptic elements. J Neurocytol 2004;33:517–33.

[103] Harrison PJ, Eastwood SL. Preferential involvement of excitatory neurons in medial temporal lobe in schizophrenia. Lancet 1998;352:1669–73.

[104] Eastwood SL, Burnet PW, Harrison PJ. Expression of complexin I and II mRNAs and their regulation by antipsychotic drugs in the rat forebrain. Synapse 2000;36:167–77.

[105] Eastwood SL, Cotter D, Harrison PJ. Cerebellar synaptic protein expression in schizophrenia. Neuroscience 2001;105:219–29.

[106] Eastwood SL, Harrison PJ. Decreased expression of vesicular glutamate transporter 1 and complexin II mRNAs in schizophrenia: further evidence for a synaptic pathology affecting glutamate neurons. Schizophr Res 2005;73:159–72.

[107] Sawada K, Barr AM, Nakamura M, Arima K, Young CE, Dwork AJ, Falkai P, Phillips AG, Honer WG. Hippocampal complexin proteins and cognitive dysfunction in schizophrenia. Arch Gen Psychiatry 2005;62:263–72.

[108] Basso M, Giraudo S, Corpillo D, Bergamasco B, Lopiano L, Fasano M. Proteome analysis of human substantia nigra in Parkinson's disease. Proteomics 2004;4:3943–52.

[109] Tannenberg RK, Scott HL, Tannenberg AE, Dodd PR. Selective loss of synaptic proteins in Alzheimer's disease: evidence for an increased severity with APOE varepsilon4. Neurochem Int 2006;49:631–9.

[110] Qiao LY. Neurotrophin signaling and visceral hypersensitivity. Front Biol 2014;9(3): 216–24.

Chapter 5

Posttraumatic Stress Disorder Biomarker — p11

Lei Zhang, Xian-Zhang Hu, He Li, Xiaoxia Li,
Stanley Smerin, Dale W. Russell, Angela Boutte,
Berwin Yuan, Nora Wang, Ze Chen and
Robert J. Ursano

Additional information is available at the end of the chapter

http://dx.doi.org/10.5772/61073

Abstract

Post-traumatic stress disorder (PTSD) is a chronic and disabling anxiety disorder associated with a traumatic event [1]. It is linked to increased risk of suicide and deficits in social functioning [2, 3]. Despite extensive study in psychiatry, the underlying mechanisms of PTSD are still poorly understood [4, 5]. Currently, the diagnosis for PTSD is based on clinical observation and symptom checklist [4, 6-8] and no laboratory blood-based tests. Although biomarker discovery for PTSD is not easy [8], a reliable biomarker would significantly impact the diagnosis and therapeutic monitoring of PTSD. Developing interventions to identify and treat PTSD requires objective approaches to determining the presence of PTSD [8]. Substantial data indicate several potential biomarkers for PTSD. Of these candidate markers, p11 (S100A10) has been studied in PTSD animal models [7] and in human subjects with PTSD [6]. We found that p11 is over-expressed in both animal models and post-mortem brains of subjects with PTSD [7]. Incorporating testing of p11, a novel biomarker for PTSD, into clinical practice, along with more subjective measures, such as participants' medical history, mental status, duration of symptoms, and symptom checklist or self-report, would provide additional power to predict impending PTSD. In this chapter, we discuss the biomarker concept and the potential clinical utility of PTSD biomarkers. We further discuss the potential of p11 as a PTSD biomarker and as a tool that may enhance PTSD diagnosis and intervention in health care practice.

Keywords: PTSD, p11, biomarker

1. Introduction

Post-traumatic stress disorder (PTSD) is a chronic and disabling anxiety disorder which is a result of exposure to a traumatic event and is associated with an increased risk of suicide and marked deficits in social dysfunction [2, 3]. Currently, a PTSD diagnosis is made based on clinical observation, symptoms, and the duration of symptoms. In 2013, the American Psychiatric Association's *Fifth Edition of the Diagnostic and Statistical Manual of Mental Disorders* (DSM-5) revised PTSD diagnostic criteria to better codify it to adults, adolescents, and children over age six. The criteria currently include exposure to a traumatic event and symptoms of four symptom clusters: intrusion, avoidance, negative alterations in cognitions and mood, and alterations in arousal and reactivity. Additional criteria include the duration of symptoms [9]. Given that there are currently no laboratory biomarker tests for PTSD, this chapter will discuss the concept of using biomarkers to diagnose the potential for the existence of PTSD. Specific focus will be given to the potential of biomarker p11.

2. Biomarker concept

Biomarkers are defined as "cellular, biochemical, or molecular alterations that are measurable in biological media such as human tissues, cells, or fluids" [10-12]. Biomarkers can be measurable and quantifiable biological parameters, such as levels of protein or enzyme and hormone in the cerebrospinal fluid, saliva and blood, or mRNA specimen levels [10-12]. Those markers may be related to health and physiological conditions, metabolic processes, disease risk, psychiatric disorders, and environmental exposure, as well as disease diagnosis [13]. Biological changes, which link mechanism of drug action to clinical effectiveness, are also considered biomarkers [14]. Therefore, biomarkers may be considered as any substance, structure of molecule, or biological process that are measurable, influential and/or able to predict the incidence of outcome of disease (WHO International Program on Chemical Safety).

3. Biomarker classification and application

Biomarker research has advanced substantially as part of the Human Genome Project [15]. Initially, potential gene biomarkers were screened using high-throughput analytical instruments. Those markers were classified into four subgroups: type 0 biomarkers; type 1 biomarkers; surrogate end point-type (type 2 biomarkers); and risk markers (http://en.wikipedia.org/wiki/Human_Genome_Project). Depending on the function of those markers, they may be called imaging biomarkers (CT, PET, MRI), molecular biomarkers, or genetic markers. Molecular biomarkers include the markers in biological specimens (plasma, serum, saliva, cerebrospinal fluid, bronchoalveolar lavage, and biopsy). They can be peptides, proteins, lipids metabolites, enzymes, and other small molecules (http://en.wikipedia.org/wiki/Human_Genome_Project). Genetic markers are micromRNA, mRNA and DNA mutations, or polymorphisms. Finally, these markers may also be used for diagnosing the disease, determining the stage of the disease, monitoring the outcome of the treatment, and evaluating the disease prognosis.

4. Potential PTSD biomarkers

For the last 10 years, researchers have been focusing on developing a single test, such as a blood or genetic test, which may determine PTSD and simplify its treatment. In other medical fields, biomarkers have already been developed and used for diagnosis. For example, cholesterol measurements and genetic tests have been used for predicting the risks for heart attacks and Huntington's disease, respectively. In psychiatry, researchers hope to use the same strategies to identify and implement the biomarkers for predicting PTSD risk(s). However, the searching for such a test is still ongoing, though scientists are closer than ever to achieve this goal. Why is the search for biomarkers for PTSD needed when the disorder has been diagnosed by clinical-interview-based DSM diagnostic criteria for decades. Because, at least in part, biomarkers can help us better understand PTSD, its etiology and its pathologies, which in turn can lead to the development of more successful therapeutic approaches. It may help psychiatrists make faster and more effective decisions on the treatments based on the individual's pathology. In addition, biomarkers might identify high-risk populations that had not manifested any symptoms met in PTSD diagnostic criteria. To search for PTSD biomarkers, high-throughput omic approaches are required. The approaches used in biomarker studies of other diseases [16, 17] have just begun to be used in PTSD research. Although potential biomarker(s) for PTSD have been reported in the animal research [8] and human subjects research [6], the confirmation and validation of their clinical utility have not been accomplished. In PTSD biomarker studies, gene expression, metabolite levels and protein concentration in saliva [18], blood [19], cerebral spinal cord fluid [20], urine [21], and tissues [7] are compared between PTSD patients and healthy control subjects. In addition, physiological parameters (blood pressure [22], ECG [23], heartbeat [24], neurotransmitters [25-27], and brain imaging [28] are considered as biomarkers for PTSD.

PTSD biomarkers can be associated with PTSD-related behavioral characteristics (e.g., hypervigilance), the level or type of exposure to traumatic stress, genetic susceptibility, conditions of response to traumatic stress exposure, subclinical or clinical state, and conditions of response to therapy. During the course of PTSD, or after single or multiple traumatic stresses, the biomarkers can be identified. It also can be a predictor for PTSD-related risk, state, or progression. Like biomarkers identified in cancer research, PTSD biomarker research may be used for antecedent, screening, diagnostic, monitoring stage, and prognosis. One biomarker may be associated with a single or multiple phenotypes of PTSD, while a single symptom can be associated with multiple PTSD biomarkers.

Few studies have evaluated the use of multiple biomarkers for patients' risk stratification [29]. The desirable properties of biomarkers for PTSD vary with their different usages. For example, a screening test requires having high sensitivity, specificity, predictive values, large likelihood ratios, and low cost to test a large population including normal and high-risk subjects. A diagnostic biomarker may be chosen for testing stages of the disease (acute and chronic). In those tests, sensitivity or specificity of monitoring biomarkers are less important because the marker from the same individual serves as his or her own control. The ability to monitor intra-individual variation is more important. Costs may be less important for prognostic markers since only those diagnosed with PTSD are subjects of focus.

In PTSD biomarker research, the sample size is often critical. A standard diagnostic biomarker test requires a relatively smaller sample size and a cross-sectional design. However, PTSD biomarker research requires a larger sample size and a prospective design. Although all biomarker features can be shown in one biomarker, a specific biomarker feature for use is the ultimate goal in the search for PTSD biomarkers. It would be ideal to have all the features to test PTSD and to help clinicians optimally manage PTSD patients with specific therapeutic targets. For example, the level of glucocorticoid [30] and/or concentration of epinephrine in the blood could be an indicator of responding to traumatic stress, or a plasma GABA level may evaluate whether or not the subject is recovering from trauma [31]. It is important that a biomarker test is an accurate, reproducible, standardized and acceptable procedure for PTSD diagnosis.

4.1. A strategy to identify a PTSD biomarker

The development of PTSD biomarker(s) for clinical utility is a process from preclinical development (potential biomarker identification) to clinical validation (clinical utility approval) [8]. This long process includes three major steps: screening, analytical validation, and clinical validation. In the initial stage of screening, the high-throughput approaches are used to search for the potential biomarker(s). Analytical validation is laboratory or bench work, which involves sample selection, collection, storage, and determination of the optimum analytical procedure that provide high reproducibility and accuracy. Clinical validation (clinical utility) is the final step of the development of an accurate biomarker test, including testing sensitivity and specificity of the diagnosis [8].

4.2. Screening biomarker(s) for PTSD

Biomarker screening is the first step in identifying a potential PTSD biomarker. During the screening stage, researchers can start the study from animal models or human subjects. In general, animal models needs to be validated [29]. If human subjects are used, the bias should be avoided in the sample selection process. Since current animal models of PTSD have used different stress paradigms, a wide range of behavioral responses is obtained. In many prior studies, the data are presented by the mean values (with the standard deviation or the standard error) of the entire study group. It is known that only a proportion of individuals (20%–30%) who are exposed to a traumatic event will eventually develop PTSD [29]. Therefore, it is key to identify a marker for those subjects who are in the risk population to provide a solid basis for biomarker validation research [29].

Unlike the research in other medical fields, PTSD biomarker study provides little information about the molecular mechanisms of post-traumatic psychopathology. Previously, a genome-wide screen in a validated animal model showed the possible biomarkers for PTSD [29]. A genomic analysis requires pure samples, which are identified by highly stringent criteria. The subjects are validated along three dimensions—analogous (similarity of phonotype), predictive (predictability of drug response or stress), and biological mechanism (regulation of gene expression and brain function). Once a potential biomarker is identified in the screening stage, an analytical validation is considered.

4.3. Analytical validation of the PTSD biomarker assay

A standardized biomarker validation process used in oncology has been considered for use in PTSD biomarker research. Adaptation of this methodological approach includes a rigorous definition and evaluation of the whole process of PTSD biomarker determination (analytical validation), and an assessment of the impact of PTSD biomarker on clinical practices (clinical validation).

Here, we briefly discuss three of the several terms that relate to analytical validation of the biomarker assay for PTSD. The first term is **precision**, which relates to reproducibility in that others should obtain similar results when following the original protocol procedures [32, 33]. Precision includes repeatability, intermediate precision, and reproducibility. Repeatability indicates the levels of the precision under the same operating conditions over a short interval of time and is referred to as intra-assay precision. Intermediate precision is within laboratory variations (different days, analysts, equipment, etc.). The second term is **accuracy**, which relates to the closeness of agreement between the value that is accepted either as a conventional true value or an accepted reference value(http://www.fda.gov/downloads/Drugs/GuidanceComplianceRegulatoryInformation/Guidances/ucm073381.pdf). The third term is **detection limit**, which refers to the lowest quantity of a substance relative to a blank value within a stated confidence limit (generally 1%) (http://en.wikipedia.org/wiki/Detection_limit). A signal-to-noise ratio between 3:1 to 2:1 is generally acceptable for estimating the detection limit (http://www.fda.gov/downloads/Drugs/GuidanceComplianceRegulatoryInformation/Guidances/ucm073381.pdf).

There are four major phases in the analytical validation stage, including setting up and standardizing operating procedures, and obtaining an internal quality control and external quality assessment. In phase one, operating procedures are established for PTSD biomarker determination. Phase two entails the validation of the operating procedures in terms of precision and accuracy according to the standards definition of operating procedures. Phase three obtains an internal quality control by evaluation of the validated standards within the laboratory. The final phase of the analytical validation is to conduct an external quality assessment comparison and assessment of their accuracy between laboratories.

In summary, analytical validation is to examine whether the procedure is suitable for testing PTSD. The analytical procedures in the protocol should be clearly defined. Thus, analytical validation should be done in different testing sites (Lab) using the same protocol. Validation includes the biomarkers' specificity, linearity, accuracy, precision (repeatability, intermediate precision, and reproducibility), range quantitation limit, and detection limit. Analytical validations must be completed prior to their use in clinical sites. In 1999, the United States Food and Drug Administration established final guidelines for the industry validation of analytical procedures and terminology (http://www.fda.gov/downloads/Drugs/GuidanceComplianceRegulatoryInformation/Guidances/ucm073381.pdf) [32, 33], which provides guidance on the validation of analytical procedures.

In the screening stage, high-throughput approaches, such as gene microarray and proteomics, are the important formats for simultaneous analyses of tens of thousands of molecules in a sample. These approaches require quality control and quality assurance. Many factors, including changes in the reaction conditions and calibration, influence the results in the analytical phase. Furthermore, since high-throughput approaches use many reagents or samples together in a single device, it makes the process more complex. Therefore, it is important to control analytical factors at different strategies by replicating analysis and normalization. The data with analytical validation for each operator and instrument can be provided to the next step, clinical validation.

4.4. Clinical validation of the PTSD biomarker assay

The development of a new PTSD biomarker test terminates with clinical validation that includes five phases: preclinical exploratory, clinical assay and validation, retrospective longitudinal, prospective screening, and PTSD control. Preclinical exploratory involves using a case-control approach to identify promising PTSD biomarker candidates. The second phase of clinical validation is to determine if a clinical biomarker assay can detect PTSD (population-based). The third phase uses a nested case-control approach in a population cohort; retrospective longitudinal study is conducted to verify if the biomarker is able to detect PTSD before it clinically manifests. In phase four, prospective screening is performed to determine the extent and characteristics of PTSD detected by tests in the subjects of cross-sectional cohort. Finally, if feasible, a randomized trial is conducted to examine the effect of test screening on reducing the burden of PTSD.

Clinical validation entails testing the ability of the markers to distinguish PTSD from non-PTSD cases, and to test the sensitivity and specificity. In this stage, it needs to find the true-positive rate (TPR), the proportion of PTSD cases who are biomarker-positive; the false-positive rate (FPR), and the proportion of non-PTSD subjects who are biomarker-positive. Then, a receiver operating characteristic (ROC) curve should be plotted. In this plot, the TPR versus the FPR can be used as the discrimination threshold. During clinical validation, it is important to assess factors associated with the biomarker, including demographic details such as age, gender, and race.

Clinical validation of PTSD biomarkers should include both retrospective and prospective analyses. Using stored samples, a retrospective analysis can be used to determine the detective ability of the potential biomarker(s) and the cut-point. If it involves multiple potential PTSD biomarkers, those PTSD markers can be compared and developed to algorithms together. Longitudinal observation will examine the variability within-subjects and compare the time-specific ROC. Again, the cut-off for a biomarker is determined by a ROC curve.

Longitudinal observation provides data from the sequential testing point, which may add additional power to the PTSD biomarker. The key issue is how to obtain the appropriate and well-characterized samples from each collecting point. Sometimes the subjects cannot be identified again or have dropped out from the study. In addition, we found that PTSD biomarkers in the brain and in the blood are not necessarily altered in the same direction. Therefore, determining the relationship between biomarkers in the peripheral nervous system and central nervous system could be more important in the clinical validation study for PTSD, though sometimes those study designs are a challenge. Finally, clinical validity of PTSD biomarker test, including its rates of false negatives and false positives, should be well established before the tests enter clinical use. Meanwhile, bridging studies are required if changes of platform device occurred after clinical validation.

5. P11 as a potential PTSD biomarker

Given that current diagnosis for PTSD rely on a clinician-administered interview, the development of a biomarker test for PTSD would be useful [7, 8]. There are no available laboratory blood biomarker tests for PTSD. We have pioneered the use of our patented blood p11 mRNA as a biomarker to differentiate PTSD from control and from other mental disorders. Our previous study demonstrates that p11 mRNA levels can be differentially detected in human blood from subjects with or without PTSD [7]. We, and others, found that p11 mRNA expression is significantly changed in post-mortem cortex of patients with PTSD [7] and depression [34]. That suggests that p11 mRNA levels in the peripheral blood cells can serve as a biomarker for PTSD.

P11, annexin light chain [35], is a member of the S100 protein family. It is one of the proteins within the EF-hand super-family of Ca^{2+} binding proteins [36]. The p11 gene is located in chromosome 1q21 in humans and expressed in many types of cells and tissues, such as in the lungs, intestines, kidneys, brain, and blood of many species [37]. P11 protein was originally identified in a complex with the Ca^{2+}/lipid-binding protein annexin A2 [36]. It regulated the function of exocytosis and endocytosis. Unlike other S100 proteins, it has crucial amino acid substitutions and deletions in the two EF-hand loops that render both Ca^{2+}-binding sites inactive [36, 37]. It is locked in the equivalent of a Ca^{2+}-loaded structure and in a permanently activated state. P11 binds to the target protein on hydrophobic cellular surfaces without Ca^{2+}. Thus, p11 regulates the function of several membrane proteins, such as annexin II and the 5-HT_{1B} receptor, which are associated with mental disorders [34]. In the nucleus, p11 participates in the regulation of the stress response. P11 is up-regulated by stress or stress hormones in the brain [7]. Stress-induced p11 overexpression is mediated by the glucocorticoid receptor (GR), which interacts with glucocorticoid receptor response elements (GREs) in the p11 promoter region [7]. These observations have received support from our data showing that mRNA levels of p11 increased in the post-mortem prefrontal cortex (area 46) of PTSD patients. Furthermore, in rats we showed that three days of inescapable shock induced over expression of p11 mRNA in the prefrontal cortex (PFC) and elevated corticosterone levels in the plasma [7]. This up-regulation of p11 expression can be countered by either a glucocorticoid receptor antagonist, RU486, or by mutating two of the three GREs (GRE2 and GRE3) [7]. Our preliminary data (Fig. 1, unpublished data) also demonstrated that p11 was significantly over-expressed in the blood of soldiers with PTSD who were deployed, compared to deployed soldiers who did not have

PTSD (Fig. 1a and 1b). Such overexpression is significantly associated with the severity of PTSD symptoms (Fig. 1c). Our results warrant further exploration of p11 as a potential biomarker for PTSD in a large sample size.

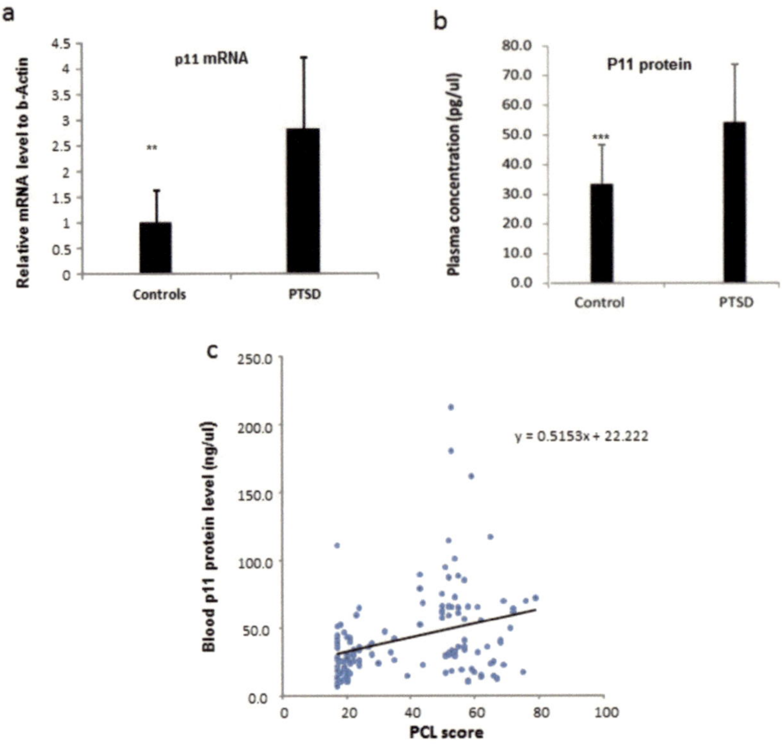

Figure 1. P11 mRNA and protein levels were significantly higher in subjects with PTSD (n=67) than that in the non-PTSD controls (n=67), and the relationship between blood p11 levels and PTSD symptom severity (unpublished data). (a) P11 mRNA level was significantly higher in subjects with PTSD than that in the non-PTSD controls (**$p<0.01$). (b) P11 protein level was significantly higher in subjects with PTSD than that in the non-PTSD controls (***$p<0.001$). (c) The relationship between blood p11 protein levels and PTSD checklist (PCL) score ($p<0.0027$).

6. Biorepository or biobank in biomarker study

To obtain a large quantity of good quality samples is a challenge. It requires developing a standardized protocol for sample collection, storage, and quantitative control. A biobank will provide such opportunity. A preliminary type of biobank, a biorepository can store biological samples (usually human) for use in PTSD biomarker research. The biobank market is expanding with a significant increase in using human tissues, blood, and other biomaterials to do biomarker research, and pharmaceutical and diagnostic tool development [38]. In 2008, there were 270 million specimens in biobanks. Each year, about 20 million samples have been collected for research, including biomarker studies [39], indicating worldwide changes in the nature of biomedical research. In general, more and more biobanks have been established.

They are established by multiple research centers, leading to an infrastructure of next-generation research demand [40]. A typical example is the Psychiatric Genomics Consortium (PGC) that is comprised of more than 80 institutions. The PGC has samples from more than 150,000 people; of which, 36,989 samples are from subjects with diagnosed schizophrenia [41]. Recently, using the PGC samples, researchers have spotted 108 genetic loci in the DNA sequence of schizophrenia. The large PGC sample has also allowed for the development of an algorithm to calculate a 'risk score' for each variant's contribution to schizophrenia. PGC plans to sequence 100,000 subject samples with mental illnesses in an effort to identify the meaningful biomarker associations [41].

However, there are many issues for biobanks ahead, including ethical, legal, and social issues pertaining to their existence, the fairness of collecting donations from vulnerable populations, providing informed consent to donors, the logistics of data disclosure to participants, the right to ownership of intellectual property, and the privacy and security of donors who participate [39]. Nevertheless, biobanks will provide a great opportunity to researchers in the PTSD biomarker study.

7. Our biorepository and biomarker study, including p11 research

Since 2009, we have collected blood and saliva samples from soldiers who were deployed to Iraq and Afghanistan. To date, over 2,000 blood and 5,000 saliva samples have been collected. This study was initiated at Fort Bragg in 2009 and expanded to multiple Army National Guard units throughout California, Pennsylvania, and Guam in 2011. Biological samples and detailed mental health data, using DSM driven surveys, were voluntarily collected from soldiers, including ~500 before, during, and following a deployment to Iraq or Afghanistan, to allow for a longitudinal assessment. The mental health surveys contained established self-report inventories (e.g., PCL, GAD, and PHQ). Using our biorepository dataset to examine p11 as a potential PTSD biomarker may help scientists discover why some people, particularly those in the military, develop PTSD, depression, and suicidal behaviors while others do not.

Author details

Lei Zhang[1*], Xian-Zhang Hu[1], He Li[1], Xiaoxia Li[1], Stanley Smerin[1], Dale W. Russell[1], Angela Boutte[2], Berwin Yuan[1], Nora Wang[1], Ze Chen[1] and Robert J. Ursano[1]

*Address all correspondence to: Lezhang@usuhs.edu

1 Uniformed Services University of the Health Sciences, Department of Psychiatry, Bethesda, MD, USA

2 Brain Trauma, Neuroprotection, and Neurorestoration Branch, Center for Military Psychiatry and Neuroscience Research, Walter Reed Army Institute of Research, Silver Spring, MD, USA

References

[1] Kessler, R.C., et al., *Posttraumatic stress disorder in the National Comorbidity Survey.* Arch Gen Psychiatry, 1995. 52(12): p. 1048-60.

[2] Brockie, T.N., et al., *The Relationship of Adverse Childhood Experiences to PTSD, Depression, Poly-Drug Use and Suicide Attempt in Reservation-Based Native American Adolescents and Young Adults.* Am J Community Psychol, 2015. 55(3-4): p. 411-21.

[3] Gupta, M.A., *Suicide attempt and externalizing behaviours in posttraumatic stress disorder (PTSD): possible role of the activating effect of antidepressants.* Aust N Z J Psychiatry, 2015. 49(1): p. 89-90.

[4] Zhang, L., et al., *P11 (S100A10) as a potential biomarker of psychiatric patients at risk of suicide.* J Psychiatr Res, 2011. 45(4): p. 435-41.

[5] Zhang, L., R.J. Ursano, and H. Li, *P11: a potential biomarker for posttraumatic stress disorder.* Methods Mol Biol, 2012. 829: p. 453-68.

[6] Su, T.P., et al., *Levels of the potential biomarker p11 in peripheral blood cells distinguish patients with PTSD from those with other major psychiatric disorders.* J Psychiatr Res, 2009. 43(13): p. 1078-85.

[7] Zhang, L., et al., *p11 is up-regulated in the forebrain of stressed rats by glucocorticoid acting via two specific glucocorticoid response elements in the p11 promoter.* Neuroscience, 2008. 153(4): p. 1126-34.

[8] Zhang, L., et al., *A strategy for the development of biomarker tests for PTSD.* Med Hypotheses, 2009. 73(3): p. 404-9.

[9] Bisson, J.I., *What happened to harmonization of the PTSD diagnosis? The divergence of ICD11 and DSM5.* Epidemiol Psychiatr Sci, 2013. 22(3): p. 205-7.

[10] Hulka, B.S. and B.H. Margolin, *Methodological issues in epidemiologic studies using biologic markers.* Am J Epidemiol, 1992. 135(2): p. 200-9.

[11] Hulka, B.S. and T. Wilcosky, *Biological markers in epidemiologic research.* Arch Environ Health, 1988. 43(2): p. 83-9.

[12] Lee, L.W., et al., *Human tissue monitoring and specimen banking: opportunities for exposure assessment, risk assessment, and epidemiologic research.* Environ Health Perspect, 1995. 103 Suppl 3: p. 3-8.

[13] *Biomarkers and surrogate endpoints: preferred definitions and conceptual framework.* Clin Pharmacol Ther, 2001. 69(3): p. 89-95.

[14] Jain, K.K., *The Handbook of Biomarkers.* 2010, Springer Science + Business Media: London.

[15] DeLisi, C., *Meetings that changed the world: Santa Fe 1986: Human genome baby-steps.* Nature, 2008. 455(7215): p. 876-877.

[16] Kohn, E.C., et al., *Proteomics as a tool for biomarker discovery.* Dis Markers, 2007. 23(5-6): p. 411-7.

[17] Zhou, J.Y., J. Hanfelt, and J. Peng, *Clinical proteomics in neurodegenerative diseases.* Proteomics Clin Appl, 2007. 1(11): p. 1342-50.

[18] Young, E.A. and N. Breslau, *Saliva cortisol in posttraumatic stress disorder: a community epidemiologic study.* Biol Psychiatry, 2004. 56(3): p. 205-9.

[19] Spitzer, C., et al., *C-reactive protein, pre- and postdexamethasone cortisol levels in posttraumatic stress disorder.* Nord J Psychiatry, 2014. 68(5): p. 296-9.

[20] Bremner, J.D., et al., *Elevated CSF corticotropin-releasing factor concentrations in posttraumatic stress disorder.* Am J Psychiatry, 1997. 154(5): p. 624-9.

[21] Yehuda, R., et al., *Urinary catecholamine excretion and severity of PTSD symptoms in Vietnam combat veterans.* J Nerv Ment Dis, 1992. 180(5): p. 321-5.

[22] Kibler, J.L., K. Joshi, and M. Ma, *Hypertension in relation to posttraumatic stress disorder and depression in the US National Comorbidity Survey.* Behav Med, 2009. 34(4): p. 125-32.

[23] Falconer, E.M., et al., *Developing an integrated brain, behavior and biological response profile in posttraumatic stress disorder (PTSD).* J Integr Neurosci, 2008. 7(3): p. 439-56.

[24] Bryant, R.A., et al., *A multisite study of initial respiration rate and heart rate as predictors of posttraumatic stress disorder.* J Clin Psychiatry, 2008. 69(11): p. 1694-701.

[25] Kovacic, Z., et al., *Platelet serotonin concentration and suicidal behavior in combat related posttraumatic stress disorder.* Prog Neuropsychopharmacol Biol Psychiatry, 2008. 32(2): p. 544-51.

[26] Hamner, M.B. and P.B. Gold, *Plasma dopamine beta-hydroxylase activity in psychotic and non-psychotic post-traumatic stress disorder.* Psychiatry Res, 1998. 77(3): p. 175-81.

[27] Geuze, E., et al., *Reduced GABAA benzodiazepine receptor binding in veterans with posttraumatic stress disorder.* Mol Psychiatry, 2008. 13(1): p. 74-83, 3.

[28] Morey, R.A., et al., *The role of trauma-related distractors on neural systems for working memory and emotion processing in posttraumatic stress disorder.* J Psychiatr Res, 2009. 43(8): p. 809-17.

[29] Zhang, L., et al., *Identification of gene markers based on well validated and subcategorized stressed animals for potential clinical applications in PTSD.* Med Hypotheses, 2006. 66(2): p. 309-14.

[30] Yehuda, R., *Advances in understanding neuroendocrine alterations in PTSD and their therapeutic implications.* Ann N Y Acad Sci, 2006. 1071: p. 137-66.

[31] Vaiva, G., et al., *Relationship between posttrauma GABA plasma levels and PTSD at 1-year follow-up.* Am J Psychiatry, 2006. 163(8): p. 1446-8.

[32] Goodsaid, F. and F. Frueh, *Process map proposal for the validation of genomic biomarkers.* Pharmacogenomics, 2006. 7(5): p. 773-82.

[33] Downs-Kelly, E., et al., *Analytical validation and interobserver reproducibility of EnzMet GenePro: a second-generation bright-field metallography assay for concomitant detection of HER2 gene status and protein expression in invasive carcinoma of the breast.* Am J Surg Pathol, 2005. 29(11): p. 1505-11.

[34] Svenningsson, P., et al., *Alterations in 5-HT1B receptor function by p11 in depression-like states.* Science, 2006. 311(5757): p. 77-80.

[35] Grabarek, Z., *Structural basis for diversity of the EF-hand calcium-binding proteins.* J Mol Biol, 2006. 359(3): p. 509-25.

[36] Rety, S., et al., *The crystal structure of a complex of p11 with the annexin II N-terminal peptide.* Nat Struct Biol, 1999. 6(1): p. 89-95.

[37] Harder, T., E. Kube, and V. Gerke, *Cloning and characterization of the human gene encoding p11: structural similarity to other members of the S-100 gene family.* Gene, 1992. 113(2): p. 269-74.

[38] Hewitt, R.E., *Biobanking: the foundation of personalized medicine.* Curr Opin Oncol, 2011. 23(1): p. 112-9.

[39] Haga, S.B. and L.M. Beskow, *Ethical, legal, and social implications of biobanks for genetics research.* Adv Genet, 2008. 60: p. 505-44.

[40] Fullerton, S.M., et al., *Meeting the governance challenges of next-generation biorepository research.* Sci Transl Med, 2010. 2(15): p. 15cm3.

[41] Reardon, S., Gene-hunt gain for mental health. Nature, 2014. 511(7510): p. 393.

Chapter 6

Anxiety Disorders and Suicide: Psychiatric Interventions

Cicek Hocaoglu

Additional information is available at the end of the chapter

http://dx.doi.org/10.5772/60594

Abstract

A universal phenomenon equally ancient as the history of mankind, suicide is defined as the willful and intentional ending of one's own life. Risk factors for suicidal behavior are traumatic childhood and adulthood experiences, negative interfamily interactions, social isolation, decreased social solidarity, financial troubles, losses, despair, impulsivity, and migration. Recognized as a critical public health problem, preliminary causes of suicide are financial, religious, political, social, cultural, and medical in addition to mental disorders like depression and alcohol addiction. It has been proven in a number of researches till today that there is a correlation between major depression, bipolar disorder, schizophrenia, borderline personality disorder, alcohol-drug use, and suicidal behavior. Nonetheless, the relation between anxiety disorders and suicidal behavior has not been clearly defined to date. The evidences gathered so far reveal that panic disorder is only an independent risk factor for suicide attempt. The limited number of studies on this domain provided nonhomogenous results. It is however a point to keep in mind that if anxiety disorders are codiagnosed with mental disorders, they pose risk for suicidal behavior. In different studies with a wider sampling in this domain, analyzing the effect of specific anxiety disorders on suicidal behavior might be useful for suicide prevention programs.

Keywords: Anxiety disorders, suicidal thoughts, suicide attempts, comorbid psychiatric disorders, suicidal behavior

1. Introduction

Nowadays, suicide is a major public health issue worldwide. Suicide is undoubtedly the most tragic event in human life. Globally speaking, around one million people commit suicide each year. Suicide is possibly witnessed among a wide range of population extending from normal individuals reacting differently to stress-triggering life conditions to people diagnosed with a mental disorder. Mental disorders as suicide causes have been studied in numerous researches and the correlation between depression and suicide has been particularly emphasized because major depression disorder comes first among the mental disorders that are related to both completed suicide and also suicidal ideation and attempt. The relation between anxiety disorders and suicidal behavior has been examined in limited numbers of studies with differing results. Some studies posited that there might be a relation between anxiety disorder and suicidal behavior, while in other studies it was posited that anxiety disorders on their own cannot be effective in triggering suicidal behavior. Anxiety disorders often cooccur with depression, and this may be masking a risk of suicidal behavior specifically related to anxiety. This higher likelihood was seen despite controlling for current depression, highlighting the importance of clinicians considering suicidal risk when working with anxiety patients who do not necessarily also have a diagnosis of depression. Although anxiety has been proposed to be a potentially modifiable risk factor for suicide, research examining the relationship between anxiety and suicidal behaviors has demonstrated mixed results. Until recently, anxiety disorders were not regarded as an independent risk factor for suicidal behavior which in turn limited the number of studies focusing on the significant relation between anxiety disorder and suicidal behavior. In a different saying, suicidal ideation in anxiety-diagnosed patients went unnoticed. Strong evidences have been gathered proving that panic disorder is an independent risk factor for suicide. There are uncertain findings about the possibility that specific anxiety disorders such as generalized anxiety disorder, obsessive-compulsive disorder, and posttrauma stress disorder may be independent risk factors for suicide. There are, however, stronger evidences that when anxiety disorder is codiagnosed with comorbid depression, bipolar disorder, schizophrenia, drug use, and personality disorders the risk may be substantially higher. In other words, controversy exists whether anxiety disorders are independently associated (i.e., after adjusting for comorbid mental disorders) with suicidal ideation and suicide attempts. Despite the existence of literature studies providing nonhomogenous findings, it is of great importance that clinicians focus more eagerly and attentively on suicide behavior in patients with anxiety disorder – particularly in patients codiagnosed with mental-disorder – to provide assistance to suicide prevention attempts. In this chapter, the relation between suicidal behavior and the anxiety disorder will be discussed.

2. Anxiety disorders

Anxiety disorders belong to the most frequent mental disorders and are often characterized by an early onset and a progressive, persistent/chronic, or recurrent course. Several individual, familial, and environmental risk factors for adverse course characteristics of anxiety disorders (including higher persistence, lower probability of remission, and increased risk of recurrence) have been identified, and previous research suggests that clinical features of anxiety (e.g., higher severity, duration, and avoidance) as well as comorbid other mental disorders are particularly useful for predicting an unfavorable course of anxiety disorders [1]. The literature reviewed here is consistent in showing that anxiety disorders are common psychiatric disorders that typically has an early age of onset, a chronic course, and a high degree of comorbidity with mood disorders and other psychiatric disorders [2]. Anxiety disorders are one of the most prevalent of all psychiatric disorders in the general population [3-5]. Phobias are the most common with the highest rates for simple phobia (SP) and agoraphobia. For example, SP is the most common anxiety disorder, with up to 49% of people reporting an unreasonably strong fear. Among general population, prevalence of social anxiety disorder (SAD) meeting DSM-IV diagnosis criteria is circa 13%. Among general population, prevalence of posttraumatic stress disorder (PTSD) is 7.8%; however among particular groups (war veterans with 20%, domestic violence victim women 12%), higher prevalence of PTSD has been reported [6]. Panic disorder (PD) and obsessive-compulsive disorder (OCD) are less frequent, and there are discordant results for SAD and generalized anxiety disorder [7]. The epidemiological studies have shown that anxiety disorders are highly prevalent and important causes of functional impairment [2, 8]. However, due to their methodic differences, epidemiologic studies fail to adequately explain the effects of anxiety disorders on functionality since the high frequency of confusing sociodemographic variables (gender, age, race, ethnic structure, education, and marital status) can play different roles in the symptom severity and course of anxiety disorders [7]. Agoraphobia, SP, and generalized anxiety disorder (GAD) are more common in female, while there is no gender difference for SAD, PD, and OCD [6]. Anxiety disorders are more common among separated, divorced, or widowed people between ages 25 and 44. Anxiety disorders are rare among age 65 and above. Start age for anxiety disorders however varies for specific anxiety disorders. For instance, phobic disorders start at early age, while panic disorder is witnessed during early adulthood stage. Rather than epidemiological studies, stressful life events, childhood experiences, and familial factors as risk factors have been examined in clinical researches. Anxiety disorders are usually chronic and persistent and are generally accompanied with other psychiatric disorders such as other anxiety disorders, depressive disorders, personality disorders, and drug use. These codiagnosed conditions may negatively affect functionality and life quality. Further study is needed to better understand the comorbidity between anxiety disorders, the consistently higher rates of anxiety disorders, and the differential effects of socioeconomic and cultural factors on anxiety disorders.

3. Suicidal behaviors

The currently accepted nomenclature of suicide-related behaviors identifies suicide, nonfatal suicide attempts, and suicidal ideation [9]. Suicidal ideation is verbally expressing one's ideas about killing himself/herself. Suicide attempt is performing behaviors with the intention of killing oneself not ending with death but potentially causing major injuries. Completed suicide is dying as a result of the behavior performed to kill oneself. It is a requirement to make such classification for suicidal behaviors since for three different groups risk factors and clinical presentations vary. Hence this classification is needed in the prevention of suicides likewise. Global estimates suggest that each year there are 10–20 million suicide attempts and one million completed suicides [10]. Suicide attempts are costly in terms of occupational and interpersonal disruption [11]. Moreover, substantial financial costs are associated with the intensive psychiatric resources devoted to these patients [12]. Suicide is a multivariate phenomenon occurring with the combined effect of a multitude of factors such as psychological, sociological, economical, and cultural. That explains the reason why suicide can be witnessed among a vast sampling group ranging from normal individuals to patients with severe mental disorders. Mood disorders and personality disorders (borderline personality disorder in particular) are psychiatric problems most frequently associated with suicide. Besides, there have been striking findings recently that point to the increasing effect of anxiety disorders on suicide. On that account this relation should definitely be analyzed in the prevention of suicide, which is a crucial public health problem. In cases with anxiety disorder, analyzing suicidal ideation and suicide attempt may prevent completed suicides hence lower the ratios of completed suicide; because suicidal ideation and preattempted suicide are the biggest risk factors for a completed suicide [10, 13, 14]. Studying such thoughts and behaviors, therefore, may increase our understanding of who is likely to attempt or complete suicide, potentially informing suicide risk management and prevention efforts. Psychiatric disorders are one the primary risk factors for suicidality, with up to 95% of suicides committed by individuals with one or more disorders.

4. Anxiety disorders and suicidal behaviors

Patients with anxiety disorders are at high risk for suicidal ideation, regardless of whether the suicidal ideation is due to anxiety disorders itself or to cooccurring conditions. In evaluating the literature, it is necessary to review general requirements for establishing anxiety as a risk factor for suicidal behaviors [9]. In addition to establishing a meaningful and consistent interrelation of anxiety with suicidal behavior, the other requirement is the absence of a third variance (mixing factor) between suicidal behaviors and anxiety. Besides, anxiety must have existed before suicidal behavior and in suicidal behaviors anxiety must act as the independent risk factor. Psychiatric disorders are one of the primary risk factors for suicidality, with up to 95% of suicides committed by individuals with one or more disorder [15]. In particular, the mood and anxiety disorders are associated with suicide ideation and attempts [16-19]. The relationship between anxiety disorders and suicide-related behaviors has received a modest amount of attention. However, research has also accumulated over the past several years indicating that anxiety disorders confer unique risk of suicide [20, 21]. The presence of current or lifetime anxiety disorders, including panic disorder, social phobia, generalized anxiety disorder, and posttraumatic stress disorder, are associated with increased suicide risk [10, 18, 22, 23]. Individuals with anxiety disorders demonstrate increased suicidal ideation and rates of self injury and more frequent suicide attempts than those without mental health disorders [10, 16, 17]. For this reason, it is of vital importance to comprehend and manage the risk factors for suicide among individuals with anxiety disorders. Despite the prevalence of high risk for suicide within cases with anxiety disorder, the determinants of suicide risk in this group have not yet been clearly established. In other words, anxiety disorders are very common and increase risk for suicide attempts. Little is known about predictors of increased risk specifically among individuals with anxiety disorders [19]. Studies of individuals with specific anxiety disorders including panic disorder, social phobia, and posttraumatic stress disorder indicate that the additional presence of depression and substance use disorders increases suicide risk

[10, 24]. Severity and aspects of functional impairment are also related to suicide risk in patients with anxiety disorders. For example, anxiety symptom severity is associated with increased suicidal ideation and attempts in patients with PD and patients with PTSD [10, 25, 26]. Associations between suicide risk and impairment in general functioning in PTSD and social functioning in both PTSD and PD are also documented [27, 28]. Twelve-month prevalence rates of suicidal ideation in patients with obsessive-compulsive disorder (OCD, 27.3%), the prevalence rate of suicide attempts in panic disorder (3.6%) and the prevalence rate of suicide attempts in OCD (3.3%) were the highest [21]. The overall 12-month and lifetime prevalence of GAD was 0.8% and 1.2%, respectively. Being older than 25 years and female, lower education level, unemployed status, and lower monthly income were associated with increased risk of GAD in China [29]. It remains unclear whether certain anxiety disorders are risk factors for suicide. For instance, Uebelacker et al. [19] have reported that PTSD, major depressive disorder (MDD), intermittent depressive disorder, epilepsy, pain and low social functionality are, according to univariate analysis, predictors of suicide attempt. In the same study, the findings of multivariate analysis showed that, even when the suicide attempts of the past are controlled, MDD and intermittent depressive disorder are independent risk factors in current attempts for suicide. However, it was concluded in this research that except panic disorder, no other specific anxiety disorder constituted an independent risk factor for suicide attempt. Mood disorders and past history of suicide attempts are the most powerful predictors of a future suicide attempt. Particularly, the patients with comorbid major depressive disorder anxiety are at higher risk for suicide. Thereby primary care health service doctors, emergency and mental health professionals, and clinicians who frequently come across with anxiety disordered cases should be alerted and attentive against potential suicidal ideation and suicide attempts among these patients.

4.1. Anxiety disorders and completed suicide: Associated factors

The presence of anxiety disorder is frequently associated with suicide ideation and behaviors. Considering the high costs of suicidal behaviors for the individuals and also the society, it is a foremost priority to prevent suicide. Grasping the factors related to increased risk for suicide among people with anxiety disorders may be contributive to suicide prevention attempts [10]. Anxiety disorders are independent risk factors for suicide attempts and underscore the importance of anxiety disorders as a serious public health problem [17]. The relationship between anxiety disorders and completed suicide is not known exactly. There are a limited number of studies on this subject [30, 31]. It is unclear whether clinical and behavioral suicide risk factors, identified primarily among men, can be extended to women. Personality variants and gender differences among suicide completers with psychopathological autopsy method were investigated. Among women, the ratio of completed suicides is lower than men. Impulsivity and alcohol use are risk factors for completed suicides. It is less common among women to see lifelong alcohol consumption, and among women with alcohol addiction, there is less prevalence of comorbid depression when compared to men. There exists a correlation between alcohol consumption and impulsivity. The low ratio of impulsivity among women triggers alcohol consumption as well. Furthermore, when the relation between impulsivity and applied suicide method is examined, it surfaces that among cases with high ratio of impulsivity, the tendency to apply violence methods is more common. It is argued that women prefer non-violent suicide methods less pain causing but regardless of their sex, cases with anxiety disorder apply to nonviolent methods more frequently. On the other hand, when high ratio of impulsivity is combined with alcohol consumption, there may occur an elevated risk of suicide for both sexes [30].

4.2. Anxiety disorders and attempted suicide: Associated factors

The relationship between anxiety disorders and racial and ethnic differences has been studied in several research. For instance, Vanderwerker et al. [32] examined in their study covering 131 adults from different ethnic and racial origins (more than half of the cases with African American roots) the differences of risk factors for suicidal ideation and suicide attempts. They have detected that among young white adults, anxiety disorder (not depression) has an independent relation with suicide tendency, while there is no such relationship for African-Americans among whom there is a significant relation between suicidal behavior and social support could be identified. These findings clearly prove that suicide risk factors vary among races and ethnicities [32]. The results suggest that race/ethnicity-specific risk profiles may improve the detection of suicidality in vulnerable populations. But, Beautrais et al. [33] were found no ethnic differences in suicidal ideation. Risks of suicidal ideation, plan, and attempt were associated with mood disorder, substance use disorder, and anxiety disorder. Major depression was the specific disorder most strongly associated with suicidal ideation, plan, and attempt [33]. In a different study based on society sampling, a number of variables (demographic, work status, mental and physical health condition, personality features, stressful life experiences, and social environment) impacting the suicide-attempt speed in cases with suicidal ideation have been examined. Among age groups between 20–24 and 40–44 having committed suicide attempt, it has been seen that there was a higher ratio of suicidal ideation with respect to age-matched groups and higher levels of anxiety and depression. Upon checking the remaining variables, it has been reported that in cases between ages 20–24, rather than suicidal ideation but anxiety itself constituted a risk factor for suicide attempt. Particularly among men between ages 40–44, physical diseases and unemployment, rather than anxiety and depression, posed greater risks for suicide attempt. In a different saying, Fairweather et al. [34] found that ideators and attempters experience comparable levels of depression and anxiety. Rates of self-harm and associations between self-harm and suicidal behaviors, anxiety, hostility, and paranoid ideas were reported by Fliege et al. [35]. Although there has been significant interest in whether anxiety disorders are risk factors for suicidal behavior, this remains a controversial area. Cross-sectional community and clinical studies have repeatedly demonstrated in univariate models that anxiety disorders are associated with suicidal ideation, attempted suicide, and completed suicides. In multivariate models, it has been questioned whether panic disorder is associated with suicidal behavior after adjusting for other anxiety and psychiatric disorders. Because anxiety disorders are highly comorbid with other anxiety disorders and tend to cluster together, it is important to address whether anxiety disorders as a group of psychiatric disorders have an impact on suicidal behavior after adjusting for other types of other psychiatric disorders (especially mood and substance use disorders) [16].

http://dx.doi.org/10.5772/60594

5. Specific anxiety disorders and suicidal behaviors

The relationship between anxiety disorders and suicidal behaviors has not received sufficient amount of interest till present age. Literature review shows that when there is a definite result for a single anxiety disorder, anxiety disorders in general have high frequency relation with suicidal ideation; however its relationship with suicide attempt is not definite [9, 18, 36]. General tendency indicates that for each anxiety disorder there is a similar risk for suicide primarily obsessive-compulsive disorder, generalized anxiety disorder, and social anxiety disorder are associated with suicide ideation. The only specific anxiety disorder related most with suicide attempt is panic disorder [37]. In addition, a clear relationship was reported between PTSD and suicidal thoughts and behaviors, irrespective of the type of trauma experienced. It has been suggested that PTSD has a strong association with suicidality, predicting subsequent suicidal attempts [28, 38].

5.1. Panic disorder and suicide

Suicidal behaviors are multifactorial behaviors. While, historically, anxiety has been regarded as an important risk factor in suicidal behaviors, epidemiological studies carried out on general population or panic patients have evidenced the possible links between suicidal behaviors and the occurrence of panic attacks [39, 40]. Both panic attacks and panic disorders are, in the society and primary health care service, independently related with the increased suicide attempt risk. In epidemiologic samplings, panic disorder is, like major depressive disorder, a risk factor for lifelong suicide ideation and suicide attempt [40-42]. For example, an association between panic and suicidal ideation has been reported by Goodwin and Roy-Byrne [43]. Epidemiologic catchment area (ECA) studies indicate that, when contrasted with other psychiatric disorders, panic disorder is associated with increased suicide ideation and suicide attempt risk [40]. Additionally, epidemiologic data show that when panic disorder is codiagnosed with major depression, alcohol addiction, personality disorders, and cocaine use, there is higher risk for suicide attempt [44, 45]. For instance, Goodwin and Roy-Byrne report that despite the vital role comorbid depression and drug abuse play, attempts for the last one year (not lifelong) are independently related to panic disorder [43]. It has been suggested that panic disorder may not increase past suicide attempt systematically but may climb the suicide attempt in the future. In a vast majority of the monitoring studies of patients with anxiety disorder, there was 20% ratio of suicide caused deaths like the results in major depressive disorder. Similarly, the ratios in suicide attempts have been similar to major depressive disorder and panic disorder [40, 46]. Existing findings are quite remarkable. Patients who suffered from major depressive disorder with related panic disorder were given to more impulsive suicide attempts, even if the difference with depressed patients without panic disorder was statistically insignificant [39]. Primary care patients with PD are at high risk for suicidal ideation, and patients with PD and cooccurring MDD are at especially high risk. Patients with PD in primary care thus should be assessed routinely for suicidal ideation and depression [42]. Although in society-based studies it is indicated that there is a strong relation between PD and suicide ideation, in many other studies with clinic sampling (receiving psychiatric treatment and hospitalized in psychiatry clinic or hospital), no statistically significant relation between PD and suicidal ideation could be detected [24, 47]. For example, Warshaw et al. [24] reported that there was no association between PD and suicidal ideation after controlling for common comorbid psychiatric disorders. In another study, it was revealed that suicidal behavior risk in panic disorder is not higher than the risk in major depressive disorder [42]. Dammen et al. [47] could not find any difference in terms of suicidal ideation between patients with or without panic disorder. Several mental disorders, such as personality disorders, and life events that that have been associated with suicidality, e.g., early childhood abuse, were not assessed and may account partially for the observed association between PD and suicidal ideation [48, 49]. In some clinical studies, patients with PD and borderline personality disorder were at significantly higher risk of suicidal behavior than were PD patients with panic disorder alone [24]. To sum up, there is still an ongoing discussion about the relation between panic disorder and suicide behavior. It is not yet identified if panic disorder singly or when comorbid with other mental disorders like major depressive disorder is effective in suicidal behavior [24, 40, 50]. Thus, the data indicate that the risk of suicide in panic disorder is substantial. As a consequence, clinicians should alert themselves to this preventable outcome and approach treatment with added caution.

5.2. Posttraumatic stress disorder and suicide

Posttraumatic stress disorder (PTSD) is frequently associated with suicidal ideation and suicide attempts. Suicide is an important cause of death in veterans, and the risk for intentional death continues to be high many years after service [51]. Suicidal behavior is a critical problem in war veterans. Combat veterans are not only more likely to have suicidal ideation, often associated with PTSD and depression, but they are more likely to act on a suicidal plan [52]. Citizen soldiers (National Guard and Reserves) represent approximately 40% of the two million armed forces deployed to Afghanistan and Iraq. Twenty-five to forty percent of them develop PTSD, clinical depression, sleep disturbances, or suicidal thoughts [53]. Veterans reporting subthreshold PTSD were three times more likely to endorse these markers of elevated suicide risk relative to the veterans without PTSD [54]. They found no significant differences in likelihood of endorsing hopelessness or suicidal ideation comparing subthreshold and threshold PTSD groups, although the subthreshold PTSD group was less likely to report prior mental health treatment [54]. Major depressive disorder cooccurs frequently with PTSD, and both disorders are linked to suicidal ideation. For the war veterans with depression symptoms, there is a strong relation between PTSD symptoms and suicidal ideation. According to these findings, when analyzing PTSD-diagnosed war veterans, depression symptoms of suicidal ideation must be taken into account [55]. Of those veterans diagnosed with PTSD, many have comorbid psychiatric disorders, typically major depressive disorder, substance use disorders, and other anxiety disorders [56]. Veterans with PTSD are also more likely to have social, occupational, and functional difficulties, including social isolation, frequent interpersonal altercations, and suicidal ideation [28]. PTSD and MDD occur together frequently, and both disorders have been separately linked to the increased risk of suicidal ideation [57, 58]. It is unclear, however, whether the combination of comorbid MDD and PTSD confers an increased risk for suicidal ideation beyond the risk presented by either diagnosis alone. Several studies of veteran samples have found that the combination of PTSD and MDD did not place individuals at greater risk for suicidal ideation than did a single diagnosis [54, 55, 59]. Conversely, Oquendo et al. [60] found that individuals with current MDD and comorbid PTSD were more likely to endorse suicidal ideation compared to those without a current PTSD diagnosis. In a different study, it was determined that among veterans with schizophrenia and schizoaffective disorder, there is an independent relation between comorbid PTSD suicidal ideation risk but no such risk could be detected for suicide attempt [61]. Suicide has huge effect on public health but despite efficient interventions, a great number of people with suicide risk cannot benefit from these interventions and lose their lives. Until now, a huge number of programs and strategies named as "suicide prevention" have been developed. Recent interventions about exercise give hope in the prevention of suicide thanks to its ease of application because exercise mitigates depression symptoms. Alleviating depression symptoms may provide lessened suicidal ideation and attempt but no study has so far indicated a direct relation between exercise and suicidal behavior. Davidson et al. [62] analyzed in veteran sampling a number of variables (sleep disorders, PTSD, and depression) that might be associated with suicidal risk. In this study, it has been emphasized that there may exist an indirect relation between exercise and suicide. It has also been suggested that exercise is also connected with low depression symptoms and a better sleep pattern, which might in effect lead to lower suicidal risk. A high prevalence of all types of violence is associated with the highest prevalence of depression and PTSD [63]. It is well established that intimate male partner violence (IPV) has a high impact on women's mental health. Compared to women in control group, among women subjected to physical and psychological IPV, there is higher ratio of depression and anxiety disorders, PTSD, and suicidal ideation. Among women exposed to sexual abuse and sexual violence, there is high ratio of depression symptoms, physical/ psychological abuse, and suicide attempt. In reality, PTSD on its own is quite hard to see. Depression symptoms are present either singly or codiagnosed with PTSD. Anxiety ratios are higher among women with comorbidite or abused women with depression symptoms. This may explain the high ratio of suicide attempts and anxiety among physically/psychologically abused women [64, 65]. Recovery from depressive symptoms, state anxiety, and posttraumatic stress disorder in women exposed to physical and psychological but not to psychological intimate partner violence alone. A metaanalysis with 50-article examining the relation among PTSD and past and present suicidal ideation and behavior has been conducted. There is no evidence showing that among PTSD patients there is a risk for completed suicide risk. A relation has been found among presuicide attempt and past and present suicidal ideation. Upon checking other psychiatric disorders (including depression), the relation between PTSD and suicide attempt has been examined but no sufficient data could be detected, but it was also reported that comorbidity depression and pretraumatic psychiatric state may have been a mediator. It is seen that a relation exists among various factors and PTSD and suicidal tendency [66]. In a different study, it was seen that among women patients with comorbid PTSD and drug addiction, suicide behavior varies according to drug addiction type and presence of preventive factors (for instance, worries about kids, will to live, and coping skill) [67]. Clinicians should be attentive to suicide risk in returned veterans and in women exposed to physical/psychological and psychological IPV. For future studies, assessing suicide risk in PTSD and identifying risk factors shall assist in better understanding the topic and preventing suicidal behavior.

5.3. Obsessive-compulsive disorder and suicide

Suicidal thoughts and behaviors, also known as suicidality, are a fairly neglected area of study in patients with obsessive-compulsive disorder. Patients with obsessive-compulsive disorder (OCD) have historically been considered at low risk for suicide, but recent studies are controversial. Torres et al. [68] found thirty-six percent of the patients reported lifetime suicidal thoughts, 20% had made suicidal plans, 11% had already attempted suicide, and 10% presented current suicidal thoughts. The sexual/religious dimension and comorbid substance use disorders remained associated with suicidal thoughts and plans, while impulse-control disorders were associated with current suicidal thoughts and with suicide plans and attempts [68]. The risk of suicidal behaviors must be carefully investigated in OCD patients, particularly those with symptoms of the sexual/religious dimension and comorbid major depressive disorder, PTSD, substance use disorders, and impulse-control disorders [69]. Lester and Abdel-Khalek [70] reported that there is no relation between OCD and suicidal ideation but a relation between OCD and suicide attempt. However, there are certain limits such as the smallness of sampling group and failure to control depression. In a different study conducted with same research group in 2002, it was reported that there is a significant relation between OCD and suicidal ideation but again depression was not controlled in another study [71]. Obsessive-compulsive personality disorder is a factor increasing risk for nonfatal suicidal behavior independently of risk conferred by depressive disorders. For example, Diaconu and Turecki [72] reported that the comorbid obsessive-compulsive personality disorder depression group presented increased current and lifetime suicide ideation compared to the groups with depression alone or without depression, or personality disorders they also had increased history of suicide attempts which were often multiple attempts. OCD is associated with a high risk for suicidal behavior. Depression and hopelessness are the major correlates of suicidal behavior [73]. Suicidal behavior is not a common phenomenon in OCD, but among single patients in particular, accompanying depression, symmetry/order obsession, and compulsions are high risk factors for suicide [74]. In patients with OCD, risk factors for suicidal behavior have been left ignored when compared to other anxiety disorders. However, a high ratio as 10–27% was reported for suicidal behavior. This condition shows that OCD patients may commit suicide attempt at least once in their life [16]. Besides as in OCD assistance-seeking ratio is comparatively lower than assistance search in comorbid OCD, it becomes evident that in OCD patients assistance-seeking methods should be increased in suicide prevention strategies. Suicidality has been underestimated in OCD and should be investigated in every patient, so that appropriate preventive measures can be taken.

5.4. Generalized anxiety disorder and suicide

Generalized anxiety disorder (GAD) is a chronic general disease among adult population but it is comparatively a less understood clinical state. Clinicians may have knowledge about the characteristics of GAD such as over anxiety, anxiety, and hypervigilance, but such symptoms may fall short in distinguishing GAD from other psychiatric disorders, because in the course of several mental diseases these symptoms are frequently observed. Interestingly enough, despite the changes in diagnosis criteria, prevalence predictions for GAD are quite consistent among epidemiologic studies. It is predicted that among general population, lifelong prevalence is 5% (DSM-III and/or DSM-IV-R criteria). GAD is common in different levels among gender, ethnics, and social groups. Among age 40 and above women, in addition to high ratio as 10%, in the cases applying to primary care service, GAD is 8%. Again in the first primary care service, GAD is the most widely diagnosed anxiety disorder. GAD's age of onset is different than other anxiety disorders. Prevalence ratios are low among teenagers and young adults but age is a remarkably triggering effect. Women are, compared to men, at higher risk. GAD is more frequent among unemployed housewives with chronic medical diseases [75]. GAD is frequently associated with accompanying depression, other anxiety, and somatoform disorders [76]. Weak family relations, codiagnosed C group personality disorders in stressful life events and codiagnosed Axis 1 disorders, are the increasing factors of GAD's effects [77]. GAD is quite prevalent all over the world but the relation between GAD and suicidal behavior has not been investigated. There are a limited number of studies on this topic. In another study, it was detected that there is a relation between impairment and suicidal ideation and GAD [29]. Zimmerman and Chelminski [78] found that depressed patients with GAD had higher levels of suicidal ideation when compared to patients with depression only. In future studies, analyzing the impact of GAD on suicidal behavior may be illuminating on the potential risk factors.

5.5. Social anxiety disorder (social phobia) and suicide

Life-long prevalence of social anxiety disorder is 13%, which is a quite high ratio among general public. Not only it leads to a major loss of ability but it is often associated with increased suicide ratios and codiagnosed drug abuse; but the relation between social anxiety disorder and suicidal behaviors has not been analyzed adequately so far. The characteristics of patients with social anxiety disorder are that they unrealistically fear that others will constantly and persistently criticize their acts. Social anxiety disorder usually springs up during puberty and it really emerges for the first time after age 25 [79]. Rates of social anxiety disorder were highest among women and persons who were younger, less educated, single, and of lower socioeconomic class. SAD is a common illness often followed by comorbid MDD and alcohol dependence. SAD with comorbid MDD predicts a substantially elevated risk of alcohol dependence and suicide-related symptoms, stressing the need for early SAD detection [80]. It has been reported that despite the high frequency of suicidal ideation among patients with anxiety disorder, the level of suicide attempt is low. Furthermore, the data show that in social anxiety disordered cases, the ratio of lifelong suicide attempt is 12–18% but this condition is associated with codiagnosed depression symptoms [81]. It is also reported that 69% of patients with social anxiety disorder are afflicted with other lifelong comorbid mental disorders and with the occurrence of social anxiety usually, they are added into clinical picture. Once contrasted with people having no mental disorder, uncomplicated social anxiety disorder is found to be connected with increased suicidal ideation, financial dependency, and having sought medical treatment. Nonetheless, no connection was established between social anxiety disorder and suicide attempt and psychiatric treatment. It has been reported that in social anxiety disorder there is elevated suicide attempts, but these cases are surprisingly comorbid cases. In the absence of comorbidity, social anxiety disorder is still a problem that spoils the functionality, but patients rarely seek psychiatric treatment; hence large numbers of cases cannot be examined well by the clinicians [82]. The effect of anxiety disorder alone on suicide behavior has not yet been established but when social anxiety disorder's chronic course and adverse impact on functionality are considered, particular attention needs to be paid in the assessment of patients in this group.

Comparison of the suicidal behaviors of the specific anxiety disorders is given in Table 1.

Specific anxiety disorders	**Suicide ideation**	**Suicide attempt**	**Completed suicide**
Panic disorder	++++	++++	?
Posttraumatic stress disorder	+++	+++	?
Obsessive-compulsive disorder	+/?	?	?
Social anxiety disorder	?	?	?
Generalized anxiety disorder	?	?	?
Simple phobia	?	?	?

Strong evidence: ++++, Evidence: +++, No clear evidence +/?, No data: ?

Table 1. Specific anxiety disorders and suicidal behaviors

6. The comorbidity of anxiety disorders in other illnesses and suicide

Anxiety disorders, when accompanied with other comorbid mental disorders, may affect the course and treatment of disease. Comorbid conditions may occasionally lead to diagnostic ambiguity, and in a number of cases, multiple comorbid mental disorder may accompany the present clinical picture. In a research conducted by Sanderson et al. [83], it was reported that among 70% of patients with anxiety disorder, there is minimum one additional Axis 1 diagnosis. In present study, the highness of comorbidity ratio draws attention. However, once considered that current diagnosis systems are largely consisting of joint symptom clusters, these ratios appear to be exaggerated predictions. Nevertheless, mental disorder comorbidity is considered negative for the natural course of illness by implying additional kinds of dysfunction depending on whether it is a disorder of mood, substance abuse, or personality [84, 85]. These three are the most common comorbid disorders.

6.1. The comorbidity of anxiety disorders in mood disorders and suicide

The potential association between anxiety disorders and suicidal ideation rendered mixed results. In the researches, positive findings between anxiety and suicidal ideation may be connected to accompanying depression. In patients diagnosed with anxiety disorder not positing mood disorder story, there was no increased risk for suicidal ideation. On the other hand, in a recent study, it has been reported that among anxiety disordered cases not accompanied with mood disorder, there is an increased risk for suicidal ideation [86]. Nonetheless, in current research, subsyndromic depression symptoms have not been excluded, which puts the findings of research open to discussion. Traditionally, research on suicide has emphasized relationships with mood disorders, psychotic disorders, and some personality disorders. Although certain features of anxiety have been incorporated into models of suicide, anxiety-related conditions such as severe psychic anxiety, agitation, and panic have typically been examined as predictors of suicidal behaviors only to the extent that they overlap with mood disorders. Sareen et al. [16] in their 3-year long monitoring studies probed into the relation between anxiety and mood disorder–diagnosed cases and lifelong suicide ideation and suicide attempt, and they found out that in the presence of an anxiety disorder not positing a mood disorder story, there is a significant relation between lifelong suicidal ideation and suicide attempt. However, the main limitation of their study is that while analyzing particular anxiety disorders, probable mixing factors (syndromal depressive symptoms, etc.) have not been excluded. Despite this, there is fairly strong evidence that even subthreshold depressive symptoms are associated with increased psychosocial impairment, higher rates of comorbid substance use problems, and greater risk for future syndromal depressive episodes [87]. Further, studies provide strong evidence for an additive and interactive relative risk conveyed by cooccurring anxiety and depression. Consequently, comprehensive suicide assessment plans are strongly recommended when evaluating or treating individuals with an anxiety disorder, and especially individuals with comorbid anxiety and depressive disorders [88].

6.2. The comorbidity of anxiety disorders in bipolar disorder and suicide

Clinical and epidemiological studies have provided convincing evidence that comorbid anxiety disorders are relatively prevalent among patients with bipolar disorder (BD), found in up to 65% of cases [89]. Henry et al. [90] studied 318 inpatients including bipolar I and found that 24% had at least one lifetime anxiety disorder and 11% of the patients had more than one such disorder. Comorbidity of anxiety disorders may be associated with greater suicidality, substance abuse, resistance to pharmacological treatment, and poor outcome [91-93]. Altındag et al. [94] studied 70 outpatients including bipolar I and found that 27.1% had at least one lifetime anxiety disorder, and most common anxiety disorders in this sample were obsessive-compulsive disorder (12.8%) and specific phobia (12.8%), followed by panic disorder (5.7%). Anxiety disorder comorbidity appears to be associated with greater number of hospitalizations, psychotic symptoms, and suicide attempts in patients with bipolar disorder type I. Bipolar subjects with anxiety disorders were younger, had earlier age at onset of illness, and were overrepresented by female subjects and those with earlier onset illness compared to those without anxiety disorder [95]. Panic disorder, which also confers an independent risk of suicide and psychiatric comorbidity, in general has been found to amplify suicidality in mood-disordered patients [96]. The presence of comorbid panic disorder in individuals with bipolar disorder may confer an increased risk of suicide risk. Some papers' reviewed have conflicting conclusions but the majority of papers support an increased risk. Future research should study specific bipolar subgroups, focus on anxiety and panic symptoms rather than diagnosis, and look at the role of specific pharmacological treatment in patients with comorbid mood and anxiety disorders. Among anxiety disorders, only social phobia (SP) was significantly associated with history of suicide attempt in BD. In other words, SP is an important risk factor for suicidal behavior in BD [97]. Suicide takes significantly different forms within different stages of behavioral bipolar disorder. Suicide attempts and suicidal ideation have been found to be most closely connected to the depressive periods of disease. Severity of despair and depression are the key indicators of risk for all stages [98]. Previous studies have shown a significant relationship between suicide ideation and mixed depression. The rates of mixed depression among bipolar and nonbipolar depressive suicide attempters were much higher than previously reported among nonsuicidal bipolar II and unipolar depressive outpatients, suggesting that suicide attempters come mainly from mixed depressives with predominantly bipolar II base. Irritability and psychomotor agitation were the strongest predictors of suicide attempt [99]. Although anxiety may be a modifiable suicide risk factor among bipolar patients, anxiety disorder comorbidity has not been highlighted as critical in identification of high-risk individuals nor has its treatment been integrated into suicide prevention strategies. Although lifelong anxiety disorders are related to past suicide attempts, current comorbid anxiety disorders are found to be connected to suicidal ideation. In anxiety disordered individuals, suicidal ideation is a risk factor for suicide behaviors in future. The early onset of polar disorder and frequent appearance of rapid cycling and mixed periods constitute great risk for suicidal behavior. All in all, both bipolar disorder and anxiety disorder bear risks for suicidal behavior. In the presence of comorbid anxiety disorders, suicide behavior risk may gain even further impetus in bipolar disorder cases. To put differently, anxiety disorders (social anxiety disorder at most) may play active role in developing suicidal ideation and suicide attempt among bipolar disordered cases [100]. In the presence of comorbid anxiety disorders in bipolar disordered cases, patients must be attentively monitored against suicidal risk. Further studies shall contribute to better comprehending suicide behavior in bipolar disorder patients with anxiety disorder.

6.3. The comorbidity of anxiety disorders in substance abuse and suicide

The high prevalence of comorbid drug abuse in anxiety disorders is attributed to patients' relief seeking in alcohol and/or drugs for alleviating the emotional stress they cope with (self-medication). Regardless of the high ratios of alcohol and drug use in anxiety disorders, self-medication has been discussed in limited numbers of studies. Likewise although in mood disorders there is high frequency of alcohol and drug abuse, there is a limited body of research on this domain. The use of alcohol and drugs to relieve affective symptoms is common among individuals with mood disorders in the general population [101]. Comorbid specific mood and anxiety disorders and specific drug use are widely common in American society. Among women in particular comorbid psychiatric disorders may lead to critical use of illegal drugs. In present study, it was reported that among female cases diagnosed with comorbid mood and anxiety disorder, in comparison to postdrug-alcohol addicted men, medical prognosis of disease is affected more negatively [102]. Among cases with anxiety disorder self-medication has been associated with accompanying mood disorders, drug abuse, anxiety, suicidal ideation, and increased risk for suicide attempt. Even after controlling sociodemographic and psychiatric variances self-medication remained to be related to suicidal ideation and increased risk for suicide attempt. Bolton et al. [103] reported that individuals with anxiety disorders who self-medicate their symptoms with alcohol or drugs may be at increased risk for mood and substance use disorders and suicidal behavior. In this study covering a wide sampling of society, self-medication prevalence varied between 7.9% (social phobia and speech subtype) and 35.6% (GAD). Multivariate analyses put forth that self-medication is independently related to lifelong suicidal ideation and attempts and also to an increased comorbid mood disorder and drug abuse tendency. Alcohol use disorders and suicidal ideation cooccur, yet few studies have investigated the risk and protective factors that influence their comorbidity. The comorbidity between alcohol use disorders and suicidal ideation is characterized in young women by cooccurring psychopathology, drinking to cope, and negative life events [104].

6.4. The comorbidity of anxiety disorders in schizophrenia and suicide

Among schizophrenic patients, there is a considerably high ratio of suicidal behavior. It is particularly noteworthy that among schizophrenic cases with suicide attempt story and suicidal ideation in the past, there is also comorbid OCD. Also the ones with suicide story are significantly higher in patients with OCD-schizophrenia than in patients with non-OCD schizophrenia. Compulsive symptoms were significant predictors of suicide attempt among patients with schizophrenia [105]. The obsessive-compulsive symptoms may account for the emergence of suicidality in patients with OCD-schizophrenia. In schizophrenia suicidal ideation has been auspicated with depressive mood, anxiety, low self esteem, negative disease perceptions, negative assessments of the self and others, and daily alcohol consumption. The frequency of coping with audio hallucinations and delusions has no connection with suicidal ideation but distress caused by positive symptoms was found to be related to suicidal ideation [106]. Affective dysfunction, including distress in response to hallucinations and delusions, was a key factor associated with suicidal ideation in individuals with psychotic relapse.

6.5. The comorbidity of anxiety disorders in major depression and suicide

In elderly persons with major depressive disorder, coexisting generalized anxiety disorder or panic disorder is associated with more severe symptoms and poorer short-term treatment outcomes. De Luca et al. [107] found evidence that comorbid generalized anxiety disorder or panic disorder is associated with a greater decline in memory in late-life MDD and suicidal ideation. The clinical correlates of comorbid anxiety and depression in a sample of older patients with major depression. In elderly patients with anxious depression, psychosocial support and suicidal ideation should be assessed [108]. Anxiety symptoms are the frequent comorbids of old-age depression; hence MDB comorbid with subsyndromal anxiety symptoms is termed as "anxious depression." In reality, MDD is generally comorbid with specific anxiety disorders but there is no definite information on the frequency, diagnosis, clinical course, and treatment approaches for anxiety disorders among elderly group. It is acknowledged that specific anxiety disorders, anxiety disorders comorbid with MDD, are less common among the elderly. Still, in aged people with anxious depression, particularly in complex cases comorbid with chronic physical disease, there is a heightened risk for suicidal ideation, disability, and poor prognosis. Standard pharmacotherapy could be sufficient for depression but among many older people with anxious depression. Standard pharmacotherapy on its own may fail to be sufficient. There are a number of psychosocial treatments but they are not specific for old-age anxious depression. However, psychosocial interventions may be a major constituent in the treatment of these patients [109]. In the elderly group, ratios of completed suicide are significantly higher than the other age groups, thus in preventing old-age suicides, the elderly cases diagnosed with "anxious depression" must be studied attentively.

6.6. The comorbidity of anxiety disorders in physical illness and suicide

Suicidal ideation and behavior have been associated with a variety of neurological illnesses. There are important linkages between suicidal ideation and behavior and neurological conditions, including epilepsy, multiple sclerosis, and amyotrophic lateral sclerosis [110]. Anxiety disorders are common in patients with multiple sclerosis, but are frequently overlooked and undertreated. Korostil and Feinstein [111] studied 140 outpatients including multiple sclerosis and found that 35.7% had at least one lifetime anxiety disorder, and most common anxiety disorders in this sample were panic disorder (10%) and obsessive-compulsive disorder (8.6%), followed by generalized anxiety disorder (18.6%). Subjects with an anxiety disorder were more likely to be female, have a history of depression, drink to excess, report higher social stress, and have contemplated suicide. Risk factors include being female, a comorbid diagnosis of depression, and limited social support. Clinicians should evaluate all multiple sclerosis subjects for anxiety disorders, as they represent a treatable cause of disability in multiple sclerosis. The studies have observed a strong relationship between coronary artery disease (CAD) and psychiatric disorder, notably depression, anxiety, and panic attacks. A significant positive relation was observed between CAD and lifelong prevalence of suicide attempts. Suicide attempts were found to be connected with major depression and comorbid anxiety disorder but no relation was detected between suicide attempts and anxiety singly. At the end of logistic regression analysis, the relation between suicide attempt and CAD continued after making correction for depression and anxiety. In a different saying, CAD is an independent risk factor more powerful than depression for suicide behavior [112]. Acne is a common disease in adolescence with female preponderance. It could cause poor self-esteem and social phobia. Previous studies based on questionnaires from several thousands of adolescents showed that acne is associated with major depression and suicide [113, 114]. However, the gender- and age-specific risk of depression and suicide in patients with acne remain largely unknown. The risk is additive in women with acne. Similar additive risk of suicide was noticed in women with acne. In recently, Yang et al. [115] reported that acne and gender, independently and jointly, were associated with major depression and suicide. Special medical support should be warranted in females with acne for the risk of major depression and suicide. It has been demonstrated that a correlation exists between an extensive scope of physical diseases and increased ratios of suicide. As the studies on particular topic are examined, it surfaces that medical diagnoses alone are not sufficient causes to lead a person to suicide. Comorbid mental disorders are equally responsible in the development of suicide. It is thus important to train the clinicians on identifying not only physical symptoms but mental symptoms too and the ways to determine their effects on the treatment and the course of disease. To have a lifesaving effect, particular attention to crisis periods, stages of physical illness, and postdischarge period should be monitored attentively on accounts of being risk-posing periods for suicide behavior. It is thus obviously crucial to monitor physically sick patients to stay alert against suicide behavior.

6.7. The comorbidity of anxiety disorders in personality disorders and suicide

A comprehensive metaanalysis to identify the proportions of comorbid personality disorders (PD) across the major subtypes of anxiety disorders has not previously been published. Friborg et al. [85] reported that the rate of any comorbid PD was high across all anxiety disorders. The findings reveal that Group C personality disorders are two times more common compared to Group A and B personality disorders, and within Group C personality disorders, the highest ratio was seen in avoidant PD, followed alternately by obsessive-compulsive and the dependent personality disorder. In cases where personality disorders are codiagnosed with anxiety disorders, the course and treatment response of the disease may alter. It has, for instance, been reported that in social anxiety disorder where PTSD provides a heterogeneous clinical picture, there is a high ratio of comorbid with avoidant PD. Except early onset, avoidant PD rendered insignificant or minor impacts on social anxiety disorder. No relation could be established between gender or length of anxiety disorder and personality disorder comorbidity. Patients with social phobia (61%) and generalized anxiety disorder (49%) were most often diagnosed with a personality disorder. Patients with simple phobia were rarely diagnosed with a personality disorder (12%) [83]. In a different study, it has been illustrated that present or lifelong panic disorders are related with borderline, avoidant, and dependent personality disorders; social anxiety disorder connected with avoidant personality disorder; and obsessive-compulsive disorder associated with obsessive-compulsive and avoidant personality disorders. In anxiety disorders comorbid with personality disorders, unlike anxiety disorders with no personality disorder, there has been a more chronic course, increased suicidal behavior, and low level of functionality [116]. The relationship between cooccurring personality disorders and anxiety disorders (panic disorder with or without agoraphobia, social phobia, and generalized anxiety disorder) was examined, taking into account the effect of major depression. Generalized anxiety disorder, social phobia, and major depression were positively associated with the occurrence of one or more personality disorders, whereas panic disorder with agoraphobia was not associated [117]. The effect of comorbid personality disorders in obsessive-compulsive disorder is unclear. Baer and Jenike [118] in their research covering 96 OCD adult patients detected that in patients with mixed personality disorder, the length of OCD is longer compared to the ones with no OCD. The authors argued that the impacts of personality disorders on behavior and life style can be secondary OCD. The studies indicate that most individuals with OCD have comorbid personality disorders (PDs), particularly from the anxious cluster. However, the nature and strength of this association remains unclear, as the majority of previous studies have relied heavily on clinical populations. Personality pathology is highly prevalent among people with OCD who are living in the community and should be routinely assessed, as it may affect help-seeking behavior and response to treatment [119]. Latas and Milovanovic [120] in a recent study proved that in anxiety disorder cases, personality disorders exhibit quite a high prevalence as 35% in posttraumatic stress disorder, 47% in panic disorder with agoraphobia and generalized anxiety disorder, 48% in social phobia, and 52% in OCD. In anxiety disorder cases, the highest ratio (39%) was found in Group C personality disorders. Also in samplings with personality disorders, high ratio of anxiety was detected particularly among borderline personality disorder cases. It is agreed that borderline personality disorder is a high risk factor for recurrent suicidal behavior. Personality disorders comorbid with anxiety disorder display a number of clinical outcomes such as suicide risk and more severe and less treatable anxiety disorders, thereby clinicians should place particular emphasis on identifying potential personality disorders in patients with anxiety disorder. Further studies should focus on the causes and risk factors for suicidal behavior particularly in patients with anxiety disorders comorbid with personality disorders.

7. Treatment studies

The basic principles of treatment of anxiety disorders in major depression involve longer treatment and higher doses than are usually required for major depression. The impact of psychosocial disability and severity of depressive symptoms can be ameliorated with appropriate treatment. Screening for depressive symptoms as well as administering an appropriate therapy seems the best way to prevent suicide attempts [121]. Newer treatments, such as the combination of psychotherapy and pharmacotherapy, may prove to be of greatest benefit for individuals with comorbidity of anxiety disorders in psychiatric disorders [122]. For the recent 25 years, much progress has been made in the treatment of five specific anxiety disorders such as social phobia, obsessive-compulsive disorder, generalized anxiety disorder, and posttraumatic stress disorder. Placebo-controlled evidences suggest that pharmacological and psychological treatments offer substantially effective solutions [21, 123]. Treatment of anxiety disorders involve antidepressants (selective serotonin reuptake inhibitors (SSRI) mostly) and cognitive behavioral therapy. Among patients diagnosed with mood disorder and comorbid anxiety disorders, it is advisable to administer higher doses of SSRI [124]. Besides, a long-term discussion has been going on about the use of SSRIs (paroxetine, fluoxetine, and citalopram) which, as some argue, may have a triggering/stipulating effect on adult suicides since 1991 and children since 2002. Apter et al. [125] stated that paroxetine taking adult patients with major depression are at higher risk for suicidal ideation and behavior, and the same authors also claimed that there was no attempt in OCD and social phobia cases. In sync with this finding, the benefits of sertraline outweigh its potential risks in suicidal behavior among OCD patients, and OCD's effects are, in contrast to its effects in major depression, further positive [126]. In younger patients diagnosed with major depression, the risk of suicidal behavior uncovered with treatment is even higher. It is suggested that the rise in suicidal ideation and attempt parallel to the use of antidepressants is more risky for children and teenagers [21, 123]. Rickels et al. [127] in their two randomized controlled studies reported the positive effects of long-released venlafaxine on GAD. Among children and teenagers major depression and in GAD patients with venlafaxine, there might be a stage between suicidal behaviors and hostile behaviors. Antidepressant drugs play a vital role in the treatment of anxiety disorders and preventing suicidal behaviors among adult patients. Selective serotonin reuptake inhibitors are the first-line pharmacological treatment for these disorders, and that newer serotonin and norepinephrine reuptake inhibitors show significant promise, especially for comorbid cases. In the treatment of anxiety disorders, cognitive behavior therapy (CBT) can be applied in combination with pharmacotherapy or independently. For instance, in the treatment of panic disorder, CBT aims to control agoraphobic symptoms in panic disorders comorbid with agoraphobia, to inhibit adverse effect of medicine deduction and treatment and prevention of panic attacks. Not much study has been made on the effects of CBT applications in anxiety disorders on suicidal behavior, but when anxiety disorder cases are successfully treated with CBT there is likelihood to witness fewer ratios of suicide [128]. When anxiety disorders are comorbid with depression, disease symptoms are likely to be more severe; hence symptom severity should be taken into account while making treatment plan. Particularly speaking, patients diagnosed with panic disorder, PTSD, and comorbidity of anxiety disorders in major depression bear higher risks for suicide. The cases bearing potential risks for suicide should be kept and monitored under strict scrutiny by clinicians. In order to assess and monitor these patients, there is a need for relevant measurement tools of which reliability and validity tests have been confirmed. In suicide behavior treatment studies among anxiety disorders, ethic limitations have restricted the participation of individuals with acute suicidal tendency. In relevant studies, the lowness of suicidal behavior and restricted volume of samplings inhibited a precise detection of the real effect of treatments. As we consider the fact that various factors interact in the emergence of suicidal behavior, it is probable that drug effect may be regulated in the same way with the interactions among such factors. The fact that no treatment study manages to equally control the risk factors among treatment groups makes it hard to identify the causal factors in suicide-relevant cases. Furthermore, in the analysis of SSRIs, short-term risks alone were examined; hence it is a requirement to detect long-term risks and create future-oriented study designs with wider databases and closer monitoring procedures. There is a need for more research to develop a guideline/protocol exclusively for suicide prevention in patients with anxiety disorders.

8. Conclusion

Traditionally, anxiety disorders have not been viewed as independent risk factors for suicidal behavior, and therefore assessment of anxiety disorders has not been particularly emphasized in clinical enquiries, and suicide screening tools specific anxiety disorders (e.g., generalized anxiety disorder, panic disorder, and obsessive-compulsive disorder) may be independently associated with suicidality, to which they particularly contribute when they are comorbid with bipolar disorder, personality disorders, depression, schizophrenia, and substance use disorders. Despite methodological issues, these findings should prompt clinicians to evaluate more specifically the impact of anxiety disorders on suicidal behavior, particularly when they are comorbid. Further research into treatment of anxiety disorders in relation to preventing suicide is required.

Acknowledgements

I offer thanks to our team for suggesting that we write a book about anxiety disorders and suicide.

Author details

Cicek Hocaoglu*

Address all correspondence to: cicekh@gmail.com

Recep Tayyip Erdogan University, Rize, Turkey

References

[1] Asselmann E, Beesdo-Baum K. Predictors of the course of anxiety disorders in adolescents and young adults. Cur Psychiatry Rep. 2015; 17: 543–548. doI: 10.1007/s11920-014-0543-z.

[2] Bruce S, Yonkers K, Otto M. Influence of psychiatric comorbidity on recovery and recurrence in generalized anxiety disorder, social phobia, and panic disorder: A 12 year prospective study. Am J Psychiatry. 2005; 162: 1179–1187.

[3] Lepine J. The epidemiology of anxiety disorders: Prevalence and societal costs. J Clin Psychiatry. 2002; 63: 4–8.

[4] Kessler R, Berglund P, Demler O. Lifetime prevalence and age-of-onset distributions of DSM-IV disorders in the National Comorbidity Survey replication. Arch Gen Psychiatry. 2005a; 62: 593–602.

[5] Kadri N, Agoub M, El Gnaoui S, Berrada S, Moussaoui D. Prevalence of anxiety disorders: A population-based epidemiological study in metropolitan area of Casablanca, Morocco. Ann Gen Psychiatry. 2007; 6: 6. Doı: 10.1186/1744-859X-6-6.

[6] Hettema J, Prescott C, Meyers J. The structure of genetic and environmental risk factors for anxiety disorders in men and women. Arch Gen Psychiatry. 2005; 62: 182–189. DOI: 10.1001/archpsyc.62.2.182.

[7] Martin P. The epidemiology of anxiety disorders: A review. Dialogues Clin Neurosci. 2003; 5: 281–298.

[8] Kessler R, Demler O, Frank R. Prevalence and treatment of mental disorders 1990–2003. N Eng J Med. 2005b; 352: 2515–2523. DOI: 10.1056/NEJMsa043266.

[9] Hill R.M, Castellanos D, Pettit JW. Suicide-related behaviors and anxiety in children and adolescents: A review. Clin Psychol Rev. 2011; 31: 1133–1144. DOI: 10.1016/j.cpr. 2011.07.008.

[10] Bomyea J, Lang AJ, Craske MG, Chavira D, Sherbourne CD. Suicidal ideation and risk factors in primary care patients with anxiety disorders. Psychiatry Res. 2013; 209: 60–65. DOI: 10.1016/j.psychres.2013.03.017.

[11] American Foundation for Suicide Prevention. Suicide prevention priorities for health reform. 2009. http://healthyamericans.org/assets/files/Suicideprevention.pdf. Accessed 15 October 2010.

[12] Rissmiller DJ, Steer R, Ranieri WF. Factors complicating cost containment in the treatment of suicidal patients. Hosp Community Psychiatry. 1994; 45: 782–788.

[13] Kuo W, Gallo JJ, Tien AY. Incidence of suicide ideation and attempts in adults: The 13-year follow-up of a community sample in Baltimore, Maryland. Psychol Med. 2001; 31: 1181–1191.

[14] Joiner TE, Steer RA, Brown G, Beck AT. Worst-point suicidal plans: A dimension of suicidality predictive of past suicide attempts and eventual death by suicide. Behav Res Ther. 2003; 41; 1469–1480. DOI: 10.1016/S0005-7967(03)00070-6.

[15] Stevens D, Wilcox HC, MacKinnon DF, Mondimore FM. PTSD increases risk for suicide attempt in adults with recurrent major depression. Depress Anxiety. 2013; 30: 940–946. DOI: 10.1002/da.22160.

[16] Sareen J, Cox B, Afifi T. Anxiety disorders and risk for suicidal ideation and suicide attempts. Arch Gen Psychiatry. 2005; 62: 1249–1257. DOI: 10.1001/archpsyc. 62.11.1249.

[17] Bolton JM, Cox BJ, Afifi TO. Anxiety disorders and risk for suicide attempts: Findings from the Baltimore epidemiologic catchment area follow-up. Depress Anxiety. 2008; 25: 477–481. DOI: 10.1002/da.20314.

[18] Cougle JR, Keough ME, Riccardi CJ, Sachs-Ericsson N. Anxiety disorders and suicidality in the National Comorbidity Survey-replication. J Psychiatr Res. 2009; 43: 825–829. DOI: 10.1016/j.jpsychires.2008.12.004.

[19] Uebelacker LA, Weisberg R, Millman M, Yen S. Prospective study of risk factors for suicidal behavior in individuals with anxiety disorders. Psychol Med. 2013; 43: 1465–1474. DOI: 10.1017/S0033291712002504.

[20] Khan A, Leventhal R, Khan S, Brown W. Suicide risk in patients with anxiety disorders: A meta-analysis of the FDA database. J Affect Disorder. 2002; 68: 183–190. DOI: http://dx.doi.org/10.1016/S0165-0327(01)00354-8.

[21] Hawgood J, De Leo D. Anxiety disorders and suicidal behaviour: An update. Curr Opin Psychiatry. 2008; 21: 51–64. DOI: 10.1097/YCO.0b013e3282f2309d.

[22] Nepon J, Belik S. Bolton J, Sareen J. The relationship between anxiety disorders and suicide attempts: Findings from the national epidemiologic survey on alcohol and related conditions. Depress Anxiety. 2010; 279: 791–798. DOI: 10.1002/da.20674.

[23] Lopez-Castroman J, Perez-Rodriguez MDIM, Jaussent I, Alegria AA. European Research Consortium for Suicide (EURECA) distinguishing the relevant features of frequent suicide attempters. J Psychiatric Res. 2011; 45: 619–625. DOI: 10.1016/j.jpsychires.2010.09.017.

[24] Warshaw M, Dolan R, Keller M. Suicidal behaviour in patients with current or past panic disorder five years of prospective data from the Harvard/Brown Anxiety Research Program. Am J Psychiatry. 2000; 157: 1876–1878.

[25] Freeman TW, Moore WM. A comparison of chronic combat-related posttraumatic stress disorder (PTSD) patients with and without a history of suicide attempt. J Nerv Ment Dis. 2000; 188: 460–463.

[26] Huang M, Yen C, Lung F. Moderators and mediators among panic, agoraphobia symptoms, and suicidal ideation in patients with panic disorder. Compr Psychiatry. 2010; 51: 243–249. DOI: 10.1016/j.comppsych.2009.07.005.

[27] Tarrier N, Gregg L. Suicide risk in civilian PTSD patients: Predictors of suicidal ideation, planning and attempts. Soc Psychiatry Psychiatr Epidemiol. 2004; 39: 655–661. DOI: 10.1007/s00127-004-0799-4.

[28] Pangioti M, Gooding P, Tarrier N. Post-traumatic stress disorder and suicidal behaviour: A narrative review. Clin Psychol Rev. 2009; 29: 471–482. DOI: 10.1016/j.cpr.2009.05.001.

[29] Ma X, Xiang YT, Cai ZJ, Lu JY. Generalized anxiety disorder in China: Prevalence, sociodemographic correlates, comorbidity, and suicideattempts. Perspect Psychiatric Care. 2009; 45: 119–127. DOI: 10.1111/j.1744-6163.2009.00212.x.

[30] McGirr A, Séguin M, Renaud J, Benkelfat C, Alda M. Gender and risk factors for suicide: Evidence for heterogeneity in predisposing mechanisms in a psychological autopsy study.J Clin Psychiatry. 2006; 67: 1612–1617.

[31] Poorolajal J, Rostami M, Mahjub H, Esmailnasab N. Completed suicide and associated risk factors: A six-year population based survey. Arch Iran Med. 2015; 18: 39–43. DOI: 0151801/AIM.0010.

[32] Vanderwerker L, Chen J, Charpentier P. Differences in risk factors for suicidality between African American and White patients vulnerable to suicide. Suicide Life Threat Behav. 2007; 37: 1–9.

[33] Beautrais A, Wells J, McGee M, Oakley BM. Suicidal behaviour in Te Rau Hinengaro: The New Zealand Mental Health Survey. Aust N Z J Psychiatry. 2006; 40: 896–904.

[34] Fairweather A, Anstey K, Rodgers B, Butterworth P. Factors distinguishing suicide attempters from suicide ideators in a community sample: Social issues and physical

health problems. Psychol Med. 2006; 36: 1235–1245. DOI: http://dx.doi.org/10.1017/S0033291706007823.

[35] Fliege H, Kocalevent R, Walter O. Three assessment tools for deliberate self-harm and suicide behaviour: Evaluation and psychopathological correlates. J Psychosom Res. 2006; 61: 113–121. DOI: http://dx.doi.org/10.1016/j.jpsychores.2005.10.006.

[36] Blasco-Fontecilla H, Baca-García E, Díaz-Sastre C. Anxiety disorders and suicide behavior: An update. In: Velotis CM (Ed.), New developments in anxiety disorder research. Hauppauge: Nova Biomedical Books; 2006. pp. 1–39.

[37] Lönnqvist J. Major psychiatric disorders in suicide and suicide attempters. In: Wasserman D, Wasserman C, (Eds.), Oxford textbook of suicidology and suicide prevention. Oxford: Oxford University Press; 2009.

[38] Steyn R, Vawda N, Wyatt GE. Posttraumatic stress disorder diagnostic criteria and suicidal ideation in a South African Police sample. Afr J Psychiatry (Johannesbg). 2013; 16: 19–22. DOI: http://dx.doi.org/10.4314/ajpsy.v16i1.3.

[39] Florequin C, Hardy P, Messiah A, Ellrodt A. Suicide attempts and panic disorder: A study of 62 hospitalized suicidal patients. Encephale. 1995; 21: 87–92.

[40] Weissman MM, Klerman GL, Markowitz JS. Suicidal ideation and suicide attempts in panic disorder and attacks. N Eng J Med. 1989; 321: 1209–1214.

[41] Diaconu G, Turecki G. Panic disorder and suicidality: Is comorbidity with depression the key? J Affect Disord. 2007; 104: 203–209. DOI: http://dx.doi.org/10.1016/j.jad.2007.03.006.

[42] Pilowsky D, Olfson M, Gameroff M. Panic disorder and suicidal ideation in primary care. Depress Anxiety. 2006; 23: 11–16. DOI: 10.1002/da.20092.

[43] Goodwin R, Roy-Byrne P. Panic and suicidal ideation and suicide attempts: Results from the National Comorbidity Survey. Depress Anxiety. 2006; 23: 124–132. DOI: 10.1002/da.20151.

[44] Anthony JC, Tien AY, Petronis KR. Epidemiologic evidence on cocaine use and panic attacks. Am J Epidemiol. 1989; 129: 543–549.

[45] Petronis KR, Samuels JF, Moscicki EK. An epidemiologic investigation of potential risk factors for suicide attempts. Soc Psychiatry Psychiatr Epidemiol. 1990; 25: 193–199.

[46] Noyes R. Suicide and panic disorder: A review. J Affect Disord. 1991; 22: 1–11.

[47] Dammen T, Bull Bringager C, Arnesen H. A 1-year follow- up study of chest-pain patients with and without panic disorder. Gen Hosp Psychiatry. 2006; 28: 516–524. DOI: http://dx.doi.org/10.1016/j.genhosppsych.2006.08.005.

[48] Birchall H, Brandon S, Taub N. Panic in a general practice population: Prevalence, psychiatric comorbidity and associated disability. Soc Psychiatry Psychiatr Epidemiol. 2000; 35: 235–241.

[49] Ystgaard M, Hestetun I, Loeb M, Mehlum L. Is there a specific relationship between childhood sexual and physical abuse and repeated suicidal behavior? Child Abuse Negl. 2004; 28: 863–875. DOI: 10.1016/j.chiabu.2004.01.009.

[50] Weissman MM, Klerman GL, Johnson J. Panic disorder and suicidal ideation. Am J Psychiatry. 1992; 149: 1411–1412.

[51] Pompili M, Sher L, Serafini G, Forte A. Posttraumatic stress disorder and suicide risk among veterans: A literature review. J Nerv Ment Dis. 2013; 201: 802–812. DOI: 10.1097/NMD.0b013e3182a21458.

[52] Sher L, Braquehais MD, Casas M. Posttraumatic stress disorder, depression, and suicide in veterans. Clev Clin J Med. 2012; 79: 92–97. DOI: 10.3949/ccjm.79a.11069.

[53] Greden JF, Valenstein M, Spinner J. Buddy-to-Buddy, a citizen soldier peer support program to counteract stigma, PTSD, depression, and suicide. Ann N Y Acad Sci. 2010; 1208: 90–97. DOI: 10.1111/j.1749-6632.2010.05719.x.

[54] Jakupcak M, Hoerster KD, Varra A. Hopelessness and suicidal ideation in Iraq and Afghanistan War Veterans reporting subthreshold and threshold posttraumatic stress disorder. J Nerv Ment Dis. 2011; 199: 272–275. DOI: 10.1097/NMD.0b013e3182124604.

[55] Pukay-Martin ND, Pontoski KE, Maxwell MA. The influence of depressive symptoms on suicidal ideation among U.S. Vietnam-era and Afghanistan/Iraq-era Veterans with posttraumatic stress disorder. J Trauma Stress. 2012; 25: 578–582. DOI: 10.1002/jts.21741.

[56] Mills KL, Teesson M, Ross J. Trauma, PTSD, and substance use disorders: Findings from the Australian National Survey of Mental Health and Well-Being. Am J Psychiatry. 2006; 163: 652–658.

[57] Bryan CJ, Corso KA. Depression, PTSD, and suicidal ideation among active duty veterans in an integrated primary care clinic. Psychol Services. 2011; 8: 94–103. DOI: 10.1037/a0023451.

[58] Rudd MD, Goulding J, Bryan CJ. Student veterans: A national survey exploring psychological symptoms and suicide risk. Professional Psychol Research Pratice. 2011; 42: 354–360.

[59] Guerra VS, Calhoun PS. Mid-Atlantic mental illness research, education clinical center workgroup. Examining the relation between posttraumatic stress disorder and suicidal ideation in an OEF/OIF veteran sample. J Anxiety Disord. 2011; 25: 12–18. DOI: 10.1016/j.janxdis.2010.06.025.

[60] Oquendo MA, Friend JM, Halberstam B. Association of comorbid posttraumatic stress disorder and major depression with greater risk for suicidal behavior.Am J Psychiatry. 2003; 160: 580–582.

[61] Strauss JL, Calhoun PS, Marx CE, Stechuchak KM. Comorbid posttraumatic stress disorder is associated with suicidality in male veterans with schizophrenia or schizoaffective disorder. Schizophr Res. 2006; 84: 165–169. DOI: http://dx.doi.org/10.1016/j.schres.2006.02.010.

[62] Davidson CL, Babson KA, Bonn-Miller MO. The impact of exercise on suicide risk: Examining pathways through depression, PTSD, and sleep in an inpatient sample of veterans. Suicide Life Threat Behav. 2013; 43: 279–289.

[63] Dutton MA, Kaltman S, Goodman LA. Patterns of intimate partner violence: Correlated and outcomes. Violence Vict. 2005; 20: 483–497.

[64] Pico-Alfonso MA, Garcia-Linares MI, Celda-Navarro N. The impact of physical, psychological, and sexual intimate male partner violence on women's mental health: Depressive symptoms, posttraumatic stress disorder, state anxiety, and suicide. J Womens Health. 2006; 15: 599–611. DOI: 10.1089/jwh.2006.15.599.

[65] Blasco-Ros C, Sánchez-Lorente S, Martinez M. Recovery from depressive symptoms, state anxiety and post-traumatic stress disorder in women exposed to physical and psychological, but not to psychological intimate partner violence alone: A longitudinal study. BMC Psychiatry. 2010; 10: 98. DOI: 10.1186/1471-244X-10-98.

[66] Krysinska K, Lester D. Post-traumatic stress disorder and suicide risk: A systematic review. Arch Suicide Res. 2010; 14: 1–23. DOI: 10.1080/13811110903478997.

[67] Harned MS, Najavits LM, Weiss RD. Self-harm and suicidal behavior in women with comorbid PTSD and substance dependence. Am J Addict. 2006; 15: 392–395.

[68] Torres AR, Ramos-Cerqueira AT, Ferrão YA. Suicidality in obsessive-compulsive disorder: Prevalence and relation to symptom dimensions and comorbid conditions. J Clin Psychiatry. 2011; 72: 119–120. DOI: 10.4088/JCP.09m05651blu.

[69] Torres AR, de Abreu Ramos-Cerqueira AT, Torresan RC. Prevalence and associated factors for suicidal ideation and behaviors in obsessive-compulsive disorder. CNS Spectr. 2007; 12: 771–778.

[70] Lester D, Abdel-Khalek AM. Manic-depression, suicidality, and obsessive-compulsive tendencies. Psychol Rep. 1999; 85: 1100.

[71] Abdel-Khalek A, Lester D. Manic-depressiveness, obsessive-compulsive tendencies, and suicidality in Kuwaiti college students. Psychol Rep. 2002; 90: 1007–1008.

[72] Diaconu G, Turecki G. Obsessive-compulsive personality disorder and suicidal behavior: Evidence for a positive association in a sample of depressed patients. J Clin Psychiatry. 2009; 70: 1551–1556. DOI: 10.4088/JCP.08m04636.

[73] Kamath P, Reddy YC. Suicidal behavior in obsessive-compulsive disorder. J Clin Psychiatry. 2007; 68: 1741–1750.

[74] Alonso P, Segalàs C, Real E, Pertusa A. Suicide in patients treated for obsessive-compulsive disorder: A prospective follow-up study. J Affect Disord. 2010; 124: 300–308. DOI: 10.1016/j.jad.2009.12.001.

[75] Wittchen HU. Generalized anxiety disorder: Prevalence, burden and cost to society. Depress Anxiety. 2002; 16: 162–171.

[76] Wittchen HU, Hoyer J. Generalized anxiety disorder: Nature and course. J Clin Psychiatry. 2001; 62: 15–19.

[77] Weisberg RB. Overview of generalized anxiety disorder: Epidemiology, presentation, and course. J Clin Psychiatry. 2009; 70: 4–9.

[78] Zimmerman M, Chelminski I. Generalized anxiety disorder in patients with major depression: Is DSM-IV's hierarchy correct? Am J Psychiatry. 2003; 160: 504–512.

[79] Bandelow B, Wedekind D. Social phobia. Nervenarzt. 2014; 85: 635–644. DOI: 10.1007/s00115-013-3955-9.

[80] Nelson EC, Grant JD, Bucholz KK, Glowinski A. Social phobia in a population-based female adolescent twin sample: Co-morbidity and associated suicide-related symptoms. Psychol Med. 2000; 30: 797–804.

[81] Cox BJ, Direnfeld DM, Swinson RP, Norton GR. Suicidal ideation and suicide attempts in panic disorder and social phobia. Am J Psychiatry. 1994; 151: 882–927.

[82] Schneier FR, Johnson J, Hornig CD, Liebowitz MR. Social phobia: Comorbidity and morbidity in an epidemiologic sample. Arch Gen Psychiatry. 1992; 49: 282–288.

[83] Sanderson WC, Wetzler S, Beck AT. Prevalence of personality disorders among patients with anxiety disorders. Psychiatry Res. 1994; 51: 167–174.

[84] Ansell EB, Pinto A, Edelen MO. The association of personality disorders with the prospective 7-year course of anxiety disorders. Psychol Med. 2011; 41: 1019–1028. DOI: 10.1017/S0033291710001777.

[85] Friborg O, Martinussen M, Kaiser S, Overgård KT, Rosenvinge JH. Comorbidityofpersonality disorders in anxiety disorders: A meta-analysis of 30 years of research. J Affect Disord. 2013; 145: 143–155. DOI: 10.1016/j.jad.2012.07.004.

[86] Van Orden KA, Witte TK, Cukrowicz KC. The interpersonal theory of suicide. Psychol Rev. 2010; 117: 575–600. DOI: 10.1037/a0018697.

[87] Lewinsohn PM, Solomon A, Seeley JR, Zeiss A. Clinical implications of "subthreshold" depressive symptoms. J Abnorm Psychol. 2000; 109: 345–351.

[88] Joiner TE, Walker RL, Rudd MD, Jobes DA. Scientizing and routinizing the assessment of suicidality in outpatient practice. Professional Psychol Res Practice. 1999; 30: 447–453.

[89] Abreu LN, Lafer B, Baca-Garcia E, Oquendo MA. Suicidal ideation and suicide attempts in bipolar disorder type I: An update for the clinician. Rev Bras Psiquiatr. 2009; 31: 271–280. DOI: http://dx.doi.org/10.1590/S1516-44462009005000003.

[90] Henry C, Van den Bulke D, Bellivier F. Anxiety disorders in 318 bipolar patients: Prevalence and impact on illness severity and response to mood stabilizer. J Clin Psychiatry. 2003; 64: 331–335.

[91] Lee J, Dunner D. The effect of anxiety disorder comorbidity on treatment resistant bipolar disorders. Depress Anxiety. 2007; 1: 1–7.

[92] Kauer-Sant'Anna M, Frey B, Andreazza A. Anxiety comorbidity and quality of life in bipolar disorder patients. Can J Psychiatry. 2007; 52: 175–181.

[93] Tamam L, Ozpoyraz N. Comorbidity of anxiety disorder among patients with bipolar I disorder in remission. Psychopathology. 2002; 35: 203–239. DOI: 10.1159/000063824.

[94] Altindag A, Yanik M, Nebioglu M. The comorbidity of anxiety disorders in bipolar I patients: Prevalence and clinical correlates. Isr J Psychiatry Relat Sci. 2006; 43: 10–15.

[95] Okan Ibiloglu A, Caykoylu A. The comorbidity of anxiety disorders in bipolar I and bipolar II patients among Turkish population. J Anxiety Disord. 2011; 25: 661–667. DOI: 10.1016/j.janxdis.2011.02.008.

[96] Kilbane EJ, Gokbayrak NS, Galynker I, Cohen L. A review of panic and suicide in bipolar disorder: Does comorbidity increase risk? J Affect Disord. 2009; 115: 1–10. DOI: 10.1016/j.jad.2008.09.014.

[97] Perroud N, Baud P, Preisig M, Etain B. Social phobia is associated with suicide attempt history in bipolar inpatients. Bipolar Disord. 2007; 9: 713–721.

[98] Valtonen HM, Suominen K, Mantere O, Leppämäki S. Suicidal behaviour during different phases of bipolar disorder. J Affect Disord. 2007; 97: 101–107. DOI: http://dx.doi.org/10.1016/j.jad.2006.05.033.

[99] Balázs J, Benazzi F, Rihmer Z, Rihmer A. The close link between suicide attempts and mixed (bipolar) depression: Implications for suicide prevention. J Affect Disord. 2006; 91: 133–138.

[100] Simon N, Zalta A, Otto M. The association of comorbid anxiety disorders and suicide attempts and suicidal ideation in outpatients with bipolar disorder. J Psychiatr Res. 2007; 41: 255–264. DOI: http://dx.doi.org/10.1016/j.jpsychires.2006.08.004.

[101] Bolton JM, Robinson J, Sareen J. Self-medication of mood disorders with alcohol and drugs in the National Epidemiologic Survey on alcohol and related conditions. J Affect Disord. 2009; 115: 367–375. DOI: 10.1016/j.jad.2008.10.003.

[102] Conway KP, Compton W, Stinson FS. Lifetime comorbidity of DSM-IV mood and anxiety disorders and specific drug use disorders: Results from the National Epide-

miologic Survey on alcohol and related conditions. J Clin Psychiatry. 2006; 67: 247–257.

[103] Bolton J, Cox B, Clara I. Use of alcohol and drugs to self-medicate anxiety disorders in a nationally representative sample. J Nerv Ment Disord. 2006; 194: 818–825.

[104] Agrawal A, Constantino AM, Bucholz KK. Characterizing alcohol use disorders and suicidal ideation in young women. J Stud Alcohol Drugs. 2013; 74: 406–412.

[105] Sevincok L, Akoglu A, Kokcu F. Suicidality in schizophrenic patients with and without obsessive-compulsive disorder. Schizophr Res. 2007; 90: 198–202. DOI: http://dx.doi.org/10.1016/j.schres.2006.09.023.

[106] Fialko L, Freeman D, Bebbington PE, Kuipers E. Understanding suicidalideation in psychosis: Findings from the psychological prevention of relapse in psychosis (PRP) trial. Acta Psychiatr Scand. 2006; 114: 177–186. DOI: 10.1111/j.1600-0447.2006.00849.

[107] De Luca AK, Lenze EJ, Mulsant BH, Butters MA. Comorbid anxiety disorder in late life depression: Association with memory decline over four years. Int J Geriatr Psychiatry. 2005; 20: 848–854. DOI: 10.1002/gps.1366.

[108] Jeste ND, Hays JC, Steffens DC. Clinical correlates of anxious depression among elderly patients with depression. J Affect Disord. 2006; 90: 37–41. DOI: http://dx.doi.org/10.1016/j.jad.2005.10.007.

[109] Diefenbach GJ, Goethe J. Clinical interventions for late-life anxious depression. Clin Interv Aging. 2006; 1: 41–50.

[110] Coughlin SS, Sher L. Suicidal behavior and neurological illnesses. J Depress Anxiety. 2013; 18: 12443. DOI: 10.4172/2167-1044.S9-001.

[111] Korostil M, Feinstein A. Anxiety disorders and their clinical correlates in multiple sclerosis patients. Mult Scler. 2007; 13: 67–72. DOI: 10.1177/1352458506071161.

[112] Artero S, Astruc B, Courtet P, Ritchie K. Life-time history of suicide attempts and coronary artery disease in a community-dwelling elderly population. Int J Geriatr Psychiatry. 2006; 21: 108–112. DOI: 10.1002/gps.1429.

[113] Cheng TA, Chen THH, Chen CC. Psychosocial and psychiatric risk factors for suicide: Case-control psychological autopsy study. Br J Psychiatry. 2000; 177: 360–365. DOI: 10.1192/bjp.177.4.360.

[114] Poli F, Dreno B, Verschoore M. An epidemiological study of acne in female adults: Results of a survey conducted in France. J Eur Acad Dermatol Venereol. 2001; 15: 541–545. DOI: 10.1046/j.1468-3083.2001.00357.x.

[115] Yang YC, Tu HP, Hong CH, Chang WC. Female gender and acne disease are jointly and independently associated with the risk of major depression andsuicide: A national population-based study. Biomed Res Int. 2014; 2014: 504279. DOI: 10.1155/2014/504279.

[116] Skodol AE, Oldham JM, Hyler SE, Stein DJ. Patterns of anxiety and personality disorder comorbidity. J Psychiatr Res. 1995; 29: 361–374.

[117] Dyck IR, Phillips KA, Warshaw MG. Patterns of personality pathology in patients with generalized anxiety disorder, panic disorder with and without agoraphobia, and social phobia. J Pers Disord. 2001; 15: 60–71.

[118] Baer L, Jenike MA. Personality disorders in obsessive compulsive disorder. Psychiatr Clin North Am. 1992; 15: 803–812.

[119] Torres AR, Moran P, Bebbington P, BrughaT. Obsessive-compulsive disorder and personality disorder: Evidence from the British National Survey of psychiatric morbidity 2000. Soc Psychiatry Psychiatr Epidemiol. 2000; 41: 862–867.

[120] Latas M, Milovanovic S. Personality disorders and anxiety disorders: What is the relationship? Curr Opin Psychiatry. 2014; 27: 57–61. DOI: 10.1097/YCO.0000000000000025.

[121] Glaesmer H, Braehler E. The differential roles of trauma, posttraumatic stress disorder, and comorbid depressive disorders on suicidal ideation in the elderly population. J Clin Psychiatry. 2012; 73: 1141–1146. DOI: 10.4088/JCP.11m07598.

[122] Dunner D. Acute and maintenance treatment of chronic depression. J Clin Psychiatry. 2001; 62: 10–16.

[123] Ballenger J. Current treatments of the anxiety disorders in adults. Biol Psychiatry. 1999; 46: 1579–1594.

[124] Kaufman J, Charney D. Comorbidity of mood and anxiety disorders. Depress Anxiety. 2000; 12: 69–76.

[125] Apter A, Lipschitz A, Fong R, Carpenter DJ, Krulewicz S. Evaluation of suicidal thoughts and behaviors in children and adolescents taking paroxetine. J Child Adolesc Psychopharmacol. 2006; 16: 77–90.

[126] March J, Klee B, Kremer C. Treamtent and benefit and the risk of suicidality in multicenter, randomized, controlled trials of sertraline in children and adolescents. J Child Adolesc Psychopharmacol. 2006; 16: 91–102. DOI: 10.1089/cap.2006.16.91.

[127] Rickels K, Etemad B, Khalid-Khan S, Lohoff FW, Rynn MA. Time to relapse after 6 and 12 months' treatment of generalized anxiety disorder with venlafaxine extended release. Arch Gen Psychiatry. 2010; 67: 1274–1281. DOI: 10.1001/archgenpsychiatry.2010.170.

[128] Gelder, M. Combined pharmocotherapy and cognitive behavior therapy in the treatment of panic disorder. J Clin Psychopharmacol. 1998; 18: 2S–5S.

Chapter 7

Comorbid Anxiety in Schizophrenia and Schizoaffective Disorder

Delia M. Podea, Aurora I. Sabau and Karol J. Wild

Additional information is available at the end of the chapter

http://dx.doi.org/10.5772/60643

Abstract

There is some evidence that antipsychotic medication (Quetiapine) is somewhat efficient in reducing anxiety in schizophrenic patients.

This study compared the efficacy of Olanzapine and Quetiapine versus Risperidone, Aripiprazole, and Haloperidolum in reducing the anxiety symptoms in patients diagnosed with schizophrenia and schizoaffective disorder hospitalized in the Psychiatry Department of Arad between 2013–2014.

Considering the treatment, 63 subjects were divided in two groups: T1 (treated with Olanzapine and Quetiapine) and T2 (treated with Haloperidolum, Risperidone, and Aripiprazol).

Anxiety is frequent in the course of schizophrenia and schizoaffective disorder with significant differences among the two groups. After treatment, the level of anxiety reduced with significant improvement of total score of PANSS; the effect is higher in group T2 compared to T1. Before treatment, anxiety is positively correlated with scores of PANSSN ($r=.285$; $p=0.010$), PANSST ($r=.260$; $p=0.040$), and HAM-D ($r=.455$; $p<0.0001$).YMRS is negatively correlated with negative items of PANSSN scale ($r=-.321$; $p=0.010$). IQ (intelligence quotient) was decreased posttreatment for both treatments, but T1 had had a higher effect on it.

Some antipsychotics have been reported to be successful in reducing the anxiety level in psychotic patients: in group T2 the treatment has a higher effect on anxiety and lower size effect on intelligence.

Keywords: Anxiety, Schizophrenia, Schizoaffective Disorder, Antipsychotics

1. Introduction

Anxiety disorders are serious, debilitating conditions, with wide discrepancies being found in the reports of the prevalence rates, in clinical and epidemiological studies.

Based on the literature, the rate of prevalence of anxiety disorder in patients with schizophrenia or schizoaffective disorder remains uncertain due to limiting factors: the definitions of the disorders themselves the sample size, the study procedures and the utilization of different measures and clinical assessments.

A meta-analysis by Achim et al., in 2011, found a prevalence rate for anxiety disorder of 38.3% in the schizophrenic population, compared with 28.8% reported for the general population [1].

Seedat et al., in 2007, in a study of hospitalized schizophrenic patients, found that 25% suffered from anxiety disorder [2]. In 2007, using a sample of inpatients, Ciapparelli et al. found anxiety disorders in 74% of the subjects [3].

In a study conducted by Braga et al., in 2004, 42% of schizophrenic outpatients presented anxiety disorders [4].

In schizoaffective disorder, the rates of anxiety disorders range from 32% in outpatients [3] to 45% in inpatients [5].

Schizophrenia is a common, chronic and severe mental illness defined by the presence of delusions, hallucinations, and disorganized behavior (positive symptoms); by the presence of apathy, social withdrawal, and involution (negative symptoms); and by cognitive disorganization [6].

It has long been known that anxiety has an important role in the psychopathology of schizophrenia. However, the nature of the development of anxiety disorder in psychosis is not well understood.

The presence of the comorbidity of anxiety in major psychotic disorders (schizophrenia, schizoaffective disorder) results in reduced cognitive functioning, increases the severity of comorbid medical conditions, increases the risk of reoccurrence, adds to internalized stigma, reduces functioning, and has a negative impact on the overall outcome for the patient.

Comorbid anxiety in schizophrenia and schizoaffective disorder is associated with the more positive symptoms: extrapyramidal symptoms suggesting more severe medication side effects [6], an increase in drug/alcohol abuse, a worsening of social and professional functioning, and in the quality of life [7].

Anxiety is common among patients with schizophrenia or schizoafective disorder, and it may also manifest itself as a symptom during an acute psychotic episode [8], as a result of the side effects of medication or as a symptom of a comorbid anxiety disorder. Patients are generally discharged as soon as their psychotic episode is resolved, with little recognition of the presence of an anxiety disorder [9].

It is difficult to evaluate the relation of anxiety to psychotic symptoms since it is not clear which anxiety symptoms the disorder is associated with. Furthermore, the operational criteria developed for the assessment of the level of anxiety found in the nonpsychotic population (Hamilton Anxiety Rating Scale, Yale Brown Obsession Compulsion Rating) may themselves be problematic. Extrapyramidal symptoms which develop secondary to neuroleptic treatment may coincide with anxiety symptoms [7].

Progress in understanding the etiology of comorbid anxiety in major psychotic disorders such as schizophrenia or schizoaffective disorder has been made. For example, in the field of genetics, two basic genetic strategies have been developed, enabling a better understanding of the etiology of anxiety: the linkage approach and the polymorphism or susceptibility allele, which associates different genes (e.g., dysbindin, the gene for the dystrobrevin-binding protein 1, located within the linkage peak on chromosome 6 p; or chromosomal regions, e.g., 6p22.3) with traits or illness [10].

Generally, anxiety disorders are relatively responsive to treatment so greater awareness should be paid to their comorbidity with psychosis in order to obtain clinical benefits.

Comorbid anxiety may have implications for treatment choice. Generally, anxiety is considered to be secondary to the psychotic condition and it is expected to improve simultaneous with an improvement in the schizophrenic symptoms. There is some evidence that antipsychotic medication (such as Quetiapine) has some degree of efficacy in reducing anxiety in schizophrenic patients [11].

The treatment for acute schizophrenia involves one of the newer generation antipsychotic drugs which is well-tolerated and can be used for maintenance therapy. In particular, it is desirable to use drugs with little sedative effect in order to optimize functioning and to preserve the quality of life [12,13]. However, lack of compliance with antipsychotics must be taken in consideration as it is known that nonadherence plays a significant role in psychotic relapse. In these cases, long-acting injectable antipsychotics (administered at two to four week intervals) are preferable as they may result in a lower risk of dose-related adverse effects (because of lower peak antipsychotic plasma levels) and lower rates of hospitalization due to acute exacerbations. These factors contribute to improving the individual quality of life.

A personalized treatment approach is necessary in the management of comorbid anxiety with schizophrenia which should be based on the pathogeneses and the clinical assessments.

In clinical practice, in those patients with significant agitation and anxiety, drugs with low sedative potential are not sufficient for the reduction of these symptoms. In these patients, anxiety may interfere with compliance to medication. So, benzodiazepines or sedative neuroleptics (levomepromazine) are often incorporated into the antipsychotic treatment [13].

In practice, two strategies are available to satisfactorily manage the severe anxiety associated with acute psychotic episodes: the use of sedative antipsychotic drugs (thioridazine, pipamperone, melperone, cyamemazine, a-flupenthixol, and levomepromazine) [14, 15, 16] or the use of adjuvant benzodiazepines therapy [17, 18, 19]. These sedative antipsychotics have been shown to have anxiolytic effects at low doses both in nonpsychotic patients and during acute psychotic episodes [18].

In order to prevent the risk of benzodiazepine dependence and rebound anxiety on the cessation of treatment, the use of benzodiazepines should be for as short a period as possible. Benzodiazepines should be prescribed in combination with nonsedative disinhibitory atypical antipsychotics.

Benzodiazepines used in psychotic episodes are drugs with potent anxiolytic action, a low propensity for pharmacokinetic drug interactions, and a long half-life to ensure uninterrupted cover [19, 20].

After the patient reaches a position where the symptoms are well-controlled, the treatment can be switched to a nonsedative antipsychotic for maintenance therapy.

Some atypical antipsychotics rely on the serotonin (5-HT) neurotransmitter system. The antagonism of 5-HT receptors permits the atypical antipsychotics to have a lower propensity to cause extrapyramidal symptoms and tardive dyskinesia.

The 5-HT actions may also result in improvements in the negative or cognitive symptoms of schizophrenia.

It has been proposed that the antagonism of 5-HT receptors and/or partial antagonism of 5-HT receptors and antihistaminic properties may play a role in the antianxiety effect of some atypical antipsychotics.

The literature indicates that Olanzapine and Quetiapine have a degree of efficacy in reducing anxiety in schizophrenic and schizoaffective patients [11, 19].

In order to explore the efficacy of atypical antipsychotics in reducing comorbid anxiety in schizophrenic and schizoaffective patients, we performed a study in our clinic.

We aimed to measure the efficacy of various antipsychotics in reducing anxiety levels in patients diagnosed with schizophrenia and schizoaffective disorder, who had been hospitalized in Arad between 2013-2014.

2. Methodology

2.1. Objectives

The aims of this study are: (a) to determine the relationship between anxiety and schizophrenia/ schizoaffective disorder, (b) to determine if the anxiety level is reduced under pharmacological treatment and to compare the efficacy in the two groups (T1- Olanzapine, Quetiapine; and T2- Haloperidolum, Risperidone, Aripiprazol), and (c) to estimate the effect of antipsychotic treatment on cognitive ability (intelligence level, IQ).

2.2. Sample

Sixty three patients diagnosed with schizophrenia, schizoaffective disorder, and anxiety were evaluated on admission and after 28 days of antipsychotic treatment. The patients were hospitalized in the Psychiatry Ward of The County Clinical Emergency Hospital in Arad, between 2013–2014. The patients were divided in two groups: T1, who receieved anthypsichotic treatment with Olanzapine or Quetiapine; and group T2, who received treatment with typical and atypical antipsychotics (Haloperidolum, Risperidone, and Aripiprazol).

The diagnoses of schizophrenia, schizoaffective disorder and anxiety disorders were established according to the ICD-10[21][and DSM-V-TM[22]] criteria.

GENDER	Females:54%	Mean: 43.27		
AGE	Mean:43.27	SD: 7.5		
EDUCATION	Secondary school: 9%	High school: 33.3%	Professional school: 46%	University: 7%
MARITAL STATUS	Never married: 7.9%	Married: 20.6%	Divorced: 20.6%	In a relationship: 7.9%
ALCHOL USE	6.3%			

Table 1. Sample characteristics

The sample (Table 1) presented the following socio-demographic characteristics: (a) gender: 54% females, 46% males; (b) age: mean = 43.27, SD = 7.5; (c) education: 9% secondary school, 33.3% high school, 46% professional school and 7% university; (d) marital status: 7.9% never married, 20.6% married, 20.6% divorced, and 7.9% in a relationship; and (e) 6.3% alcohol use.

2.3. Measures

All subjects were evaluated using the following measures:

a. **The Hamilton Anxiety Scale** (HAM-A; Hamilton, 1959) [23] is a rating scale used to quantify the severity of anxiety symptomatology. It consists of 14 items, each defined by a series of symptoms. Each item is rated on a 5-point scale, ranging from 0 (not present) to 4 (severe).

b. **Positive and Negative Syndrome Scale** (PANSS; Kay SR, Fiszbein A, Opler LA. 1987) [24] is a semistructured clinical interview scale comprising 30 items and a seven point severity rating. There are seven psychiatric parameters belonging to a positive symptoms subscale, seven parameters belonging to a negative symptoms subscale and 16 parameters belonging to a general psychopathology subscale. The interitem correlations for PANSS were significant with a Cronbach's alpha between.71 to.83.

c. **The Hamilton Depression Rating Scale** (HAMD - 17 items; Hamilton M. A Rating Scale for Depression 1960) [25] is a scale that measures the symptoms of depression experienced over the previous week, and was originally developed for hospital inpatients. One limitation of the HAMD is that atypical symptoms of depression (e.g., hypersomnia, hyperphagia) are not assessed. A score of 0–7 is generally accepted to be within the normal range (or in clinical remission), while a score of 20 or higher (indicating at least moderate severity) is usually required for entry into a clinical trial. HAMD have good internal consistency, between 0.77 to 0.91.

d. **YoungMania Rating Scale (YMRS)** [26] is a rating scale used to evaluate manic symptoms in individuals with mania. The scale has 11 items and is based on the patient's subjective report of his or her clinical condition over the previous 48 hours. The studies regarding the psychometric characteristics of YMRS report a high degree of internal consistency ($\alpha = 0.91$).

e. **Raven's Progressive Matrices** [27] is a nonverbal multiple choice measure of general intelligence; in each test item, the subject is asked to identify the missing element that completes a pattern. On the Romanian sample of 2755 subjects, RPM reported a high internal consistency (α =.91).

2.4. Procedure and design

The participants of this study filled in the tests package presented at the section work instruments. For the protection of the participants, they only noted a code on the answer papers. We shall use the variance analysis (ANOVA factorial) considering that we shall observe the simultaneous influence of two interdependent variables on the dependent variable.

We have structured our research into three studies as follows:

a. a correlation study—for which we have used Pearson correlation "r," in order to establish the relationship between all measurements in the pretreatment phase.

b. a comparative study—between pre- and postintervention, respectively, between the two treatments on the dependent variables (anxiety, mania, depression, and positive versus negative psychotic symptoms); we have calculated **ANOVA 2 x 2 - General Lineal Model for Repeated Measurements** for the cases in which there was no initial (pretreatment) difference between the dependent variables means (e.g., HAMA, YMRS, PANSS-N).

ANOVA 2 x 2 as a statistical indicator is helpful to observe as well the evolution in time, as well the effect on the dependent variables of the interaction between treatment condition and evolution in time as independent variables.

We have calculated **ANCOVA - General Lineal Model Univariate Analysis of Variance** for the cases in which we have observed an initial difference between the dependent variables means (e.g., PANSS-P, PANSS-G, PANSS-T, HAMD).

ANCOVA as a statistic indicator helps to eliminate the initial difference (preintervention) from the end-results (postintervention) in order to see if at the end the difference is significant as a result of intervention and to estimate which would be the end-results means if we wouldn't had initial differences.

c. a comparative study—on effect of the treatment on IQ as a dependent variable, for this propose we have used ANCOVA - Univariate Analysis of Variance, because we have observed a initial difference between the two groups regarding the IQ level.

3. Results

3.1. Correlations

Before treatment, anxiety is positively correlated with the total score of negative items on the PANSS scale (PANSSN: r =.285; p = 0.010); anxiety is also positively correlated with the total score on PANSS (PANSST: r =.260; p = 0.040) and the total score for depression assessed according to the Hamilton Depression Scale (HAM-D: r =.455; p<0.0001).

The score on the YMRS is negatively correlated with negative items on the PANSSN scale (r = -.321; p = 0.010). In general, it is to be expected that a subject with negative symptoms will have a lower level of mania.

The IQ was positive correlated with the total score on the PANSS scale (PANSST: r =.261; p = 0.036) suggesting, in our study, that a higher level of intelligence represents possible a risk in the development of psychotic symptoms. The observed positive correlation between PANSST and IQ accounts for approximately 9% of the variation.

Pearson	IQ	PANSSP	PANSSN	PANSSG	PANSST	HAMA	YMRS	HAMD	No. Relapse	Age
IQ initial	1	.044	.162	.233	**.261***	.108	-.015	.241	-.035	-.003
PANSS-P		1	**.272***	-.052	**.403****	.114	-.018	.053	.055	.082
PANSS-N			1	.174	**.688****	.057	**-.321***	.217	**.286***	**.352****
PANSS-G				1	**.769****	**.285***	.003	**.304***	.027	.062
PANSS-T					1	**.260***	-.155	**.332****	.171	.242
HAMA						1	.001	**.455****	.133	.240
Sample N	63	63	63	63	63	63	63	63	63	63

PANSS-P = positive items of PANSS scale; PANSS-N = negative items of PANSS scale; PANNS-G = general items of PANSS scale; PANSS-T = total score of PANSS scale; HAMA = Hamilton anxiety scale; YMRS = Young Mania Rating scale; HAMD = Hamilton Depression scale; *. Significant at the 0.05 level (2-tailed). **. Significant at the 0.01 level (2-tailed).

Table 2. Preintervention correlations between all measurements

Based on these results, there is a possibility that IQ can be a risk factor in 9% of the cases to stimulate the productivity of psychotic symptoms. Given this fact, we need to exercise a degree of caution with regard to the afore mentioned conclusion.

3.2. Comparing treatments

To assess the level of the anxiety disorders in both groups before and after 28 days of antipsychotic treatment, we used an ANOVA 2 x 2 design.

Because we expected that there would be initial differences between the two groups (T1 and T2), we also performed a t-test for independent samples (table 2) for the pretreatment values, in order to eliminate, if necessary, any initial differences from the postintervention results by calculating ANCOVA in such cases.

We obtained statistically significant difference for the PANSS-P, PANSS-G, PANSS-T, and HAM-D. To compare the efficacy of the treatment for these dependent variables between the two groups we used ANCOVA.

Pre-intervention measurments		*t-test for Equality of Means*						
		.t.	**df**	**Sig. (2-tailed)**	**Mean Difference**	**Std. Error Difference**	**95% Confidence Interval of the Difference**	
							Lower	**Upper**
PANSS-P	Equal variances assumed	**-2.800**	**61**	**.007**	-1.8589	.6638	-3.1862	-.5315
PANSS-N	Equal variances assumed	.578	61	.566	.6310	1.0926	-1.5538	2.8159
PANSS-G	Equal variances assumed	**4.302**	**61**	**.000**	6.1028	1.4187	3.2659	8.9397
PANSS-T	Equal variances assumed	**2.206**	**61**	**.031**	4.8468	2.1966	.4543	9.2392
HAMA	Equal variances assumed	1.025	61	.310	1.2319	1.2023	-1.1723	3.6360
YOUNG MANIA	Equal variances assumed	.181	61	.857	.3992	2.2024	-4.0047	4.8031
HAMD	Equal variances assumed	**3.208**	**61**	**.002**	3.4980	1.0903	1.3179	5.6781

PANSS-P = positive items of PANSS scale; PANSS-N = negative items of PANSS scale; PANNS-G = general items of PANSS scale; PANSS-T = total items of PANSS scale; HAMA = Hamilton anxiety rating scale; YMRS = Young Mania Rating SCALE; HAMD = hamilton depression rating scale;

Table 3. Preintervention differences between the two groups (in order to see if it is necessary to use ANCOVA

As the main goal of this study was to evaluate the efficacy of antipsychotic treatment for anxiety, we compared the level of anxiety pre and postintervention, by using ANOVA because there were no initial differences observed (see table 3).

Results showed that there were differences in the level of anxiety reduction between the two groups: in group T2, the efficacy of the treatment was significantly higher than that of group T1. The result obtained was confirmed by the t-test for independent samples applied postintervention at T1 and T2 ($t = 3.018$; $p = .004$).

General Lineal Model – for Repeated Measurements for Anxiety					
Source	**Sum of Squares**	**df**	**Mean Square**	**F**	**Sig.**
Time (pre – post)	574.777	1	574.777	211.821	.000
Time * Treatments (T1 vs T2)	22.904	1	22.904	8.441	.005
Error (Time)	165.524	61	2.714		

Table 4. Comparing the level of anxiety pre and postintervention and between groups

The difference in anxiety reduction between the two groups (see table 4) was also measured, by comparing T2 with T1 with Cohen's D = 0, 7583; r = 0.3545.

Using the t-test for paired samples *t* (T1) = -4.901, p<0.0001 and *t* (T2) = -9.043, p<0.001, the results obtained in our preliminary study revealed that both types of treatments are effective in significantly reducing the intensity of anxiety both for schizophrenic and schizoaffective patients.

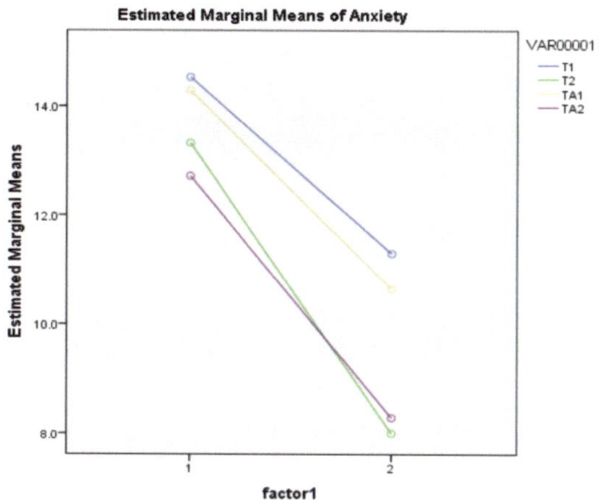

TS1= schizophrenic patients in T1 group

TA1 = schizoaffective patients in T1 group

TS2= schizophrenic patients in T2 group

TA2 = schizoaffective patients in T2 group

Figure 1. Pretreatment and posttreatment level of anxiety for both groups T1 (TS1 and TA1) and T2 (TS2 and TA2)

For both groups(Figure1), the results showed that with regard to the efficacy of the treatments for the patients diagnosed with schizoaffective disorder compared to schizophrenic patients, there was no difference, *t* (T1) = -3.94, p = 0.697 and *t* (T2) = 0.212, p = 0.933.

3.3. Comparing IQ

To eliminate the initial preintervention IQ differences between groups (*t*=5,162; p<.0001) we applied ANCOVA. In both groups of patients, antipsychotic treatment has a negative effect on cognitive functioning reducing IQ level, but the cognitive dysfunction was higher in group T1.

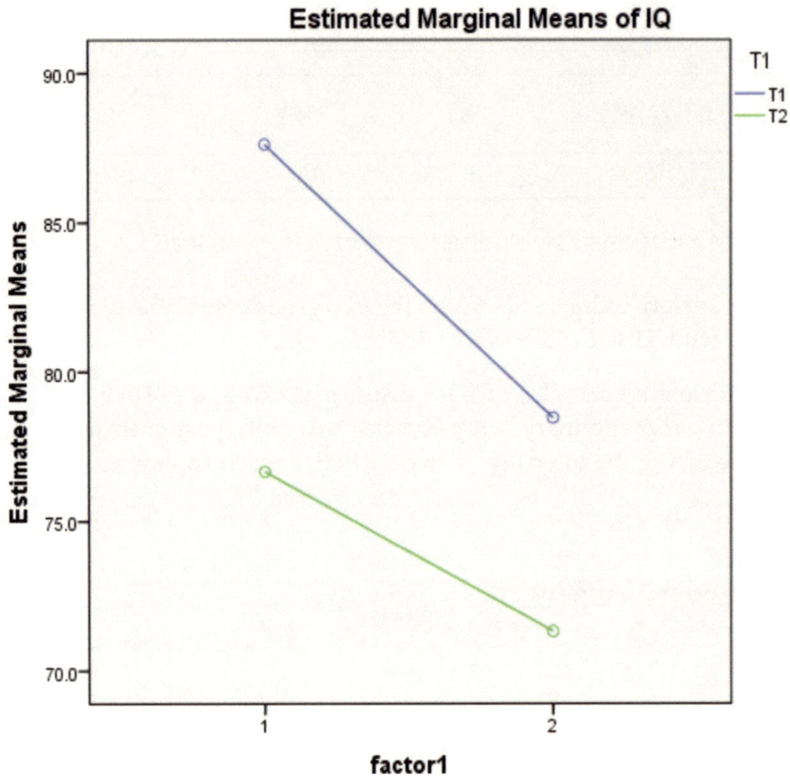

Figure 2. Evolution of the IQ levels in T1 and T2 group

The results obtained showed that in posttreatment (Figure 2) there were no statistically significant differences between the two groups, ANCOVA F = 1.085, p = 0.302. A possible explanation for these results is that the T1 treatment had a greater effect on cognitive functioning when compared with the T2 treatment, so that even if the T2 group initially had a lower intelligence level, after 28 days the difference was no longer significant (see Table 5).

Dependent Variable: IQ in evolution				
Pre-Post	**Mean**	**Std. Error**	**95% Confidence Interval**	
			Lower Bound	**Upper Bound**
T1 treatment	**74.07**[a]	.93	72.21	75.93
T2 treatment	**75.551**	.91	73.72	77.37

Note: a.Covariates appearing in the model are evaluated at the following values: IQ initial = 82.048.

Table 5. Estimated marginal means after eliminating the covariance of the Initial IQ

4. Discussions and conclusions

The study's results proved that preintervention anxiety is positively correlated with the total score on PANSSN ($r = .285$; $p = 0.010$) and PANSST ($r = 0.260$; $p = 0.040$) and the total score on HAM-D ($r = 0.455$; $p<0.0001$). Also the score on the YMRS is negatively correlated with the negative items on the PANSSN scale ($r = -0.321$; $p = 0.010$). Our results are corroborated by international studies [28, 29].

Based on the results of our study, the efficacy of Olanzapine or Quetiapine is lower than that of the typical and other atypical antipsychotics (such as Haloperidolum, Risperidone, Aripiprazol). Olanzapine or Quetiapine have a greater negative effect on cognitive functioning than other antipsychotics.

These results are contrary to the international findings [11, 19, 30, 31].

In a study by Riedl et al., 2007 [19], both Quetiapine and Olanzapine improved cognition; however, the improvement in cognitive index scores was more marked in patients receiving Quetiapine. Quetiapine produce a significantly better improvement in reaction quality/ attention than Olanzapine [11, 19].

Olanzapine, an atypical antipsychotic, has proved to be efficient in reducing the positive and negative symptoms of schizophrenia. Compared with conventional antipsychotics, it has greater affinity for serotonin 5-HT2A than for dopamine D2 receptors. In large, well-controlled trials involving patients diagnosed with schizophrenia, Olanzapine (5 to 20 mg/day) was superior to Haloperidol (5 to 20 mg/day) in the treatment of depressive and negative symptoms, comparable with effects on positive psychotic symptoms [28]. Contrary to these findings, in our study patients treated with haloperidol, Risperidone, and Aripiprazol (group T2) showed a greater reduction of symptomatology.

The 1-year risk of relapse of rehospitalisation was significantly lower with Olanzapine than with Haloperidol treatment [35].

In the first double-blind comparative study [28, 29, 33]) of Olanzapine 10 to 20 mg/day and Risperidone 4 to 12 mg/day, Olanzapine proved to be significantly more effective than Risperidone in the treatment of negative and depressive symptoms but not for overall psychopathological symptoms.

In contrast, preliminary results from an 8-week controlled study [34] suggested that Risperidone 2 to 6 mg/day was superior to Olanzapine 5 to 20 mg/day in the treatment of positive and anxiety/depressive symptoms, and that both agents demonstrated similar efficacy on overall psychopathology. These results are similar to our findings (Risperidone was superior to Olanzapine in reducing anxiety symptoms as confirmed by t-test for independent samples applied postintervention at T1 and T2: $t = 3.018$; $p = 0.004$).

However, preliminary results from an 8-week trial showed comparable cognitive enhancing effects for Olanzapine and Risperidone in patients with schizophrenia or schizoaffective disorder [30]. In our study, in both groups of patients, (T1, T2), antipsychotic treatment has a negative effect on cognition with a larger effect on group T1 treated with Olanzapine and Quetiapine.

Olanzapine demonstrated superior antipsychotic efficacy when compared to Haloperidol in the treatment of acute phase schizophrenia, and in the treatment of some patients with first-episode or treatment-resistant schizophrenia [35].

The reduced risk of adverse events and the therapeutic superiority, compared with Haloperidol and Risperidone, in the treatment of negative and depressive symptoms support the choice of Olanzapine as a first-line option in the management of schizophrenia in the acute and maintenance phase of treatment response [36].

Aripiprazole, a 5-H1A partial agonist was found to have a considerable antianxiety effect which may concur with procognitive and mood-ameliorating effects [32, 37, 38]. These are similar to our results: when comparing T2 with T1 using effect size based on differences between means (Cohen's D = 0.7583; r = 0.3545), Aripiprazol is superior to Olanzapine and Quetiapine in reducing anxiety in schizophrenic and schizoaffective disorder patients. Regarding the cognitive dysfunction, posttreatment, in both groups of patients, we noticed a negative effect on cognition, although there was no statistically significant differences between the groups as determined by analysis of covariance (ANOVA F = 1.085; p = 0.302).

One hypothesis could be that this agonism of Aripiprazole is a mechanism contributing to antianxiety effects. Case reports and studies on the antipsychotic augmentation by Aripiprazole in partial responders to Clozapine found a considerable antianxiety effect [32].

However, this could be due to external factors or to the natural evolution of the illness. A randomized controlled study is required to evaluate the efficacy of the Clozapine-Aripiprazole combination in cases of treatment-resistant schizophrenia with a predominance of anxiety [39].

Risperidone's antianxiety action was demonstrated in the study by Blider et al. in 2002 [30], conducted on 62 patients hospitalized for acute exacerbations of schizophrenia, randomly assigned to receive Risperidone (a mean dose, 7.4 mg/day), Haloperidol (7.6 mg/day), or Methotrimeprazine (100 mg/day) for 4 weeks. The antianxiety effects were significantly greater in the Risperidone patients than the Methotrimeprazine patients. The difference between Haloperidol and Methotrimeprazine was not significant.

It is concluded that Risperidone is an effective antipsychotic and anxiolytic agent in schizophrenic patients. These result are confirmed by our findings in group T2 (t = 3.018; p = 0.004).

New Drug Perspectives

It is generally agreed upon that anxiety is a frequently occurring symptom of schizophrenia, strongly associated with an increased risk of relapse and more severe symptomatology. The effects of antipsychotics in reducing anxiety in psychotic patients remain controversial and the practice of prescribing adjuvants (benzodiazepines) is unsatisfactory [17, 18].

The next clinical trials for schizophrenia with comorbid anxiety perhaps will show the efficacy of some new compounds (the anticonvulsant/anxiolytic pregabalin and the atypical antipsychotic Quetiapine) [40].

http://dx.doi.org/10.5772/60643

Consequently, we think there is a need for more research in order to obtain a clear perspective of the efficacy of Olanzapine or Quetiapine. It should also be pointed out that our findings suffer from certain limitations: such as (a) the lack of a control group, (b) the small sample size, (c) the short treatment time, and (d) the lack of a follow-up evaluation after three and six months, and after one year. Our results can serve as a guide to future studies regarding the efficacy of psychopharmacological treatment on comorbid anxiety.

Limitations

The methodological limitations of this study will be addressed in a follow-up study: this was a preliminary study with a small sample size, lacking follow up evaluations at 3 months, 6 months and 1 year. Given that some of these patients will be inevitably lost to the follow up, a large sample size will need to be used in order to ensure that sufficient numbers are available to obtain meaningful repeat measures.

Acknowledgements

This paper is partly supported by the Sectorial Operational Programme Human Resources Development (SOPHRD), financed by the European Social Fund and the Romanian Government under contract number POSDRU 141531.

Author details

Delia M. Podea[1*], Aurora I. Sabau[1] and Karol J. Wild[1]

*Address all correspondence to: deliapodea@yahoo.com

1 "Vasile Goldis" Western University of Arad, County ClinicalEmergency Hospital of Arad, Psychiatry Department, Arad, Romania

"Vasile Goldis" Western University of Arad, Psychology Department, Arad, Romania

References

[1] Achim A. M., Maziade M., Raymound E., Olivier D., Merette C., Roy M.A.: How prevalent are anxiety disorders in schizophrenia? A meta-analysis and critical review on a significant association. Schizophrenia Bulletin, 2011, 37:811-821.

[2] Seedat S., Fritelli V., Oosthuizen P., Emsley R. A., Stein D. J.: Measuring anxiety in patients with schizophrenia. Journal of Nervous Mental Disease. 2007; 1995 : 320-324.

[3] Ciapparelli A., Paggini R., Marazitti D., Carmassi C., Bianchi M., Taponecco C., Consoli G., Lombardi V., Massimetti G., Dell'Osso L.: Comorbidity with axis 1 anxiety disorders in remitted psychotic patients 1 year after hospitalization. CNNS Spectr 2007; 12:913-919.

[4] Braga R. J., Petrides G., Figuueira I.: Anxiety disorders in schizophrenia. Compr Psychiatry 2004; 45:460-468.

[5] Cosoff S.J., Hafner R.J.: The prevalence of comorbid anxiety in schizophrenia, schizoafective disorder and bipolar disorder. Aust NZJ Psychiatry 1998;32:67-72.

[6] American Psychiatric Association: The Diagnostic and Statistical Manual of Mental Disorders, 5th edition, Washington, DC. 2013.

[7] Tibbo P., Swainson J., Chue P., LeMelledo J.M.: Prevalence and relationship to delusion and hallucinations of anxiety disorders in schizophrenia. Depress Anxiety 2003;17:65-72. DOI:10.1002/da.10083.

[8] Argyle N., et al.: Panic attacks in chronic schizophrenia. Br J Psychiatry 1990;430–433.DOI: 10.1192/bjp.157.3.430.

[9] Blanchard Jack J., Mueser Kim T., Bellack Alan S.: Anhedonia, positive and negative affect, and social functioning in schizophrenia. Schizophrenia Bulletin 1998;24.3:413-424.

[10] Schwab S.G., Albus M., Hallmayer J., Honig S., Borrmann M., Lichtermann D., Ebstein R.P., Ackenheil M., Lerer B., Risch N., Maier W., Wildenauer D.B.: Evaluation of a susceptibility gene for schizophrenia on chromosome 6p by multipoint affected sibpair linkage analysis. Nature Genetics. 1995; 11:325-327.doi:10.1038/ng1195-325.

[11] Cutler Andrew J., Quetiapine, Evidence in reducing Anxiety: Clinical Evidence may suggest the atypical antipsychotic (quetiapine fumarate) tablets, is effective in reducing anxiety in patients with schizophrenia. Presented at the American Psychiatric Association annual meeting, May 5 - 10 2001; New Orleans, Louisiana 2001.

[12] Garay RP., d'Alche-Birée, Cyamémazine F.: Profil neuroleptique ou anxiolytique? L'Information Psychiatrique Lille 1995;71: 969-971.

[13] Goodwin R.D., Amador X.F., Malaspina D., Yale S.A., Goetz R.R., Gorman J.M.: Anxiety and substance use comorbidity among inpatients with schizophrenia. Schizophr Res 2003 May 1; 61(1): 89-95.

[14] Squelart P., Saravia J.: Pipamperone (Dipiperon), a useful sedative neuroleptic drug in troublesome chronic psychotic patients. Acta Psychiatr Belg. 1977;77:284-293.

[15] Meltzer H.Y., Sumiyoshi T., Jayathilake K.: Melperone in the treatment of neuroleptic-resistant schizophrenia. Psychiatry Res. 2001;105:201-209.

[16] Poldinger W. J.: Melperone in low doses in anxious neurotic patients. A double-blind placebo-controlled clinical study. Neuropsychobiology. 1984;11:181-186.

[17] Barbee J.G., Mancuso D.M., Freed C.R., Todorov A.A.: Alprazolam as a neuroleptic adjunct in the emergency treatment of schizophrenia. Am J Psychiatry 1992;149:506-510.

[18] Wolkowitz O.M., Pickar D.: Benzodiazepines in the treatment of schizophrenia: a review and reappraisal. Am J Psychiatry. 1991;148:714-726.

[19] Riedel M, Muller N, Spellmann I, Engel RR.: Efficacy of Olanzapine versus Quetiapine on cognitive dysfunction in patients with an acute episode of schizophrenia. Arch. Psychiatry Clin Neurosa 2007;402-412.

[20] Lingjaerde O.: Benzodiazepines in the treatment of schizophrenia: an updated survey. Acta Psychiatr Scand. 1991;84:453-459.

[21] World Health Organization: The ICD-10 classification of mental and behavioural disorders: Clinical descriptions and diagnostic guidelines. 1992. Geneva: World Health Organization.

[22] American Psychiatric Association: Diagnostic and statistical manual of mental disorders (4th ed., text rev.). Washington, DC: APA.2000.

[23] Hamilton M.: The assessment of anxiety states by rating. Br. J Med Psychol 195932:50-55.

[24] Kay S.R., Fiszbein A., Opler L.A.: The positive and negative syndrome scale (PANSS) for schizophrenia. Schizophrenia Bulletin 1987 ;13261-275.

[25] Hamilton M.: A rating scale for depression. J Neurol Neurosurg Psychiatry 1960; Hamilton Depression Rating Scale (HDRS).

[26] Young R.C., Biggs J.T., Ziegler V. E., Meyer D. A.: Young Mania Rating Scale. In: Handbook of Psychiatric Measures. Washington, DC: American Psychiatric Association; 2000: 540-542.

[27] Raven J.: Raven's Progressive Matrices. Journal of Psychoeducational Assessment 1998; 17,354-361. doi: 10.1177/0013164498058003002.

[28] Bhana N., Foster R.H., Olney R.: Olanzapine: an updated review of its use in the management of schizophrenia. Drugs 2011;61(1):111-161.

[29] Gao K., Muzina D., Gajwani P., Calabrese J. P.: Efficacy of typical and atypical antipsychotics for primary and comorbid anxiety symptoms or disorders: a review. Journal of Clinical Psychiatry 2006 ;67(9):1327–1340.

[30] Bilder R.M., Goldman R.S., Volavka J., Czobor P., Hoptman M., Sheitman B., Lindenmayer J.P., Citrome L., McEvoy J., Kunz M., Chakos M., Cooper T.B., Horowitz T.L., Lieberman J.A.: Neurocognitive effects of Clozapine, Olanzapine, Risperidone, and Haloperidol in patients with chronic schizophrenia or schizoaffective disorder. Am. J. Psychiatry2002;159:1018–1028.

[31] Schirmbeck F., Esslinger C., Rausch F., Englisch S., Meyer-Lindenberg A., Zink M.: Antiserotonergic antipsychotics are associated with obsessive-compulsive symptoms in schizophrenia. Psychol Med 2011;41(11):236.

[32] Chanachev A. et al.: Case Reports in Psychiatry Volume 2011. Article ID 846489, 3 pages.

[33] Moore N. A., Tye N.C., Axton M.S., Risius F.C.: The behavioral pharmacology of Olanzapine, a novel "atypical" antipsychotic agent. Journal of Pharmacology and Experimental Therapeutics1992; 262(2): 545–551.

[34] Kim S.W., Shin I.S., Kim J.M., Youn T., Yang S.J., Hwang M.Y., Yoon J.S.S.O.: The 5-HT2 receptor profiles of antipsychotics in the pathogenesis of obsessive-compulsive symptoms in schizophrenia. Clin Neuropharmacol 2009; 32(4):224.

[35] Csernansky J.G., Schuchart E.K.: Relapse and rehospitalisation rates in patients with schizophrenia: effects of second generation antipsychotics. CNS Drugs2002;16:473–484.

[36] TollefsonG.D., Sanger T.M., Lieberman J.A.: Olanzapine versus Haloperidol in the treatment of first episode psychosis. Schizophrenia Research 1997; 24.doi: 10.4103/2279-042X.128142

[37] Paton C., Whittington C., Barnes T.R.: Augmentation with a second antipsychotic in patients with schizophrenia who partially respond to Clozapine. a meta analysis. J Clin Psychopharmacol 2007; 27:198-204.

[38] Swainston Harrison T., Perry C.M.: Aripiprazole: a review of its use in schizophrenia and schizoaffective disorder Drugs 2004;64(15):1715-1736.

[39] Karunakaran K., Tungaraza T.E., Harborn G.C.: Is Clozapine-Aripiprazole combination a useful regime in the management of treatment-resistant schizophrenia? Journal of Psychopharmacology 2007; 21(4):453–456. doi: 10.1093/schbul/sbn018.

[40] Garay R.P., Samalin L., Hameg A., Llorca P. M.: Investigational drugs for anxiety in patients with schizophrenia. [Internet]. 2014, November 25. Available from http://informahealthcare.com/doi/abs/10.1517/13543784.2014.987339.[Accesed:2014-12-20].

Chapter 8

Joint Hypermobility, Anxiety, and Psychosomatics — The New Neuroconnective Phenotype

Guillem Pailhez, Juan Castaño, Silvia Rosado, Maria Del Mar Ballester, Cristina Vendrell, Núria Mallorquí-Bagué, Carolina Baeza-Velasco and Antonio Bulbena

Additional information is available at the end of the chapter

http://dx.doi.org/10.5772/60607

Abstract

In this chapter, after summarizing the concept and diagnosis of the Joint Hypermobility (Hyperlaxity), we review case control studies in two directions: Anxiety in Joint Hypermobility and Joint Hypermobility in Anxiety disorders, studies in nonclinical samples, review papers, and one incidence study. Collected evidence tends to confirm the strength of the association described two and a half decades ago. Common mechanisms involved include genetics, autonomic nervous system dysfunctions, and interoceptive and exteroceptive processes. Considering clinical and nonclinical data, pathophysiological mechanisms, and present nosological status, we suggest a new Neuroconnective phenotype in which together around a common core Anxiety-Collagen hyperlaxity, it includes five dimensions: behavioral, psychopathology, somatic symptoms, somatosensory symptoms, and somatic illnesses. Somatic illnesses include irritable bowel, dysfunctional esophagus, multiple chemical sensitivity, dizziness or unsteadiness (central vestibular pattern), chronic fatigue, fibromyalgia, glossodynia, vulvodynia, hypothyroidism, asthma, migraine, temporomandibular dysfunction, and intolerances or food and drug hypersensitivity. It is envisaged that new descriptions of anxiety disorders and also of some psychosomatic conditions will emerge and different nosological approaches will be required.

Keywords: Anxiety disorders, joint hypermobility, hyperlaxity, psychosomatic medicine, phobic disorders

1. Introduction

The strong association of a heritable collagen condition and anxiety was an unexpected finding that we first described in 1988 at the Hospital del Mar in Barcelona [1]. Ever since, several clinical and nonclinical researches have been carried out. In this chapter, after summarizing the concept and diagnosis of the Joint Hypermobility (Hyperlaxity), we review case control studies in two directions: Anxiety in Joint Hypermobility and Joint Hypermobility in Anxiety Disorders, studies in nonclinical samples, review papers, and one incidence study. Collected evidence tends to confirm that the association is strong, as described two and a half decades ago. Common mechanisms involved included genetics, autonomic nervous system dysfunctions, and also interoceptive and exteroceptive processes. Considering clinical and nonclinical data, pathophysiological mechanisms, and present nosological status, we suggest a new Neuroconnective phenotype, in which together around a common core Anxiety-Collagen hyperlaxity it includes five dimensions: behavioral, psychopathology, somatic symptoms, somatosensory symptoms, and somatic illnesses. Somatic illnesses include irritable bowel, dysfunctional esophagus, multiple chemical sensitivity, dizziness or unsteadiness (central vestibular pattern), chronic fatigue, fibromyalgia, glossodynia, vulvodynia, hypothyroidism, asthma, migraine, temporomandibular dysfunction, and intolerances or food and drug hypersensitivity. It is envisaged that new descriptions of anxiety disorders and also of some psychosomatic conditions will emerge and different nosological approaches will be required.

Although there is increasing evidence for somatic comorbidity in the major psychiatric conditions, actual psychiatric classifications do not include specific psychiatric illnesses associated to medical conditions other than organic dementias and secondary psychiatric conditions yet. Apparently two main factors concur for this. First, the current nosologies include only two conditions (psychiatric and somatic) when there is a causal connection between them, for instance, organic brain disorder (dementia) with mental symptoms. Along these lines, concepts like vascular depression or even vascular psychiatry are emerging. The reasoning behind this point of view is quite straightforward because it implies the search for etiology and therefore for treatment. Second, there is little evidence of specific somatic signs or conditions in the description of the present psychiatric illnesses. This has reduced the psychiatrists' expectancies to find the coexistence of both other than the secondary psychiatric-somatic comorbidity. There are examples of such comorbid situations like diabetes and schizophrenia already, which some have considered part of the same illness [2]. However the most studied and developed comorbid condition is the joint hypermobility syndrome in anxiety patients. Therefore, there is a need to develop clinical phenotypes containing both psychopathological and somatic features, or even proper psychiatric and somatic conditions. The new phenotype will be built around the core of the association between anxiety disorders (particularly panic, agoraphobia, and social phobia) and the Joint Hypermobility (better Hyperlaxity) syndrome.

The proposed name Neuroconnective to this new phenotype is both comprehensive and specific. It covers the neural component along with the connective dimension of the new phenotype. The prefix neuro- refers to the neural basis of the syndrome, which includes the

http://dx.doi.org/10.5772/60607

dysfunctional Autonomic Nervous System and also the enhanced "body awareness", including interoception, proprioception, and exteroception. Furthermore and, as a kind of homage, we would like to consider that the prefix neuro- also recalls the concept of neurosis in the nineteenth century which was, just in that period, a comprehensive category that included both mental and extensive physical symptoms at the same level. Concerning "connective", it refers to the relevant value of the heritable disorder of the connective tissue and also to the "connectivity" between systems, between mind and body, and actually as concept. Therefore, on the basis of the collected genetic, neurophysiological, neuroimaging, and most clinical data, several dimensions could be organized together in this neuroconnective model.

2. Historical background of the relationship between joint laxity and anxiety

The relationship between a heritable collagen condition and anxiety was a clinical observation rather than a pathophysiological reasoning. While working at the psychiatric outpatient clinic, we repeatedly found in the medical record of most of our patients suffering from anxiety, a particular rubber stamp: "Hiperlaxitud Articular." This stamp was put there by the rheumatologist, JC Duró, who was using it to systematically collect the criteria for the Joint Hypermobility syndrome described and studied by his mentor, Prof. Rotés. The reiterated coincidence of the two conditions prompted us to study this association in more detail and send a letter to The Lancet [1] with preliminary results.

Considering the high prevalence of mood disorders in patients suffering from collagenosis, psychiatrists had been closer to associate collagen conditions with these autoimmune illnesses like systemic lupus erythematosus (SLE) or rheumatoid arthritis (RA), whereas structural collagen disorders (mainly heritable) seemed to be less in mind due to the lack of knowledge of the psychiatric status of these patients [3]. However, there had been scattered observations that pointed in this new direction. In 1957, rheumatologist J. Rotés observed a remarkable degree of nervous tension suffered by patients with hypermobility [4]. To a certain extent, there were some indirect references about the relationship between "visceroptosis," in which viscera displace below their natural position due to ligamental laxity and anxiety/phobias in the classical psychosomatic literature [5]. On the other hand, in 1980, Carlsson and Rundgren [6] found higher hypermobility scores in alcoholic patients compared to controls. Although not mentioned, the case group might have consisted of a high percentage of patients with anxiety.

3. Empirical studies of the link between anxiety and collagen tissue

3.1. General diagnostic criteria of Joint Hypermobility Syndrome

In order to clarify the terminology all along this chapter, we shall use indistinctly Joint Laxity (the original name) and Joint Hypermobility (the given name). Although the second is more often used in English publications, it in fact refers to a rather unspecific consequence (increased mobility), whereas hyperlaxity refers more correctly to the intrinsic mechanism (increased laxity of fibers).

The condition was described for the first time about 60 years ago when it was properly identified and associated to pathology of the musculoskeletal system [4]. The original name proposed by Rotés was 'Joint Laxity' (Laxité Articulaire) and it was published in a French journal (Revue du Rhumatisme). In 1964, Carter and Wilkinson, also using the name of joint laxity (JL), published a relevant paper in which they proposed some diagnostic criteria [7].

In 1973, after an epidemiological study by Beighton et al. [8] using both joint laxity and joint mobility, the syndrome gained general interest in rheumatology and by then, renamed joint hypermobility (JH), began to be studied in a broader way as a separate entity [9]. Later on, the seminal work of Rodney Grahame was very important to get the Joint Hypermobility Syndrome (JHS) revisited among rheumatologists. He has produced three editions of the Beighton book [10] as well as other books about the topic and also has boosted clinical research on it [11,12]. Another prominent author who has provided insightful clinical descriptions of the JHS is Dr J. Bravo [13].

JHS is an inherited connective tissue disorder associated with a generalized collagen laxity and characterized by an increase of active or passive joint mobility in the absence of another rheumatologic disease. JHS has an estimated prevalence in the general population ranging between 10%–20%, and is one of the hereditary disorders of the connective tissue, which include other conditions such as Ehlers–Danlos syndrome, Marfan syndrome, and ostogenesis imperfecta [10]. In fact, there is an overlap with the Ehlers– Danlos type III. This condition has an autosomal dominant pattern and twin studies showed that genetics accounts for at least 70% of the phenotype variance rather than environmental factors such as training. JHS is more common in childhood and tends to decline when aging. The prevalence is higher in females and probably there are ethnic differences, which suggest genetic variations. JHS is also associated with musculoskeletal dysfunctions, possibly resulting from a glycoprotein deficiency and genetic alterations affecting the formation of collagen, which would explain tissue looseness, prolapsed organs, visceroptoses, pneumothorax, and vulnerability to trauma in these patients.

Clinical features in JHS can be articular or extra-articular and are always related to the connective tissue. Among the best known articular features of JHS are arthralgia, lumbalgia, soft-tissue rheumatism (e.g., epicondylitis, tenosynovitis, bursitis), recurrent dislocations, childhood scoliosis, or rheumatoid arthritis [13,14]. Among the best-known extra-articular features of JHS are hernias, varicose veins, "easy bruising", keloids, uterine or rectal prolapse, spontaneous pneumothorax, fibromyalgia, dysautonomia, and some other conditions also linked to panic disorder as asthma, mitral valve prolapse, thyroid dysfunction, or irritable bowel syndrome [14,15].

There are several sets of criteria that show minimal variations from the original proposed by Rotés, although new self-assessment questionnaires have been recently added to the assessment methods of JHS [16,17]. A review paper of all the available criteria showed a high degree of agreement among all of them [18]; a more comprehensive set of 10 criteria obtained by cluster analysis was also proposed. However, the most often used are the "Beighton criteria" converted to a nine point clinical scale by which subjects with a score ≥ 4 are considered as having JH. The condition is characterized through the examination of five body areas, each one receiving a separate score of hyperextension: fifth fingers, thumbs, elbows, knees, and trunk (see Figure 1).

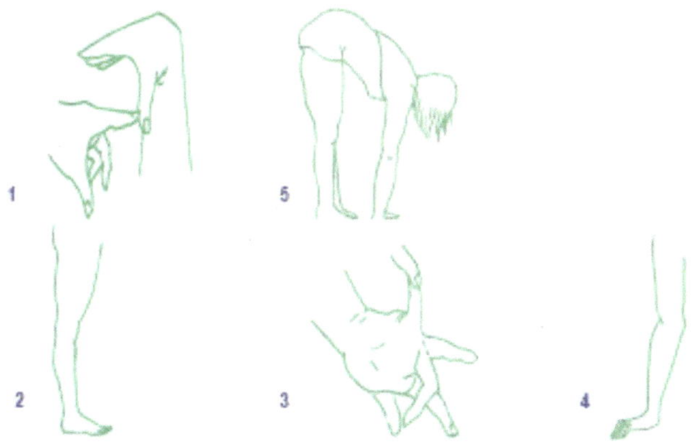

Figure 1. Joint Hypermobility criteria, taken from Beighton P, et al. 1973 [8]. Passive apposition of the thumbs to the flexor aspects of the forearm (one point for each thumb). 1. Hyperextension of the knee beyond 10º (one point for each knee). 2. Passive dorsiflexion of the little fingers beyond 90º (one point for each hand). 3. Hyperextension of the elbows beyond 10º (one point for each elbow). 4. Forward flexion of the trunk with knees fully extended so that the palms of the hands rest flat on the floor (one point).

In 1992, the Hospital del Mar criteria (Table 1) compiled all the items included in the most clinically used criteria. This new scale showed consistent indicators of reliability, internal consistency, and predictive validity and provided evidence for using different scores according to age and gender [18].

Upper extremities
1. Passive apposition of the thumb to the flexor aspect of the forearm is at a distance of less than 21 mm.
2. The passive dorsiflexion of the fifth finger is 90º or more.
3. The active hyperextension of the elbow is 10º or more.
4. External rotation of the shoulder is up to more than 85º.
Lower extremities. Supine position
5. The passive hip abduction can be taken to an angle of 85º or more.
6. Hypermobility of the rotula.
7. Hypermobility of the ankle and foot.
8. Dorsal flexion of the toe is 90º or more.
Lower extremities. Prone position
9. Hyperflexion of the knee.
10. Ecchymoses.

Table 1. Hospital del Mar criteria for JHS as mentioned in Bulbena A, et al. 1992 [18]. Male patients scoring 4 or more are considered cases; female patients are considered cases with scores 5 or over.

In 2010 Grahame [19] developed the Brighton criteria to replace the Beighton criteria for the joint hypermobility syndrome (JHS). According to these criteria, the syndrome diagnosis is made taking into account the Beighton score and also some other clinical manifestations associated with hypermobility. As it could be expected, the correlation between them is very high. They are seldom used outside of rheumatology. The main sets of criteria are included in Table 2.

Major criteria
1. A Beighton score of 4/9 or more (either currently or historically).
2. *Arthralgia* for longer than 3 months in 4 or more joints.
Minor criteria
3. *Beighton* score of 1, 2, or 3 (0, 1, 2, or 3 *if aged 50 years or older*).
4. *Arthralgia* in 1–3 joints or *lumbalgia* for more than 3 months, spondylosis or spondylolysis/spondylolisthesis.
5. *Dislocation/subluxation* in more than one joint or in one joint in more than one occasion.
6. *Soft tissue rheumatism* in three or more lesions (e.g., epicondylitis, tenosynovitis, bursitis).
7. *Marfanoid Habitus* (tall, slim, span/height ratio "/> 1.03, upper/lower segment ratio < 0.89, arachnodactily).
8. *Abnormal skin:* striae, hyperextensibility, thin skin, or papyraceous scarring.
9. *Eye signs*: drooping eyelids or antimongoloid slant.
10. Varicose veins or hernia or uterine/rectal prolapse.

Table 2. Brighton criteria, taken from Grahame R, et al. 2000 [19]. JHS is diagnosed if the patient presents 2 major criteria, 1 major and 2 minor criteria, or 4 minor criteria. 2 minor criteria will be enough when there is a first-degree relative with the syndrome clearly diagnosed. JHS is excluded by the presence of the Marfan or the Ehlers–Danlos Syndrome. The first major criterion and the first minor one exclude each other, as do the second major and the second minor.

The clinical assessment of the joint laxity syndrome is not difficult but examiners should be trained in order to ensure the reliability of the exam. Our group has developed a two-day training course with the support of a CD [20].

3.2. Comorbidity data between anxiety and JHS

Empirical history of the clinical relationship between anxiety disorders and JHS started with a case-control study conducted by our group in 1993, with rheumatologic outpatients with JHS [21]. Diagnoses of panic disorder, agoraphobia, and simple phobia were significantly more frequent among hypermobile patients. There were no significant differences in the diagnoses of generalized anxiety disorder, dysthymia, or major depressive disorder. Around 70% of rheumatologic patients with JHS had some kind of anxiety disorder. However, this only occurred in 22% of controls, a usual figure in chronic patient samples. Cases were 10 times more likely to suffer from anxiety than controls. Specifically, agoraphobia and panic disorders were, respectively, 5 and 7 times more likely (Table 3).

	% JHS	% Non-JHS	Age-Sex Adjust. Odds Ratio	95 % C. I.
Any Anxiety D.	69,3	22,0	**10.69**	4.80–23.81
Panic D.	34.2	6.8	**6.96**	2.31–20.91
Panic & Agora.	24.6	5.1	**6.40**	1.82–22.43
Simple Phobia	29.8	8.5	**5.77**	2.05–16.24
Agoraphobia	37.7	11.9	**5.08**	2.06–12.49
General.Anx.	10.5	5.1	**2.49**	0.65–9.45
Major Depress.	14.9	3.4	**4.51**	0.99–20.56
Dysthymic D.	7.9	5.1	**2.15**	0.53–8.65

Table 3. Lifetime psychiatric disorders in JHS cases (n=114) and non-JHS controls (n=59) seen at an outpatient rheumatological unit, from Bulbena A, et al. 1993 [21].

For a subsequent second study, conducted to support this hypermobility-anxiety association, outpatients with new diagnoses of panic disorder and/or agoraphobia were examined, as well as nonanxious psychiatric and nonpsychiatric outpatients as control groups [22]. Results showed that JHS was present in almost 70% of anxiety cases, versus slightly over 10% of controls. This meant that cases with panic disorders and/or agoraphobia were 17 times more likely to suffer from JHS. Conclusions were valid for women [OR=23.7; CI95% 10.6–52.9] but also for men [OR=10.5; CI95% 3.0–36.3].

Lumley et al. [23] evaluated the psychosocial functioning in patients suffering from Ehlers–Danlos Syndrome (JHS is considered EDS type III). The sample was selected from an outpatient research clinic and the results showed that EDS type III group had higher scores on anxiety, depression, and interpersonal sensitivity as well as higher scores in the symptomatology checklist and the pain scales.

Other lines of research studied possible specific somatotype characteristics in patients with panic disorder/agoraphobia [24]. Cases with panic and/or agoraphobia from an outpatient mental health clinic were compared to psychiatric and medical controls matched by age and gender. Within the entire sample, the asthenic somatotype was associated with higher JH scores. Interestingly enough, the prevalence of asthenic somatotype was at the same time significantly higher in the panic/agoraphobia group (33.3%) compared to the psychiatric (19.2%) and the medical (18.7%) controls. The authors finally concluded that the relationship between panic disorder and asthenic somatotype might be mediated through JHS.

These results were confirmed by another study carried out by the same group in 2014 [25]. They included 60 patients with Panic and Agoraphobia and 60 controls. The authors found that cases and controls differed in the percentage of ectomorphic subjects: 38.3% of cases and 13.3% of controls were categorized as ectomorphic [χ 2=8.5, df=1, p=0.004]. In order to explore the characteristics associated with the ectomorphic somatotype, the two groups were collapsed into one, and ectomorphic and nonectomorphic subjects were compared. The ectomorphic group was younger and showed significantly more hypermobility of joints and more prevalence of panic and agoraphobia. Differences in sex, intake of antidepressants, marital status, educational degree, and labour situation were minor and statistically nonsignificant (Table 4). To further clarify the relative value of previously mentioned variables in relation to somatotype, a logistic regression model was constructed with the ectomorphic somatotype as dependent variable and as independent variables, sex, age, and JH. Only the last one was independently associated with the ectomorphic somatotype [OR=3.25, 95% CI: 1.35–7.8, p=0.008]. Therefore, after adjusting for age and sex, ectomorphic somatotype was independently related to JH status (the more hypermobile, the more likely to be ectomorphic).

Characteristics	Ectomorphic group (n=31)	Nonectomorphic group (n=89)	$\chi2$ / t	p
Female	54.8	48.3	0.17	.677
Age	29.2	32.2	1.98	.050
Antidepressants	41.9	30.3	0.92	.338
Single	67.7	51.7	1.80	.180
High educated	22.6	43.8	3.53	.060
Employed	93.5	97.8	0.29	.588
Panic	64.5	41.6	3.98	**.046**
Agoraphobia	64.5	32.6	8.43	**.004**
JH status	45.2	20.2	6.09	**.014**

Table 4. Comparison of subjects with and without ectomorphic somatotype (according to the Heath-Carter method). All characteristics are expressed in %, except age expressed in mean (S.D.).

Later on, this association was studied in the general population. A two-phase cross-sectional epidemiological study was carried out in a rural town in order to establish lifetime risk for anxiety and affective disorders in subjects affected with JHS. A sample of 1,305 individuals was examined at baseline and over 500 were subsequently subjected to follow-up in a two-stage epidemiological study. Hypermobile patients were six times more likely to suffer from agoraphobia (OR 5.9; CI 95% 3 to 11.7), eight times more likely to suffer from social phobia (OR 7.8; CI 95% 2.4 to 24.8), and eight times more likely to suffer from panic disorder (OR 8.2, CI 95% 3.4 to 19.7) than non-JHS patients. Results were valid for males and females. No differences were found for other anxiety disorders or mood disorders [26].

In the same sample of general population, it was also found that hypermobiles had significantly higher scores in fear and phobia scales, strenghtening the hypothesis that intensity of fears is greater in subjects with JHS [27]. We assessed fear intensity and frequency using a modified version of the Fear Survey Schedule (FSS-III). When the groups with and without joint hypermobility were compared, the mean total scores for both genders were significantly higher for the hypermobile group. These results showed that the association of JHS and phobic anxiety is sustained for intense fears and might represent a susceptibility factor for these anxiety conditions.

The same design was replicated in 2011 in a sample of 150 nonclinical students [28]. Severe fears and daily consumption of cigarettes, alcohol, coffee, and chocolate were compared with the hypermobility scores. We found significant differences when comparing severe fears between the groups with and without hypermobility (7.6 vs. 11; p = 0.001). The frequency of chocolate intake was also significantly higher among subjects with joint hypermobility (31.2% vs. 51.2%; p = 0.038). No significant differences were found regarding cigarette (19.5% vs. 19.3%), alcohol (36.6% vs. 34.9%), and coffee (46.3% vs. 35.8%) consumption. These patterns of consumption may, therefore, be interpreted as self-treatment attempts of subsyndromal anxiety in hypermobile subjects.

In 2004, our group also assessed a nonclinical sample of subjects employed in the same company (N=526) [29]. Subjects with JHS had significantly higher scores in STAI trait anxiety [female average: 16.5 vs. 11; p<0.001] [male average: 13 vs. 11; p<0.03]. STAI state anxiety scores were also higher among hypermobile subjects, although not significantly (Figure 2).

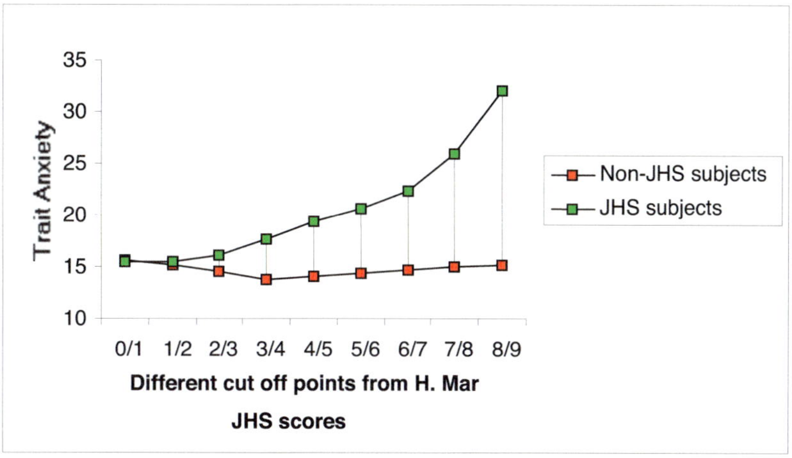

Figure 2. STAI trait anxiety scores (range: 0–60) in 203 women with or without joint hypermobility according to all possible cutoff scores on the Hospital del Mar hypermobility criteria. From Bulbena A, et al. 2004 [29].

Joint hypermobility has also been assessed in relation to psychoactive substances. Baeza-Velasco [30] designed a cross sectional study in college students to assess the use of alcohol and tobacco. The odds of being assessed with JH were greater in those who consumed tobacco and alcohol. Women with JH had higher levels of state anxiety and used emotion-focused coping (i.e., efforts to regulate affect) more than any other coping strategies to deal with stress.

The first structural neuroimaging study on the association was published in 2012 evaluating regional cerebral grey matter in regards to hypermobility status in 72 healthy volunteers [31].

Interestingly enough, bilateral amygdala volume was higher in the hypermobile group. Their findings linked hypermobility to the structural integrity of a brain center implicated in normal and abnormal emotions and physiological responses.

In 2005, we studied schizophrenic outpatients (N=124) with the hypothesis that anxiety disorders mediated by JHS were not symptoms but an independent comorbid entity in schizophrenic patients [32, 33]. Joint Hypermobility was noticeably more likely among panic disorder/phobia-clustered schizophrenic patients than among the noncomorbid group (OR = 9.35; IC = 95% [3.85–22.73]; p<0.0001). The cluster panic disorder/phobia had higher scores in fear scales and schizophrenia positive symptom scales. We are now performing a voxel-based morphometric study in order to examine brain structure, comparing magnetic resonance images of 20 schizophrenic-anxious patients and 20 schizophrenic patients. The preliminary results indicated gray matter volume differences in the schizophrenic-anxiety group in the dorsolateral prefrontal cortex related to the interaction between both conditions. Our findings suggest that the schizophrenic-anxiety group is characterized by specific neural abnormalities that cannot be explained by the presence of schizophrenia or anxiety, but by their conjunction, and this might result in a certain symptomatology [34].

The relationship between social phobia and height was studied through a cross sectional study to explore the frequency of social phobia as well as a heritable disorder of the connective tissue (HDCT) in tall people [35]. One hundred and fifty eight subjects with heights greater than 180 cm in females and 190 cm in males were included in the study; social phobia and HDCT were highly prevalent in tall subjects. JHS was associated with greater prevalence of social phobia symptoms.

The association between anxiety disorders and JHS was also assessed in a sample of university students from Chile [36]. Fifty university students with JH and 50 controls were selected to participate in this case control study. The JH group had higher use of antidepressants and anxiolytics compared to the controls. They also exhibited greater anxiety background, anxiety symptoms, and psychosomatic complaints. A similar study was carried out by Baeza-Velasco et al. in a group of undergraduates in a French university [37]. The aim of the study was to explore the Joint Hypermobility Syndrome (JHS) in the university students and also to assess a possible relationship between this collagen condition and certain psychological variables. Three hundred and sixty five undergraduates from a French University were included in the study and the researchers found that JH was present in almost 40% of the sample and it was also associated with higher levels of somatosensory amplification as well as higher scores in depression and general anxiety in females.

After a number of significant cross-sectional studies we conducted a prospective incidence analysis that assesses whether JHS could be a risk factor in developing anxiety conditions [38]. We sought to determine the cumulative incidence of anxiety disorders in a cohort of young subjects recruited from the general population who had not developed any type of anxiety condition up to the moment; consequently a scheduled 15-year follow-up covering subjects from late adolescence to adulthood was planned. The total population sample was 1,305 subjects, and in order to observe the development of anxiety disorders during the 15-year study period, only the lower age segment (at that time subjects aged between 16 and 20) included in the town's municipal registry was invited to participate. We sought to describe the occurrence of new cases of anxiety disorders during the study period, therefore the exclusion criterion for the study was having already had an anxiety disorder at baseline examination. At baseline, 158 subjects were screened for participation in the study, and after the 15-year follow-up the final sample comprised 137 subjects (86.7% retention rate). Results showed that cumulative incidence of panic/agoraphobia at follow-up was significantly higher for the JHS group (41.4%) than for the control group (1.9%) with relative risk of 22.3 (CI 95% 4.6–108.7), p<0.0001, (NNT 3, CI 95% 2.9–2.3). Incidence of social phobia (RR=6.52; CI 95% 1.7–24.2; p<0.001) and simple phobia (RR=3.31; CI 95% 1.1–9.6; p=0.02) was also significantly higher for the JHS group (Table 5). Moreover, anxiolytic drug use was nearly fourfold higher among JHS subjects compared to non-JHS.

Total Sample n = 137	JHS Status						
	JHS present *n* = 29		JHS absent *n* = 108		*RR*	**95% CI**	*P*
	n	%	*n*	%			
Anxiety Disorders							
Panic/Agoraphobia	12	41.4	2	1.9	22.3	(4.6 to 108.7)	0.0001***
Social Phobia	7	24.1	4	3.7	6.5	(1.7 to 24.2)	0.001*
Simple Phobia	8	27.6	9	8.3	3.3	(1.1 to 9.6)	0.02*
GAD	7	24.1	9	8.3	2.9	(0.97 to 8.62)	0.14 ns
Other Disorders							
Depression/Dysthymia	7	24.1	7	6.48	3.7	(1.2 to 11.7)	0.15 ns

JHS, Joint Hypermobility Syndrome according to Beighton criteria assessed at baseline.

GAD, Generalized Anxiety Disorder

Statistical significance: * p<0.05, ** p<0.001, *** p<0.0001, ns: non significant.

Table 5. Incident cases and relative risk after 15 years of follow-up according to JHS status. Taken from Bulbena A, et al. 2011 [38].

Nevertheless, some studies failed to find a significant correlation between panic disorder and JH. The study by Benjamin et al. was carried out in Israel on 101 patients with patient disorder and 39 controls [39]. The authors also attempted to examine the possible association between reactivity to carbon dioxide and JH. The rate of JH did not differ between the cases and controls neither between JH and carbon dioxide responses. However they used the crude number of hyperlax joints instead of the scoring method, which carries the cutoff point to the extreme of the distribution and therefore is not fully comparable to the rest of studies. On the other hand, the instruments used to assess anxiety in these patients (the self-rating scale of the National

Institute of Mental Health, DSM IV panic symptoms scores and 100mm visual analogue scales of anxiety) are uncommon and could explain the results of the study.

Gulpek et al. designed a study to test the association between JHS and panic disorder and also to determine whether mitral valve prolapse (MVP) accounts for or changes this association [40]. The sample consisted of 115 subjects that were divided in 3 groups. The first group (n=42) included patients with PD and MVP, the second group (n=35) consisted of patients with PD and without MVP and the third group (n=38) had patients with MVP and no psychiatric diagnosis. No significant differences were found in prevalence or severity of JH between groups according to Beighton criteria scoring. However, JH was present in 59.5% of the panic disorder patients with mitral valve prolapse, and 52.6% of the control subjects. Compared to other studies, the prevalence of JH in the control group was never found as high as in this study. Since the prevalence of JH was higher in patients with PD and MVP (59.5%), authors suggested that MVP affects the prevalence of JH in PD. The prevalence of panic disorder was also higher in the JH compared to controls.

Another research group from Turkey studied the relationship between thorax deformity, anxiety, and joint hypermobility. Fifty-two males with thorax deformity and 40 healthy controls from a general outpatient medical clinic were selected to participate in the study [41]. Twenty patients (40%) from the cases group met criteria for JH and those subjects had significantly higher scores in the anxiety scales, particularly in panic disorder. All the cases (with and without JH) had higher anxiety scores compared to controls.

Ercolani and his team designed a study to assess the psychological features of the joint hypermobility syndrome [42]. They recruited 30 JH subjects and two control groups; 25 healthy subjects and 30 fibromyalgia patients. JH group showed significant psychological distress and increased frequency and intensity of somatic symptoms compared to both control groups. A work from another Spanish group [43] has shown again a high prevalence of JHS (61.8%) among panic subjects compared with 10.9% in the healthy control group and 9% in the psychiatric control group. Interestingly, these authors found an intermediate figure among subjects suffering from fibromyalgia (25.4%).

One recent study provided insight about the importance of autonomic symptoms the hypermobility type of Ehlers–Danlos syndrome (EDS) [44]. They included 80 patients with EDS JH, as well as 11 patients with classical EDS (cEDS), seven with vascular EDS (vEDS), 38 with Fibromyalgia and 43 healthy controls. The total autonomic symptom burden was higher in EDS JH (57.9 ± 21.57) than in the other groups but comparable to FM (53.8 ± 19.85). They concluded that joint hypermobility and neuropathy may play a role in the development of autonomic symptoms. In the same line of research, another study described the lived experience of EDS JH and the impact of the symptoms in the daily functioning [45]. The most frequent physical symptoms were joint pain (99%), hypermobility (99%), and limb pain (91%). They also reported a high frequency of other conditions including chronic fatigue (82%), anxiety (73%), depression (69%), and fibromyalgia (42%). These studies are summarized in Table 6.

http://dx.doi.org/10.5772/60607

CLINICAL STUDIES

STUDY (author/year/country)	DESIGN	SETTING	SAMPLE	VARIABLES STUDIED	MAIN RESULTS
Bulbena* 1988 [1] Bulbena* 1993. [21] Spain	Case Control	Rheumatology outpatient clinic	114 JH 59 controls	Anxiety: HAD-A EPQ, SCID III JH: Beighton	Significant association between JH and PD/A [OR 10.7 (4.8-23.8)] and simple phobia [OR 5.8 (2.0-16.20]. No association with GAD [OR 2.5 (0.6-9.4)] JH patient with MVP do not present with more anxiety
Martin-Santos* 1998. [22]Spain	Case Control	Outpatient psychiatric and medical clinic	99 newly diagnosed PD/A 99 psychiatric controls 64 medical controls	Anxiety; HAM A/D, SCID III JH: Beighton Other: ECHO,	JH found on 67.7% of patients with anxiety [OR 18.6 (8.6-40.5)] (10.1% in psychiatric and 12.5% in medical control).
Lumley 1994. [23] USA	Case Control	Outpatient research clinic	21 EDS III/JH 20 controls (other EDS)	Anxiety: HAM-A JH: EDS subtypes	EDS III (JH) higher scores on anxiety, depression and interpersonal sensitivity and greater scores on symptomatology and pain.
Bulbena* 1996. [24] Spain	Case Control	Outpatient mental/medicine clinic	99 PD/A 99 psychiatric controls 64 medical controls	Anxiety JH: Beighton Other: *Quetelet index*	Significant correlation between asthenic somatotype and PD/A [OR 2.23] PD/A & asthenic somatotype may be medication through JH
Pailhez* 2014 [25]	Case Control	Outpatient clinic	60 PD/A 60 controls	Anxiety: JH: Other: somatotype, sociodemographic	Ectomorphic somatotype was independently related to JH status [OR = 3.25, 95% CI 1.35-7.8, p = 0.008].
Benjamin 2001 [39] Israel	Case Control	Anxiety outpatient clinic	101 PD/A 30 healthy controls	Anxiety: NIMH, PSS, VAS 100mm JH: Beighton	JH = in both groups No association between carbon dioxide response and JH
Gulpek 2004 [40] Turkey	Case Control	Outpatient psychiatric clinic	36 PD/A 42 PD/A + MVP 38 MVP	Anxiety: SCID IV JH Beighton Other: ECHO	JH= 3 groups PD/A higher JH MVP may affect JH prevalence in PD
Gulsun 2007 [41] Turkey	Case Control	Outpatient clinic	52 Thorax deformity 40 controls	Anxiety: SCID, HAM-A, JH: Beighton Other: Thorax diameter	21 patients with TD had JH + (40%) JH group had higher anxiety scores (specially PD). TD group higher anxiety scores (JH + and -)
Ercolani 2008 [42] Italy	Case Control	General outpatient	JH 30 30 control Fibromyalgia	Anxiety: DSM IV JH: Beighton	JH group showed psychological distress and increased frequency and intensity of somatic symptoms
		medical clinic	25 healthy control	Others: SCL-90-R, IBQ, SQ, FSF	
Garcia-Campayo 2010. [43] Spain	Case Control	Primary care clinic	55 PD/A 55 psychiatric controls 55 Fibromyalgia controls 55 healthy control	Anxiety: PAS, STAI JH: Beighton Other: SPPI	Prevalence of JH in PD was higher than in controls Prevalence of JH in PD 61.8% Significant correlation between PAS scores and Beighton criteria
De Wandele 2014 [44] Belgium	Case Control	Outpatient clinic	80 EDS-JH 11 classic EDS 7 vascular EDS 38 Fibromyalgia 43 controls	Anxiety: HADS JH: GHQ Others: ASP, QOL, SF 36, GHQ, fatigue checklist, Baecke Physical Activity	The total autonomic symptom burden was higher in EDS-HT (57.9 ± 21.57) than in the other groups but comparable to FM (53.8 ± 19.85)
Murray 2013 USA [45]	cross-sectional	Outpatient clinic	466 adults with EDS JH	237 online survey	High frequency of chronic fatigue (82%), anxiety (73%), depression (69%), and fibromyalgia (42%) among EDS JH

NONCLINICAL STUDIES

STUDY (author/year/country)	DESIGN	SETTING	SAMPLE	VARIABLES STUDIED	MAIN RESULTS
Bulbena* 2004 [26] Spain	Cross sectional	General population	1305 subjects	Anxiety: JH: Beighton MVP	Significant association between JH and PD/A [OR 10.7 (4.8-23.8)] and simple phobia [OR 5.8 (2.0-16.20]. JH patient with MVP do not present with more anxiety
Bulbena* 2004 [29] Spain	Cross sectional	Medical department of an auditing consultancy	526 subjects	Anxiety: STAI JH: Hospital del Mar	Males and females with JHS significantly higher trait anxiety scores (median scores 11 p< 0.05 and 17 p<0.001). Both trait and state anxiety showed significant correlations with JHS (Spearman's rho, 0.10–0.16; P<0.05).
Bulbena* 2006 [27] Spain	Cross sectional	General population	1305 subjects	Anxiety: FSS JH: Beighton	JH group higher fear scores and higher intensity of fears The association of JH and phobic anxiety might represent a susceptibility factor for these anxiety conditions.
Baeza-Velasco* 2009 [35] France	Cross sectional	Internet survey in tall subjects (>180cm females and >190cm males)	158 subjects	Anxiety: LSAS JH: Beighton	High rate of JH and social phobia in tall subjects JH greater social phobia symptoms
Baeza-Velasco* 2010 [36] Chile	Case control	University students	50 JH 50 Control	Anxiety: HADS, LSAS JH:	JH group had higher use of antidepressants and anxiolytics compared to the controls. They also exhibited greater anxiety background, anxiety symptoms and psychosomatic complaints

Baeza-Velasco* 2011 [37] France	Cross sectional	University students	365 subjects	Anxiety: HADS, LSAS JH: Beighton	JH was associated with higher levels of somatosensory amplification as well was higher scores in depression and general anxiety females.
Pailhez* 2011 [28] Spain	Cross sectional	High school students	150 subjects	Anxiety: FSS JH: Hackim & Grahame Others: chocolate rate	Higher fear scores in JH Frequency of chocolate intake higher in JH
Bulbena* 2011 [38] Spain	Cohort study	General population	137 subjects followed 15 years	Anxiety: SCID, STAI, ASI, FSS JH: Beighton, Hospital del Mar Other: GHQ 28	JH RR: PD/A: 22 (5-109) Social phobia: 6.5 (1.7-24.2) Simple phobia: 3.3 (1.1-9.6) GAD: 2.9 (0.97-8.6) JH score higher in social dysfunction subscale and other use of anxiolytics; - Concordance between Beighton scale and Brighton (Kappa=0.91) and Hospital del Mar (Kappa=0.61)
Baeza-Velasco* 2014 [30] France	Cross-sectional	College students	305 females	Anxiety: STAI JH: self administered JH Other: alcohol, cigarettes	More tobacco and alcohol if JHS JH higher scores on state anxiety
Eccles 2012 [31] UK	Cross sectional	General population	72 healthy volunteers	Anxiety: BAI JH: Beighton Other: Brain MRI, PBPQ	Amygdala volume greater in JH JH higher scores in interoceptive sensitivity an anxiety JH linked to brain center implicated with emotions and physiological responses,

Abbreviations

HADS Hospital anxiety and depression scale
ASI: anxiety severity index
EPQ: Eysenck Personality questionnaires
SCID: Structured clinical interview for DSM
HAM: Hamilton anxiety and depression scale
ECHO: echocardiogram
EDS: Ehlers Danlos syndrome
NIMH: self-rating scale of mental symptoms
PSS: Panic symptom scale checklist

VAS: Visual analog scale of anxiety
SCL-90: Symptom checklist 90 R
IBQ: Illness behaviour questionnaire
SQ: Symptom questionnaire
FSF: Function symptoms frequency
PAS: Panic and agoraphobia scale
STAI: state trait anxiety inventory
SPPI: Standardized polyvalent psychiatric interview
LSAS: Liebowitz social anxiety scale
ASP: autonomic symptom profile
QOL: quality of life scale
SF-96: checklist of individual strength
FSS: fear survey schedule
GHQ: general health questionnaire
BAI: Beck anxiety inventory
SSAS Somatosensory amplification scale
PBPQ: Porges body perception questionnaire

Table 6. Characteristics of the clinical and nonclinical studies on the association between joint hypermobility and anxiety. (*) Although most of papers come from the same research group, there is no study duplication. Only Bulbena et al. [26] and Bulbena et al. [27] are extracting results from the same sample but they deal with different variables.

http://dx.doi.org/10.5772/60607

4. The role of psychosomatic mechanisms involved

Once the link between anxiety and the joint laxity syndrome has been established and its association achieved validity and clinical utility, their common etiological and pathophysiological mechanisms ought to be identified. Concerning the etiology and the origin of this "new" revealed condition, so far, only the common genetic linkage has been partially proven. The fact that both conditions (anxiety disorders and joint hyperlaxity syndrome) are highly heritable provides a high likelihood to the genetic etiological pathway. In our first genetic study [46] using pedigree analysis we found duplication in chromosome 15 (15q24-q26 named "DUP25"), which appeared to be present in subjects with both conditions. Although replication studies by other research groups failed to confirm this particular duplication, recent studies of the same chromosome showed complex mental and somatic clinical conditions and also relevant clues for both, anxiety (among other features) and morphological anomalies, either in deletion studies [47] or in supernumerary chromosome markers study [48]. Furthermore, heritability is very often found in both types of patients. It is estimated to be at least 40% in anxiety patients [49] whereas 65% of the hypermobile subjects have at least one first-degree relative suffering from the same condition albeit often goes unnoticed.

In regards to the possible pathophysiology of the link JHS-Anxiety, there are two main sources of evidence. The first source is the so-called dysautonomia, a "blanket term" type of disorder, which has been related to both conditions that controversial but successful concept collects a combination of autonomic disorders, and very often, just collections of anxiety symptoms that are simply named differently [50]. On the other hand, the joint hypermobility syndrome has also been repeatedly related to dysautonomia [51, 52].

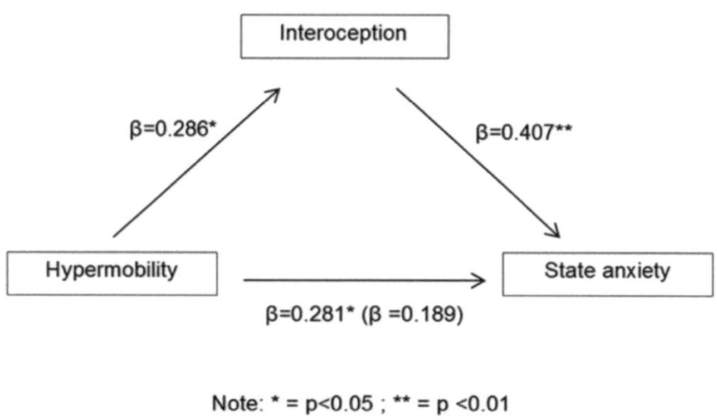

Figure 3. Schematic showing the regression coefficients, with the coefficients (β) for the effect of hypermobility on state anxiety with the latter (when entering interoception into the model) in parentheses.

The second source of evidence for common mechanisms is body awareness, particularly interoception processing. Working together with Prof. Critchley and his group of the Brighton & Sussex Universities, we could confirm a significant correlation between state anxiety score and joint hypermobility [53]. Interoceptive accuracy was associated with both state anxiety and hypermobility and was formally shown to mediate the relationship between these two conditions (Figure 3). Hypermobile participants, when compared to nonhypermobile, displayed heightened neural reactivity to sad and angry scenes in the brain regions implicated in anxiety states, notably in the insular cortex. These findings highlight the dependence of emotional state on bodily context and increase our understanding of the mechanisms through which vulnerability to anxiety disorders arises in people bearing a heritable variant of collagen.

5. The Neuroconnective Phenotype as a new psychosomatic phenotype

When talking about phenotypes in psychiatry, authors tend to include only behavioral and psychopathological traits which again, represents a bias against somatic or body characteristics. Along the first part of the twentieth century, one classic part of the clinical assessment that is currently neglected was the somatotype (i.e., Leptosomatic, Pyknic, and Athletic) after the contributions of Sheldon and Kretschmer. Nevertheless nowadays, somatotype is being used in other areas of medicine away from psychiatry, notably in Sports medicine. Our group carried out several studies assessing somatotype in psychiatric samples in which we could replicate twice the finding of the association of ectomorphic features with both Anxiety and Joint hypermobility [24,25].

The neuroconnective model is reflected in Figure 4 in which together around a common core Anxiety-Collagen hyperlaxity it includes five dimensions that allows minor overlap: behavioral, psychopathology, somatic symptoms, somatosensory symptoms, and somatic illnesses.

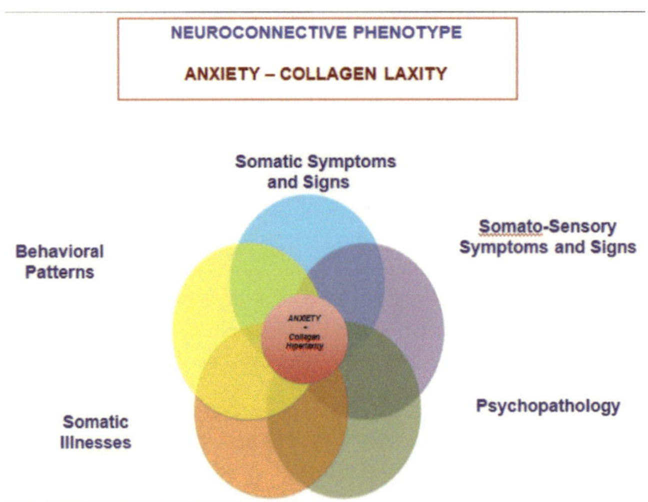

Figure 4. Neuroconnective model of anxiety-collagen laxity.

Two components appear in the core. The first is anxiety and includes any lifetime presence of panic, agoraphobia, specific, and social phobia. Generalized anxiety should be considered when it has reached great severity or when is a residual state of any of the previous disorders. The second component of the core is the Joint Hyperlaxity (hypermobility) Syndrome, which could also be classified as Ehlers–Danlos type III among the hereditary disorders of the connective tissue.

There is a common characteristic of the components of this core, as very often both go unnoticed and undiagnosed. The failure and delay in the initial treatment contact in patients with anxiety disorders is much higher and longer than in mood disorders [54]. On the other hand, the diagnosis of the joint hypermobility syndrome is very often neglected unless there are articular complaints such as pain or collateral manifestations such as sprains or repeated twisted joints. Except for somatic illnesses, which will be dealt with in the next section, we will only summarize the main characteristics of each dimension, without going into detail.

Behavioral dimensions are patterns of defensive mechanisms often identifiable at the extreme of a continuous axis. They include active flight or fight (hypervisibility), passive flight or fight (hypovisibility), trophotropism (increased appetite, sleep, social withdrawal, and rest), ergotropism (decreased appetite, weight, but increased activity, and aggressiveness), overcontrol (ritualism, compulsions), addictions (alcohol and other nonchemical), Restriction (avoidance of spaces, people, activities or delayed use of time, i.e., procrastination), and dependency (of people, spaces, activities).

Somatic symptoms include dysautonomia, asthenic somatotype, dark or "blue" sclera, easy bruising (especially in women), eczemas, esophageal dyskinesia, sprains and dislocations, visceroptosis, prolapses, allergies, dyspareunia, and hypertrophic scars or keloids.

Somatosensory symptoms include increased olfactory sensitivity (especially for negative odors), difficulties in eye contact and sensitivity to some luminous stimuli, dizziness (unsteadiness), sighing, dyspnea, dysphagia or choking, palpitations, urologic and vaginal pains (dynias), joint pain (especially cervical or lumbar) and intolerances, or enhanced sensitivities to weather, drugs (particularly psychotropic), chemicals, heat, or cold.

Psychopathology includes increased exteroception (e.g., meteorosensibility); increased interoception (visceral-body); increased and distorted proprioception; and depersonalization; high loss of sensitivity; anticipatory anxiety; high positive confrontation (high ability to deal with real acute problems); fear of annihilation or neutralization; fear of rejection, abandonment, or neglect; amplification or exaggeration; and denial or avoidance. This dimension would include fears and phobias including fear of medication (side effects or addiction), fear of illness or hypochondriasis, and mood disorder (depression and hypomanic states).

Finally, somatic illnesses include irritable bowel, dysfunctional esophagus, multiple chemical sensitivity, dizziness or unsteadiness (central vestibular pattern), chronic fatigue, fibromyalgia, glossodynia, vulvodynia, hypothyroidism, asthma, migraine, temporomandibular dysfunction, and intolerances or food and drug hypersensitivity.

6. Anxiety disorders do relate to some somatic illnesses: measuring medical conditions in anxiety patients

Patients with anxiety disorders often complain of somatic features, especially cardiac (tachycardia, chest pain), gastrointestinal (epigastric pain), and neurological complaints (headaches, dizziness, or presyncope), in emergencies and primary services [55–57]. This clinical phenomenon helped to deepen into the study of differential diagnoses: are they symptoms of the primary anxiety disorder or are they symptoms of a comorbid physical illness? [58–60]. Besides, more recent research suggests a strong association between anxiety disorders and somatic conditions, although some authors emphasize the huge amount of published research about somatic conditions and depression in contrast to a few studies about the same relationship with anxiety disorders [61–63]. Furthermore, results from the National Comorbidity Survey-Replication (NCS-R) showed that various anxiety disorders had equal or greater association than depression with four chronic physical disorders (hypertension, arthritis, asthma, and ulcers) [64].

The more recent review articles about this relationship are organized according to medical illness specifically associated to anxiety disorders in several descriptive and analytical studies with clinical samples [55,56,62,65,66]. These reviews often include the following somatic conditions: irritable bowel syndrome, asthma, cardiovascular disease, cancer, chronic pain, vestibular and thyroid dysfunction, chronic obstructive pulmonary disease, and mitral valve prolapse. Among the main general conclusions of these reviews are the following: 1) emerging evidence about the bidirectional relationship between anxiety disorders and medical illness suggests that they may be as important as depression [62]; 2) such associations provide important clues for the understanding of the neurobiology of anxiety disorders [55]; and 3) such associations are greater for panic disorder [56, 65], worsening its identification, presentation, and treatment [66].

Despite the significant prognostic and therapeutic implications derived from the comorbidity between mental disorders and medical conditions [55, 62], there is a lack of measuring instruments designed to quantify the physical health and disease in the psychiatric population. Obviously, the use of these instruments in clinical settings is virtually absent. Our group has recently developed a scale (TOPYPS scale) designed to detect and measure functional and organic diseases to be used especially in psychiatric but also in general population.

SIRSs are obtained according to the following criteria:*

Score	Limitation of activity	Treatment	Prognostic	Some examples
0	None	None	Good or mild	Absence of pathology
1	Mild	Not necessary	Mild or moderate	Skin diseases, hemorrhoids, herniae
2	Moderate	Necessary	Moderate	Some cases of diabetes, hypertension, ischemic cardiomyopathy, anxiety disorder
3	Severe	Essential (life risk)	Severe	Some cases of ischemic cardiomyopathy, heart failure, stroke, schizophrenia

*Score SIRS according to the most severe criterion

Figure 5. Criteria for obtaining the SIRS scores in each body system section.

TOPYPS yields a Cumulative Illness Rating Scale (CIRS), and detects, as well, with a high index of suspicion some functional diseases (allergies, migraine, tension-type headache, mitral valve

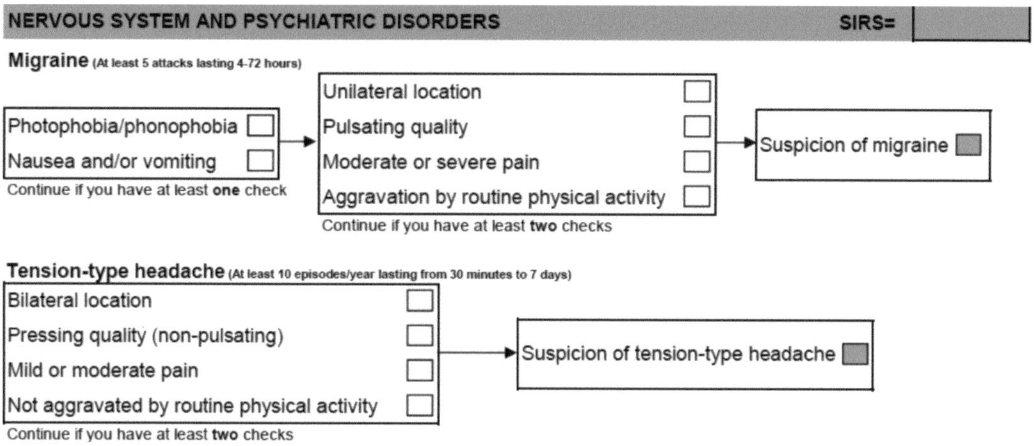

Figure 6. Example of the nervous system and psychiatric disorders section. It collects diagnostic criteria for migraine and tension-type headache.

prolapse syndrome, interstitial cystitis, sexual dysfunction, dyspepsia, functional esophageal disorder, irritable bowel syndrome, fibromyalgia, chronic fatigue, and temporomandibular joint dysfunction) by an interview according to standard diagnostic criteria. TOPYPS has six sections: 1) respiratory, eyes, ears, skin, and annexes; 2) neurological and psychiatric; 3) cardiovascular; 4) genitourinary; 5) digestive, endocrine, and metabolic; 6) musculoskeletal; each one yielding a Specific Illness Rating Scale (SIRS) scored 0–3 according to Figure 5. Figures 6 and 7 are examples of some sections (*the full version of the scale can be requested to the authors by e-mail*). CIRS is obtained at the end by the total sum of the SIRS scores in each section, rated either absent (0 points), mild (1–6), moderate (7–12), or severe (13–18).

The TOPYPS scale was administered to 67 adults randomly chosen from a primary care setting and displayed good psychometrical properties in a Spanish population [67]. Repeatability (test-retest) in each of the six sections (Kappa index) was between 0.72 (musculoskeletal) and 0.968 (respiratory), with an overall average of 0.823 (calculated in all volunteers on two occasions one week apart). Inter-rater agreement was also at its lowest value in the musculoskeletal (0.6) whereas the highest was in the respiratory section (0.78), with an overall average of 0.703. As for the total score, an intraclass correlation index of 0.923 and 0.858 was obtained for the intra- and inter-rater agreement, respectively. Validity was also acceptable (correlation coefficients between 0.726 and 1) according to the correlation of clinical assessments (gold standard) with the SIRS scores in each body system section of TOPYPS. A remarkable degree of agreement (Cohen's kappa between 0.548 and 1) between clinical assessments and diagnostic suspicion of functional diseases according to the scale was also observed. Validity was analysed by comparing the results with the clinical examination performed by two different specialists in general practice. This examination included both the application of the diagnostic criteria for the various functional diseases and the use of a clinical classification based on the same parameters of CIRS ("Gold Standard"). Therefore, TOPYPS scale appears as a suitable tool to detect and measure functional and organic diseases in general population. Our group

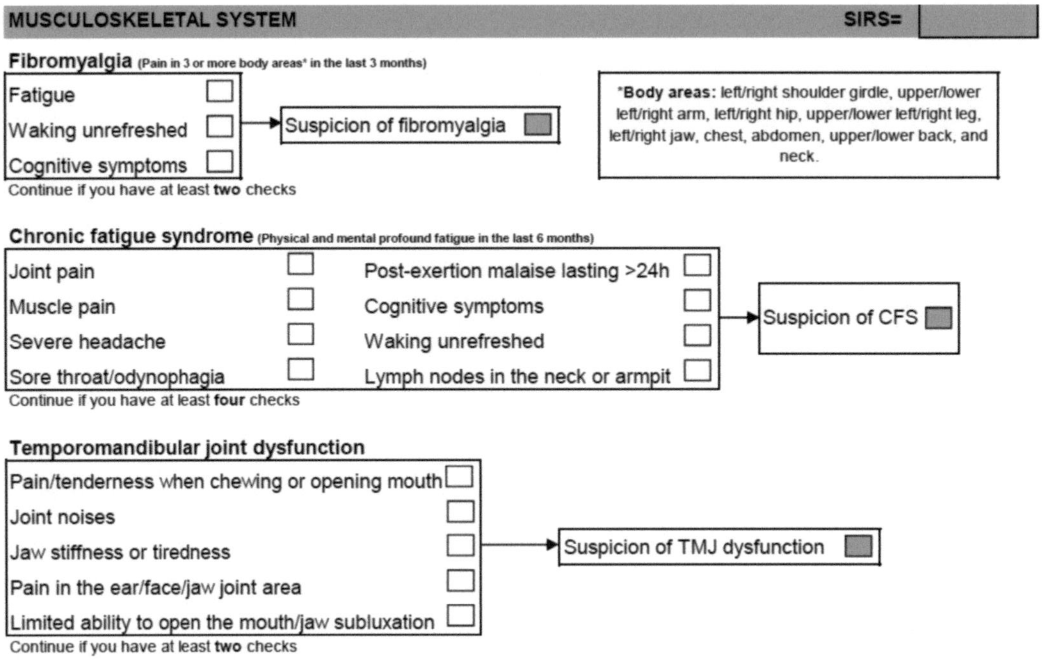

Figure 7. Example of the *musculoskeletal system* section. It collects diagnostic criteria for fibromyalgia, chronic fatigue syndrome and temporomandibular joint dysfunction.

is now actively working on evaluating if patients with panic and/or phobic disorders have a greater burden of somatic conditions than control groups with depressive disorder and with no mental illness.

7. Conclusions

Finally, a number of conclusions can be made after more than 30 years of active research and clinical work in this field. The well-established association between a collagen condition and anxiety has opened new ways to clinical and basic research. Most probably, new forms of psychosomatic conditions will emerge and different nosological approaches will be required. The Neuroconnective model is a proposal under research that may be useful for clinical practice. Nevertheless, new basic and clinical research on this reviewed association is mandatory because it might open new ways to assess, to understand, and to treat our patients.

Acknowledgements

This work was supported by grant from Instituto de Salud Carlos III FEDER (PI10/00987).

http://dx.doi.org/10.5772/60607

Author details

Guillem Pailhez[1,2*], Juan Castaño[1], Silvia Rosado[1], Maria Del Mar Ballester[3], Cristina Vendrell[3], Núria Mallorquí-Bagué[4], Carolina Baeza-Velasco[5] and Antonio Bulbena[1,2]

*Address all correspondence to: pailhezg@hospitaldelmar.cat

1 Neuropsychiatry and Addictions Institute, Hospital del Mar, Barcelona, Spain

2 IMIM (Institut Hospital del Mar d'Investigacions Mèdiques), Barcelona, Spain

3 CAP Ramon Turró, Parc de Salut Mar, Barcelona, Spain

4 Psychiatry, Psychology and Psychosomatics Department, Institut Universitari Quirón Dexeus, Barcelona, Spain

5 Université Paris Descartes - Sorbonne Paris Cité, Paris, France

References

[1] Bulbena A, Duró JC, Mateo A, Porta M, Vallejo J. Joint hypermobility syndrome and anxiety disorders. Lancet 1988;2(8612):694.

[2] Lin PI, Shuldiner AR. Rethinking the genetic basis for comorbidity of schizophrenia and type 2 diabetes. Schizophr Res 2010;123(2–3):234–43.

[3] Baeza-Velasco C, Pailhez G, Bulbena A, Baghdadli A. Joint hypermobility and the heritable disorders of connective tissue: clinical and empirical evidence of links with psychiatry. Gen Hosp Psychiatry 2014.http://dx.doi.org/10.1016/j.genhosppsych.2014.10.002

[4] Rotés-Querol J, Argany A. La laxité articulaire comme facteur des altérations de l'appareil locomoteur. Rev Rhum Mal Osteoartic 1957;24(7–8):535–9.

[5] Flanders H. Mind and Body. Psychosomatic Medicine. Boston: Random House; 1955.

[6] Carlsson C, Rundgren A. Hypermobility of the joints in women alcoholics. J Stud Alcohol 1980;41(1):78–81.

[7] Carter C, Wilkinson J. Persistent joint laxity and congenital dislocation of the hip. J Bone Joint Surg Brit Vol 1964;46:40–5.

[8] Beighton P, Solomon L, Soskolne CL. Articular mobility in an African population. Ann Rheumatic Dis 1973;32(5):413–8.

[9] Beighton P, Grahame R, Bird H. Hypermobility of Joints. 1st ed. London: Springer; 1983.

[10] Beighton P, Grahame R, Bird H. Hypermobility of Joints. 3rd ed. London: Springer; 1999.

[11] Grahame R. Hypermobility: an important but often neglected area within rheumatology. Nat Clin Pract Rheumatol 2008;4(10):524.

[12] Hakim AJ, Kerr R, Grahame R. Hypermobility, Fibromyalgia, and Chronic Pain. London: Churchill Livingstone; 2010.

[13] Bravo JF. Síndrome de Ehlers-Danlos con especial énfasis en el síndrome de hiperlaxitud articular. Rev Med Chile 2009;137:1488–97.

[14] Keer R, Grahame R. Hypermobility Syndrome: Recognition and Management for Physiotherapists. London: Butterworth – Heinemann; 2003.

[15] Mishra MB, Ryan P, Atkinson P, Taylor H, Bell J, Calver D, Fogelman I, Child A, Jackson G, Chambers JB, Grahame R. Extra-articular features of benign joint hypermobility syndrome. Br J Rheumatol 1996;35:861–6.

[16] Hakim AJ, Grahame R. A simple questionnaire to detect hypermobility: an adjunct to the assessment of patients with diffuse musculoskeletal pain. Int J Clin Pract 2003;57:163–6.

[17] Bulbena A, Mallorquí-Bagué N, Pailhez G, et al. Self-reported screening questionnaire for the assessment of joint hypermobility syndrome (SQ-CH), a collagen condition, in Spanish population. Eur J Psychiatry 2014;28(1):17–26.

[18] Bulbena A, Duró JC, Porta M, Faus S, Vallescar R, Martín-Santos R. Clinical assessment of hypermobility of joints: assembling criteria. J Rheumatol 1992;19:115–2.

[19] Grahame R, Bird HA, Child A, Dolan L, Edwards-Fowler A, Ferrell WR, et al. The revised (Brighton 1998) criteria for the diagnosis of benign joint hypermobility syndrome. J Rheumatol 2000;27:1777–177.

[20] Bulbena A, Benito P (dirs.). Pailhez G, Gago J, Carbonell J, Sperry L, Ros S. Joint Hyperlaxity: Definition and Clinical Assessment. Interactive CD Training Software. Barcelona: Almirall Prodesfarma; 2003.

[21] Bulbena A, Duró JC, Porta M, Martín-Santos R, Mateo A, Molina L, Vallescar R, Vallejo J. Anxiety disorder in the joint hypermobility syndrome. Psychiatry Res 1993;43:59–68.

[22] Martín-Santos R, Bulbena A, Porta M, Gago J, Molina L, Duró JC. Association between the joint hypermobility syndrome and panic disorder. Am J Psychiatry 1998;155:1578–83.

[23] Lumley MA, Jordan M, Rubenstein R, Tsipouras P, Evans M. Psychosocial functioning in the Ehlers-Danlos syndrome. Am J Med Genet 1994;53:149–52.

[24] Bulbena A, Martín-Santos R, Porta M, Duró JC, Gago J, Sangorrín J, Gratacós M. Somatotype in panic patients. Anxiety 1996;2(2):80–5.

[25] Pailhez G, Rosado S, Baeza-Velasco C, Bulbena A. Ectomorphic somatotype and joint hypermobility are linked in panic and agoraphobic patients: a case-control study. Int J Psychiatry Clin Pract 2014;18(2):112–7.

[26] Bulbena A, Gago J, Martín-Santos R, Porta M, Dasquens J, Berrios GE. Anxiety disorder & joint laxity a definitive link. Neurol Psychiatry Brain Res 2004;l11:137–40.

[27] Bulbena A, Gago J, Sperry L, Berge D. The relationship between frequency and intensity of fears and a collagen condition. Depress Anxiety 2006;23:412–7.

[28] Pailhez G, Rosado S, Bulbena-Cabre A, Bulbena A. Joint hypermobility fears and chocolate consumption. J Nervous Mental Dis 2011;199:903–6.

[29] Bulbena A, Agullo A, Pailhez G, Martin-Santos R, Porta M, Guitart J, Gago J. Is joint hypermobility related to anxiety in a nonclinical population also? Psychosomatics 2004; 45:432–7.

[30] Baeza-Velasco C, Stoebner-Delbarre A, Cousson-Gélie F, Pailhez G, Bulbena A, Baguet F, Gély-Nargeot MC. Increased tobacco and alcohol use among women with joint hypermobility: a way to cope with anxiety? Rheumatol Int 2015;35:177–81.

[31] Eccles JA, Beacher FD, Gray MA, Jones CL, Minati L, Harrison NA, Critchley HD. Brain structure and joint hypermobility: relevance to the expression of psychiatric symptoms. Br J Psychiatry 2012;200(6):508–9.

[32] Bulbena A, Anguiano JB, Gago J, Basterreche E, Ballesteros J, Eguiluz I, González Torres ME, Reddy DP, Coplan JD, Berrios GE. Panic/phobic anxiety in schizophrenia: a positive association with joint hypermobility syndrome. Neurol Psychiatry Brain Res 2005;12:1–6.

[33] Bulbena A, Sperry L, Anguinano B, Pailhez G, Gago J. Joint hypermobility in schizophrenia: a potential marker for co-morbid anxiety. Open Psychiatry J 2007;1:31–3.

[34] Picado M, Carmona S, Pailhez G, Cortizo R, Planet R, Bergé D, Hoekzema E, Moreno A, Rovira M, Tobeña A, Bulbena A, Vilarroya O. Specific structural abnormalities in schizophrenia anxiety and the comorbidity among them. 16th Annual Meeting of the Organization for Human Brain Mapping, June 6–10, 2010, Barcelona, Spain.

[35] Baeza-Velasco C, Bulbena A. Ansiedad social y alteración de colágeno en personas de gran estatura. C Med Psicosom 2009;89/90:40–46.

[36] Baeza-Velasco C, Bulbena A, Bravo J. Sintomatología ansiosa y sindrome de hiperlaxitud articular en un grupo de universitarios chilenos. Ansiedad y Estrés 2010; 16(1): 1–12.

[37] Baeza-Velasco C, Gély-Nargeot MC, Bulbena A, Fenetrier C, Bravo JF. Association between psychopathological factors and joint hypermobility syndrome in a group of undergraduates from a French University. Int J Psychiatry Med 2011; 41(2):187–201

[38] Bulbena A, Gago J, Pailhez G, Sperry L, Fullana MA, Vilarroya O. Joint hypermobility syndrome is a risk factor trait for anxiety disorders: a 15-year follow-up cohort study. General Hosp Psychiatry 2011;l33:363–70.

[39] Benjamin J, Ben-Zion IZ, Dannon P, Schreiber S, Meiri G, Ofek A, Palatnik A. Lack of association between joint hyperlaxity and I: panic disorder and II: reactivity to carbon dioxide in healthy volunteers. Hum Psychopharmacol 2001;16:189–192.

[40] Gulpek D, Bayraktar E, Akbay SP, Capaci K, Kayikcioglu M, Aliyev E, Soydas C. Joint hypermobility syndrome and mitral valve prolapse in panic disorder. Prog Neuropsychopharmacol Biol Psychiatry 2004;28:969–73.

[41] Gulsun M, Yilmaz MB, Pinar M, Tonbul M, Celik C, Ozdemir B, Dumlu K, Erbas M. Thorax deformity joint hypermobility and anxiety disorders. Saudi Med J 2007;28:1840–4.

[42] Ercolani M, Galvani M, Franchini C, Baracchini F, Chattat R. Benign joint hypermobility syndrome: psychological features and psychopathological symptoms in a sample pain-free at evaluation. Percept Mot Skills 2008;107(1):246–56.

[43] García-Campayo J, Asso E, Alda M, Andres EM, Sobradiel N. Association between joint hypermobility syndrome and panic disorder: a case-control study. Psychosomatics 2010;51:55–61.

[44] De Wandele I, Calders P Peersman W, Rimbaut S, De Backer T, Malfait F, De Paepe A, Rombaut L. Autonomic symptom burden in the hypermobility type of Ehlers-Danlos syndrome: a comparative study with two other EDS types, fibromyalgia, and healthy controls. Semin Arthritis Rheum 2014. doi:10.1016/j.semarthrit.2014.05.013.

[45] Murray B, Yashar BM, Uhlmann WR, Clauw DJ, Petty EM. Ehlers-Danlos syndrome, hypermobility type: a characterization of the patients' lived experience. Am J Med Genet A 2013;161A(12):2981–8.

[46] Gratacos M, Nadal M, Martín-Santos R, Pujana M, Gago J, Peral B, Armengol L, Ponsa I, Miró R, Bulbena A, Estivill X. A polymorphic genomic duplication on human chromosome 15 is a susceptibility factor for panic and phobic disorders. Cell 2001; l106:367–79.

[47] Palumbo O, Palumbo P, Palladino T, Stallone R, Miroballo M, Piemontese MR, Zelante L, Carella M. An emerging phenotype of interstitial 15q25.2 microdeletions: Clinical report and review. Am J Med Genet Part A 2012;158A: 3182–9.

[48] Kleefstra T, de Leeuw N, Wolf R, Nillesen WM, Schobers G, Mieloo H, Willemsen M, Perrotta CS, Poddighe PJ, Feenstra I, Draaisma J, van Ravenswaaij-Arts CMA. Phenotypic spectrum of 20 novel patients with molecularly defined supernumerary marker

chromosomes 15 and a review of the literature. Am J Med Genet Part A 2010;152A: 2221–9.

[49] Hettema JM, Neale MC, Kendler KS. A review and meta-analysis of the genetic epidemiology of anxiety disorders. Am J Psychiatry 2001;158:1568–78.

[50] Bulbena A, Pailhez G, Gago J. "Connective tissue" between panic disorder and dysautonomia. The American Journal of Medicine 2004;116(11):783–4.

[51] Gazit Y, Nahir AM, Grahame R, Jacob G. Dysautonomia in the joint hypermobility syndrome. Am J Med 2003;115(1):33–40.

[52] Kanjwal K, Saeed B, Karabin B, Kanjwal Y, Grubb BP. Comparative clinical profile of postural orthostatic tachycardia patients with and without joint hypermobility syndrome. Indian Pacing Electrophysiol J 2010;10(4):173–8.

[53] Mallorquí-Bagué N, Garfinkel SN, Engels M, Eccles JA, Pailhez G, Bulbena A, Critchley HD. Neuroimaging and psychophysiological investigation of the link between anxiety, enhanced affective reactivity and interoception in people with joint hypermobility. Frontiers in psychology 2014. doi: 10.3389/fpsyg.2014.01162.

[54] Wang PS, Berglund P, Olfson M, Pincus HA, Wells KB, Kessler RC. Failure and delay in initial treatment contact after first onset of mental disorders in the National Comorbidity Survey Replication. Arch Gen Psychiatry 2005;62(6):603–13.

[55] Muller JE, Koen L, Stein DJ. Anxiety and medical disorders. Curr Psychiatry Rep 2005;7:245–51.

[56] Wells KB, Golding JM, Burnam MA. Chronic medical conditions in a sample of the general population with anxiety, affective, and substance use disorders. Am J Psychiatry 1989;146:1440–6.

[57] Zaubler TS, Katon W. Panic disorder in the general medical setting. J Psychosomatic Res 1998;44:25–42.

[58] Katon W, Roy-Byrne P. Panic disorder in the medically ill. J Clin Psychiatry 1989; 50:299–302.

[59] Stein MB. Panic disorder and medical illness. Psychosomatics 1986; 27:833–40.

[60] Wise MG, Taylor SE. Anxiety and mood disorders in medically ill patients. J Clin Psychiatry 1990;51:27–32.

[61] Härter MC, Conway KP, Merikangas KR. Associations between anxiety disorders and physical illness. Eur Arch Psychiatry Clin Neurosci 2003;253:313–20.

[62] Roy-Byrne PP, Davidson KW, Kessler RC, Asmundson GJ, Goodwin RD, Kubzansky L, Lydiard RB, Massie MJ, Katon W, Laden SK, Stein MB. Anxiety disorders and comorbid medical illness. Gen Hosp Psychiatry 2008;30:208–25.

[63] Sareen J, Cox BJ, Clara I, Asmundson GJ. The relationship between anxiety disorders and physical disorders in the U.S. National Comorbidity Survey. Depress Anxiety 2005;21:193–202.

[64] Kessler RC, Ormel J, Demler O, Stang PE. Comorbid mental disorders account for the role impairment of commonly occurring chronic physical disorders: results from the National Comorbidity Survey. J Occup Environ Med 2003; 45:1257–66.

[65] Katon W. Panic disorder: Relationship to high medical utilization, unexplained physical symptoms, and medical costs. J Clin Psychiatry 1996;57:11–18.

[66] Simon NM, Fischmann D. The implications of medical and psychiatric comorbidity with panic disorder. J Clin Psychiatry 2005;66:8–15.

[67] Pailhez G, Rosado S, Castaño J, Vendrell C, Ballester M, Mallorquí-Bagué N, Baeza-Velasco C, Bulbena A. Detecting and measuring functional and organic disease in general population: validation of TOPYPS clinical scale. 14th International Forum on Mood and Anxiety Disorders, December 10–12, 2014, Vienna, Austria.

Chapter 9

Anxiety in Natural and Surgical Menopause — Physiologic and Therapeutic Bases

Juan Francisco Rodríguez-Landa,
Abraham Puga-Olguín,
León Jesús Germán-Ponciano,
Rosa-Isela García-Ríos and Cesar Soria-Fregozo

Additional information is available at the end of the chapter

http://dx.doi.org/10.5772/60621

Abstract

Generalized anxiety disorder is one of the most common psychiatric disorders, affecting a high percentage of human beings around the world. This emotional disorder possesses marked gender differences and occurs more often in women than in men, in a proportion of 2:1. Accompanying the reproductive cycle of women are significant fluctuations in plasma and brain steroid hormone concentrations, including oestradiol, progesterone, and allopregnanolone, among others. These hormonal changes are related to some illnesses and with the development of anxiety and mood swings occurring in the premenstrual and postpartum period, and particularly during the menopause. Menopause is a clinical term used to indicate the cessation of the woman's reproductive ability that occurs naturally, but also may be surgically induced by bilateral oophorectomy, with or without the removal of the Fallopian tubes and uterus. Natural menopause includes specific periods related to the physiological and hormonal changes produced by ovarian failure, it is usually a natural stage that occurs to women in midlife, during their late 40s or early 50s, indicating the end of the reproductive period in the woman. During the menopause transition years, women experience changes in the production of ovarian hormones, which are associated with significant changes in the physiological, emotional, and affective processes. Unfortunately, surgical menopause occurs at an early age, and produces similar physiological and psychiatric disorders, but they are more severe in this instance. In both cases, typical symptoms associated with menopause critically deteriorate the mental health of the women. In this way, the therapeutic management of clinical symptoms of menopause include replacement hormone therapy, the use of anxiolytic and antidepressant drugs, and other natural alternatives based on the use of chemical compounds obtained from plants such as soya. However, a general effective treatment for menopause symptoms does not yet exist. For this reason, experimental studies have proposed ovariectomy in rats as a potential tool to study the effects of a long-term absence of ovarian hormones associated with surgical menopause, which also allowed the study of substances with potential therapeutic application to ameliorate typical symptoms associated with surgical menopause. The aim of this chapter is to review the participation of ovarian hormones in the regulation of emotional and affective disorders in women with natural or surgical menopause; particularly their anatomical pathways, neurotransmission systems, and the resulting behavioural patterns. Finally, preclinical and clinical research suggested that long-term absence of ovarian hormones associated with natural or surgical menopause is the principal cause of physiological and psychiatric disorder in the women; therefore, oestrogenic compounds seem to play an important role in the maintenance of the brain structures that regulate anxiety, mood, memory, and cognitive functions in menopausal women.

Keywords: Anxiety, natural menopause, surgical menopause, oestrogens, experimental model, ovariectomy

1. Introduction

Generalized anxiety disorder is one of the most common psychiatric disorders, affecting a high percentage of the general population around the world. This psychopathology possesses marked gender differences and occurs more often in women than in men [1]. During the reproductive cycle of women, fluctuations occur in plasma and brain steroid hormone concentrations, including oestradiol, progesterone, and allopregnanolone: a reduced metabolite of progesterone. These hormonal changes are related to some illnesses and the development of anxiety and mood swings [2].

Low concentrations of steroid hormones are associated with irritability, anxiety, or depressive symptoms, and occur during the premenstrual, post-partum, and climacteric or post-menopausal periods. In particular, natural or surgical post-menopause is mainly characterized by a reduction of both oestradiol and progesterone because of failing ovarian function. These hormonal changes are associated with a major incidence of vasomotor symptoms, vaginal dryness, osteoporosis, cognitive deterioration, and hot flashes accompanied by perspiration, palpitations, irritability, anxiety, and mood swings. Unfortunately, emotional and affective alterations associated with the long-term absence of ovarian hormones are more severe in women who have undergone surgical menopause than women who experienced natural menopause. Disturbingly, surgical menopause is occurring more frequently in young women, in an economically productive stage, which impacts on the economy, on their quality of life, and, unfortunately, on their mental health [3].

Treatment of anxiety and depressive symptoms associated with the long-term absence of ovarian hormones produced by natural or surgical menopause, includes the use of benzodiazepines (i.e., diazepam), some selective serotonin reuptake inhibitors (i.e., fluoxetine or paroxetine), and hormone replacement therapy (i.e., oestrogens, or a combination of oestrogens plus progestagens), among others. Hormone replacement therapy has been used to ameliorate physiological, behavioural, and emotional alterations in post-menopausal women; for example, to reduce bone loss, hot flashes, irritability, and mood swings [4, 5]. Nevertheless, hormone replacement therapy is associated with several side-effects limiting their long-term use in vulnerable women. In this way, some investigations focusing on finding new therapeutic alternatives have explored the effects of some vegetables such as soya that contains high concentrations of the phyto-oestrogens genistein, daidzein, glycitein, and their conjugate metabolites. In some reports, there is evidence that phyto-oestrogens produces physiological effects similar to that produced by endogenous oestrogens. Apparently, these effects occur through actions on the oestradiol receptor-β [6, 7], which has been involved in the anxiolytic-like effect of endogenous and synthetic oestrogens at the experimental level.

To study the effect of the long-term absence of ovarian hormones associated with surgical menopause in the women, ovariectomy in rats has been used at a preclinical level as a potential tool to explore alterations in diverse organs and systems [8]. A rat experiencing a long-term absence of ovarian hormones induced by ovariectomy is considered as an early model of surgical menopause, which has allowed studying changes in cardiovascular, reproductive, motor, and bone systems, as well as changes in the sensitivity of neurotransmitter receptors in the brain. These changes in the brain impact negatively on the behaviour of the rats, producing higher indicators of anxiety-like behaviour and despair [6, 9]. Such facts support the hypothesis that rats with a chronic absence of ovarian hormones induced by ovariectomy could help us to understand the anxiety and mood swings typical of women who have undergone surgical menopause, as well as to screen new substances that could ameliorate anxiety symptoms in this particular group of women.

The aim of this chapter is to review the participation of ovarian hormones in the regulation of emotional and affective disorders in women experiencing natural or surgical menopause, particularly their anatomical pathways, neurotransmission systems, and the resulting behavioural patterns. Additionally, the principal pharmacological therapies used to ameliorate physiological and psychological symptoms in natural and surgical menopause will be discussed.

2. Natural and surgical menopause

Menopause is a clinical term used to indicate the cessation of a woman's reproductive ability. It may occur naturally, but also may be surgically induced by bilateral oophorectomy (removal of ovaries), with or without removal of the Fallopian tubes (salpingo-oophorectomy), and uterus (hysterectomy). Natural menopause includes specific periods (Figure 1) related with the physiological and hormonal changes produced by ovarian failure (Table 1). Menopause is usually a natural stage that occurs to women in midlife, during their late 40s or early 50s, indicating the end of the reproductive period in the woman [2]. During the menopause transition years, the women experiment fluctuations in the production and release of ovarian hormones, which produces significant changes in the physiological and affective processes. Not every woman experiences bothersome levels of these effects; it varies greatly from person to person and also depends of their lifestyles. Most women experience that their menstrual periods are gradually becoming less frequent, and that the timing of the start of the flow is usually less predictable.

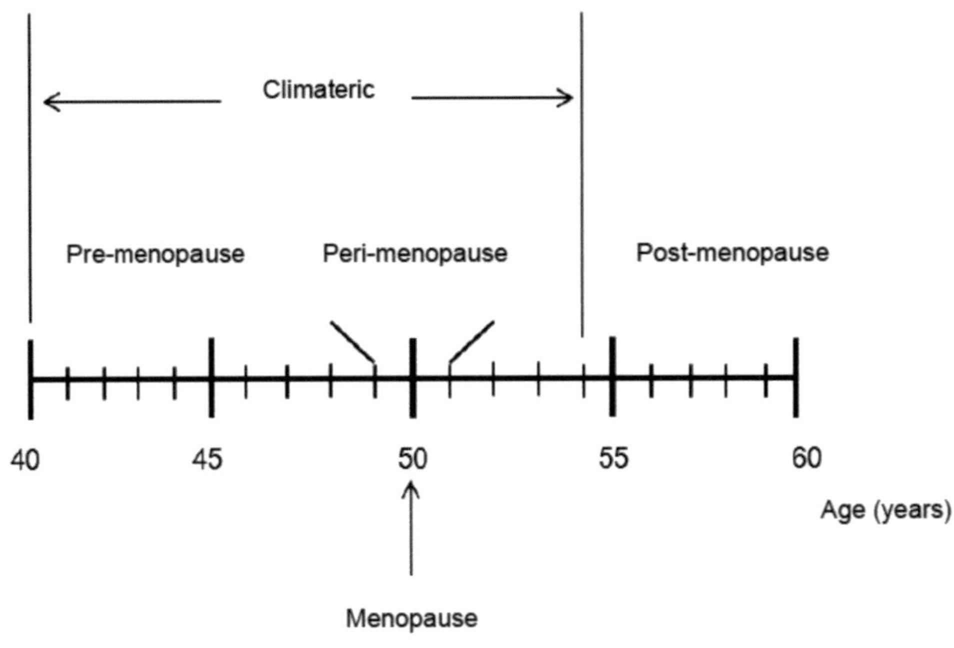

Figure 1. Scheme illustrating the different phases that characterized the end of the reproductive period in women, under natural conditions.

The beginning of menopause (the last period from natural causes) typically occurs in an age range between 40 and 61 years, [10] with an average age for the last period of 51 years [12]. The average age of natural menopause in the majority of women occurs at 51 years [11], however, in some countries (i.e., the Philippines and India), the median age of natural menopause occurs earlier, at 44 years. [13]. Nonetheless, the World Health Organization indicates that the menopause occurs at the average age of 45–55 years around the world.

During natural or surgical menopause there are significant reductions of ovarian hormones' concentrations, particularly oestradiol, progesterone, and their metabolites. This influences the beginning of menopausal symptoms, including bone density loss and vasomotor alterations, accompanied by irritability, anxiety, and depression in some cases [2, 6, 14, 15]. Natural menopause is caused by follicular atresia in which there are ovarian follicles that do not respond to gonadotrophynes; for this reason, the ovaries lose their function, ovulation ceases, and the reproductive period of the woman ends. In this state, the oestrogen concentrations are lowest, increasing the follicular stimulant hormone (FSH) and luteinizing hormone (LH) in a minor proportion [16].

Term	Description
Premenopause	Is a term used to mean the years leading up to the last menstrual period, when the concentrations of ovarian hormones are already becoming more variable and lower, and the effects of hormone withdrawal are present.
Perimenopause	It term refers to the menopause transition years, a span of time both before *and* after the date of the final menstrual period; which can last for four to eight years. It period may occur during six to ten year, ending approximately 12 months after the last menstrual period.
Menopause	Clinically, menopause is defined as the last menstrual flow period. It is necessary taken in count that this moment may only be identified retrospectively, once 12 months have gone without experiment any menstrual flow. Commonly, menopause is used to referrer to menopause transition years, but not the last menstrual period.
Postmenopause	This term include the period after 12 months without menstrual flow, assuming that women still have a uterus, and are not pregnant or lactating. Physiologically, this period is characterized by very high follicular stimulant hormone concentration (FSH) at plasma level. Thus postmenopause is all of the time that follows the point when her ovaries become inactive, evidenced by last menstrual period.

Table 1. Terms associated with natural menopause

On the other hand, surgical menopause is associated with sudden and complete reduction of oestradiol, progesterone, and testosterone plasma concentrations [17], which predisposes the appearance of physiological and psychiatric alterations, such as occur in natural menopause, but with greater intensity.

3. Anxiety disorders and mood swings associated with natural or surgical menopause in women

Menopause is a stage of biological development of women that implies physiological, psychological, and social changes. During menopause, women are vulnerable to cognitive and physical impairment as well as psychiatric illnesses as anxiety and depression. Hot flushes; night sweating; skin dryness and mucosa; even vaginal dryness; sleep disorders; and cognitive and behavioural changes are symptoms that deteriorate a woman's quality of life [18]. Mild anxiety and stress vulnerability are common in premenopause; while anxiety, depression, and irritability are more intense during perimenopause [19]. Anxiety disorders tend to be more chronic compared to mood disorders (i.e., depression) in a woman suffering during the menopause [20]. It is noteworthy that emotional and affective disorders are more severe in cases of surgical menopause compared with natural menopause, apparently due to the drastic suppression of hormonal production and the psychosocial context of the surgery and related illness.

During natural menopause, ovarian hormones biosynthesis (i.e., oestrogens and androgens) becomes gradually reduced, while surgical menopause is characterized by a drastic hormonal suppression. This reduction of hormone concentrations influences the impairment in neuronal functioning responsible for a predisposition to develop anxiety disorders and changes in general mood, mostly in woman with records of psychiatric illness. Women who had experienced disorders such as premenstrual syndrome or dysphoric premenstrual syndrome in their life, experience menopause with a certain degree of liberty and comfort with respect to their sexuality; on the other hand, women with records of psychiatric disorders can experience emotional and affective disorders more severely [21].

It has been found that between the ages of 42 to 52 years, women with high levels of anxiety during premenopause continue to experience this during menopause. Premenopausal woman with low levels of anxiety can be more susceptible to increased levels of anxiety during and after menopause transition [22]. Consistent with that findings, Jafari et al., 2014 [23], found that post-menopausal women, between the ages of 45 and 55, have high levels of anxiety compared to premenopausal women between 35 and 45.

Some authors have suggested that transition to menopause is the stage with the most risk of developing or increasing the symptoms of anxiety. Anxiety disorders such as panic disorder, social phobia, or generalized anxiety do not vary with the different stages of menopause [24]. However, studies showed that during the perimenopause, anxiety symptoms are higher than symptoms in pre- and post-menopause. Approximately 74% of women undergoing natural menopause experience hot flushes [24], which are associated with the development of anxiety symptoms. It is still controversial if anxiety develops before or in consequence of the vascular symptoms (i.e., hot flushes and night sweating) that characterized menopause.

Respecting the severity of the symptoms associated with menopause, there exists a considerable variation between samples. African-American women report similar symptoms of anxiety and panic attacks, but a higher degree of severity in vascular motor symptoms (i.e., hot flushes in the chest and head, palpitations, and sweating) when compared with Asiatic women [25]. This difference in symptoms has been associated with lifestyles and nutrition as well as particularities in metabolic activity and the disruption of some neurotransmission systems in the brain [26], but it is not yet clear if anxiety precedes vascular symptoms or vice versa. On the other hand, a close negative relation between the severity of anxiety and depression symptoms and quality of life has been reported. In this sense, post-menopausal women with a low quality of life showed a higher index of anxiety and symptoms of depression than pre-menopausal women with a good quality of life [23].

Symptoms of anxiety, irritability, depression, bluntness, mnesic disease, impairment of general capacity, and sleep disorders are the most frequent motives in women with perimenopause to attend to medical consultation [18]. It is common that women that refer to psychological discomfort in medical consultation during the whole menopause span are also the women that show less self-esteem and a low personal satisfaction [23]. Additionally, there is a relation between hormone levels and psychological wellbeing in menopausal women. For example, depression seems to increase when hormonal fluctuations occur in perimenopause, possibly as result of a lack of regulation of oestrogens over serotonergic activity and other neurotransmission systems in the brain [21]. Variations in circulating levels of androgens are related to mood disorders in young post-menopausal women, establishing a direct relation between androgen concentrations and symptoms of anxiety and depression in post-menopause [27].

Panic disorder is one of the most common anxiety disorders during menopause; it can develop once menopause has been completely established. Such disorder is more frequent in women with evident physical symptoms during menopause. In three groups of women classified in different ages (i.e., 50 to 59, 60 to 69, and 70 to 79 years old), panic attacks were more frequent in women between 50 to 59 years old. This group probably experienced perimenopause with variations in ovarian hormones production, an increased vulnerability to psychological stress, and somatic symptoms that can be more intense, which can increase the probability of developing anxiety. Other factors include negative experiences in life, general physical impairment, and comorbidity with other illness [28]. For example, women from 51 to 83 years old experienced at least one episode of panic attacks during the six months previous to suffering from a cardiovascular disorder, with a prevalence of 10%. It seems that anxiety is a risk factor that increases morbidity and mortality associated to cardiovascular illness in post-menopausal women [29].

Obsessive-compulsive disorder (OCD) is a mental illness associated with different events in the reproductive life of a woman. There are reports of a 47% of incidence of OCD during menopause while this percentage decreases considerably in post-menopausal women to 9 %. Although there are studies about the relation of menopause and OCD, the data are contradictory [30]. One research on women suffering natural or surgical post-menopause measured prevalence and comorbidity of OCD, the prevalence of OCD was about 7.1% and the more common obsessions was cleanliness, while the most common compulsions were cleanliness/washing. Comorbidity for the different disorders was 63.2 %, with comorbidity and generalized anxiety being the most frequent [31].

In relation to panic disorder (PD), some studies have related PD with vascular disturbances in perimenopausal women that attended medical consultation, with a prevalence of 18%. However, this research did not specify how it determined menopause onset; it seems the researchers used only verbal reports of patients [32], so these results must be interpreted carefully.

Concerning surgical menopause, very little literature about anxiety attacks and this kind of menopause exists. One medical case reported that a woman with a surgical extirpation of ovarian developed physiological and psychological changes similar to those of natural menopause, but also immediately developed symptoms of severe anxiety that impaired her quality of life [33]. The emotional and affective symptoms associated with surgical menopause vary between individuals, but it has been reported that bilateral extirpation of ovaries before natural menopause is related to the development of anxiety disorders and the increase of cognitive impairment risk, compared with women that experience natural menopause [34].

In summary, reported data associating anxiety disorders to natural or surgical menopause are still contradictory, perhaps due to differences between the populations of study and the variations in criteria for measuring both menopause and anxiety. Some studies report that symptoms of anxiety increase during perimenopause and decrease later in post-menopause [35]. Other studies suggest that anxiety symptoms are not directly related to a particular stage of menopause [36]. For example, Freeman et al. (2005) [37] reported that previous medical records of depression and stress vulnerability are strong predictors of anxiety during menopause, while Moilanen et al. (2010) [36] only related the lifestyle (i.e., obesity, sedentary lifestyle, and alcohol consumption) with the predisposition to suffer anxiety episodes during natural menopause. Besides, most of the investigations do not offer solid data about prevalence of anxiety disorders that fulfil the diagnostic criteria. It seems that most of the few studies comparing natural and surgical menopause have found a relation between vascular alterations and symptoms of anxiety; however, this relationship is not definitive since it must be assured that somatic and psychological symptoms were not confused with anxiety symptoms in these studies' particular populations. At the time of writing, predisposal factors of emotional and affective alterations during natural or surgical menopause have not been clearly identified, but it seems evident that during menopausal stages there is an increased vulnerability to stress which increases the prevalence of anxiety and depression symptoms that impair quality of life during natural or surgical menopause. This makes necessary specific studies with standardized criteria for measuring the factors that produce these disorders in order to design therapeutic strategies, including pharmacological treatments that improve the quality of life of women suffering natural or surgical menopause.

4. Pharmacological treatment of anxiety disorders in menopausal women: Benefits versus side-effects

Despite the evidence that in natural and surgical menopause there is a high incidence of anxiety and depression disorders, there are few controlled studies evaluating the efficacy of pharmacological treatments in this particular population, while there is a worryingly high frequency of self-medication using anxiolytic drugs in menopausal women. Treatment selection for controlling the symptoms of menopausal women requires establishing a balance between the benefits on mood and the potential risks to health. It is very important to consider the clinical background of the patient; in cases of young women who have undergone surgical menopause

http://dx.doi.org/10.5772/60621

at an early age (24 to 38 years old), efficiency of the pharmacological response can vary compared with women who experienced natural menopause.

The therapeutic treatment for the control of symptoms of anxiety includes hormonal replacement therapy, antidepressant with anxiolytic activity, and some therapies based on the use of chemical compounds isolated from vegetables (i.e., soya), which have shown certain anxiolytic potential (Table 2).

Type of Therapy	Condition (Average age)	Dosage	Therapeutic effects	Side-effects	Reference
Hormonal Ethinyl estradiol	Bilateral oophorectomy (24 year)	(3.9 mg / week; td; 3 mouth)	Without Anxiolytic effects	Increased risk of endometrial hyperplasia and cancers other, venous thromboembolic events and stroke (Hickey et al., 2005).	[34]
	Bilateral oophorectomy (46 year)	(3.9 mg / week; td; 3 month)	Anxiolytic		[34]
	Hysterectomy and bilateral oophorectomy	(3.9 mg / week; td; 6 mouth)	Anxiolytic		[41]
Tibolone	Hysterectomy and bilateral oophorectomy (47 year)	(2.5 mg/day; v. o.; 6 month)	Anxiolytic	Increased risk of stroke in women over 60 years (Cummings et al., 2008). Nausea, headache, breast tenderness, weight gain, bloating (Gupta et al., 2013).	[41, 43]
	Hysterectomy and bilateral oophorectomy (50 year)	(2.5 mg/day; v. o.; 12 month)	Anxiolytic		[87]
	Natural menopause	(2.5 mg/day; v. o.; 3 month)	Anxiolytic		[42]
Estradiol valerianate-dehydroepiandrosterone enanthate (Gynodian Depo)	Hysterectomy with bilateral oophorectomy (35-45 year)	(4 mg/200 mg/ month; i.m.; 3 month)	Anxiolytic	Pruritus, eczema, urticaria, skin reactions at the site of injection, hair loss, erythema nodosum, acne (PLM, 2015).	[86]
17β-estradiol	Natural menopause	(50 mg/day; t.d.; 3 month)	Anxiolytic	Increased risk of venous thromboembolic events (Canonico et al., 2007),	[42]

Type of Therapy	Condition (Average age)	Dosage	Therapeutic effects	Side-effects	Reference
				cerebrovascular accidents and myocardial infarction (Welty, 2003).	
	Hysterectomy and bilateral oophorectomy (48 year)	(2 mg/day; v.o. ; 6 month)	Anxiolytic		[43]
	Hysterectomy and bilateral oophorectomy (50 year)	(50 mg/day; t.d.; 12 month)	Anxiolytic		[87]
Conjugated equine estrogen (Premarin)	Total abdominal hysterectomy/ bilateral salpingo-oophorectomy (48-51 year)	(0.625 mg/day; v.o.; 12 month)	Anxiolytic	Increased risk of myocardial infarction, breast cancer and strokes, besides headache and nausea (Gupta et al., 2013).	[46]
Dehydroepiandrosterone (DHEA)	Total abdominal hysterectomy/ bilateral salpingo-oophorectomy (48-51 year)	(25 mg/day; v.o.; 12 month)	Anxiolytic	Acne and hair loss (Welty, 2003).	[46]
Testosterone (gel hidroalcoholyc TESTOGEL®)	Natural menopause (50-65 year)	(50 mg/day; t.d.; 3 month)	Anxiolytic	Headache, weight gain, facial hair, increased appetite (Nathorst-Böös et al., 2006).	[88]
Antidepressant Venlafaxine	12 month of amenorrea (45-55 year)	(450 mg/day; v.o.; 6 month)	Anxiolytic	Dry mouth, altered appetite, abdominal discomfort, decreased libido, insomnia, headache and nausea (Hickey et al., 2005; Iglesias et al., 2009; Handley et al., 2015).	[54]
Paroxetine	Natural menopause (62 year)	10 mg/day; 1 week and the subsequent dose of 20 mg/day; 6 months.	Anxiolytic	Decreased libido, insomnia, headache and nausea (Hickey et al., 2005; Handley et al., 2015).	[89]
Phytoestrogens Red clover extracts (MF11RCE,	>12 month of amenorrea (40 year)	(80 mg/day; v.o.; 3 month)	Anxiolytic	Without effects.	[38]

Type of Therapy	Condition (Average age)	Dosage	Therapeutic effects	Side-effects	Reference
containing isoflavones)					
Phytoestrogens					
PHYTO SOYA, capsules containing 17.5 mg isoflavones	Postmenopausal period	35 mg/day; v.o.; 4 months	Anxiolytic	Without severe side effects.	[59]

Table 2. Pharmacological treatment of anxiety disorders in menopausal women.

5. Hormonal replacement therapy

Reduced oestrogen concentrations during menopause impacts different biological systems, including the central nervous system. The psychiatric disorders most common during menopause include loss of motivation, lack of mental concentration, irritability, aggression, mood swings, mental tension, anxiety, and depression disorders. Anxiety in particular occurs mainly in women who have been susceptible to suffering anxiety during their whole life. It is well known that exogenous administration of oestrogens or progesterone not only prevents the common symptoms of menopause [5], but is also able to improve the mood and emotional state, and reduce the symptoms of anxiety [38, 39]. In this sense, the use of oestrogens to treat anxiety is preferable to the use of psychopharmacological drugs.

Rocca and collaborators (2008) [34] reported that women who experience surgical menopause at an early age are not responsive to the treatment with oestrogens for symptoms of generalized anxiety, while women suffering during a natural menopause but who experienced surgical extirpation of the ovaries were sensitive to treatment with ethinyl oestradiol (3.9 mg/week) which significantly decreased the symptoms of anxiety [40, 41]. This finding suggests that physiological and neurochemical conditions associated with the reduction of hormonal levels in natural and surgical menopause are age-dependent, and impacts on the establishment of anxiolytic effects of oestrogenic therapy.

Clinical studies agree that chronic administration of 17β-oestradiol to women with natural [42] or surgical menopause [43] is effective in reducing symptoms of anxiety. However, some studies relate the use of 17β-oestradiol with an increase in the risk of developing venous thromboembolism [44], strokes, and myocardial infarction in women both with and without a family history of this illness; apparently, the use of a transdermal patch with oestrogens minimizes the secondary effects but unfortunately also minimizes therapeutic effects [45].

Therapy with equine conjugate oestrogens at a dose of 0.625 mg/day also produces significant anxiolytic effects, in the same way that 25 mg/day of dehydroepiandrosterone (DHEA) does; both treatments significantly reduce genitourinary, vasomotor, psychological, vaginal dryness symptoms, and improve libido [46]. Unfortunately, the use of oestrogens alone or in combination with medroxyprogesterone acetate (synthetic progestin) used to ameliorate the symptoms associated with the menopause, also has side-effects and increases the risk of heart attacks, breast cancer, and strokes. Other symptoms include headaches, nausea, and (in the case of DHEA) secondary effects of an androgenic kind such as acne and hair loss [45, 46].

On the other hand, there are different alternative drugs for oestrogenic therapy when it is contraindicated, for example gonadomimetics such as Tibolone. This drug is a synthetic steroid from which three metabolites are produced: 3 alpha-OH-tibolone, 3 beta-tibolone with oestrogenic activity, and the isomer tibolone, which exerts a weak influence on progestegenic and androgenic activity. Tibolone, 2.5 mg/day, reduces the symptoms of generalized anxiety in menopausal women, who had undergone a hysterectomy or bilateral oophorectomy [41, 43] and in women experiencing a natural menopause [42]. It seems that these anxiolytic effects could be associated with an increase of β–endorphin concentrations in blood and the pituitary gland [47].

Collateral effects of the oestrogenic therapy include vaginal bleeding in women that still have a uterus, which in some cases determines the use of Tibolone [48], given that it not only produces anxiolytic effects but also reduce symptoms at vegetative and cardiovascular levels. Additionally, it also reduces triglyceride, total cholesterol, and bad cholesterol (LDL) levels, while increasing good cholesterol (HDL) levels, reduces loss of bone density, and increases libido in post-menopausal women [46]. Data available about the chronic use of Tibolone show that it can reduce the risk of bone fractures, and breast and colon cancers, but also increases the risk of strokes in women older than 60 [49].

Hormonal replacement therapy, in general, is contraindicated in women with hepatic and cardiovascular illness, and with records of thrombovascular or cerebrovascular disease, as well as breast and cervical cancer. Nevertheless, it exists as a treatment option with excellent clinical results.

6. Antidepressants

Women suffering during the menopause have reduced serotonergic activity associated with low concentrations of steroid hormones, which is associated with the symptoms of anxiety and depression [50]. The reduction in oestrogenic levels during menopause could alter the availability of cerebral tryptophan used in serotonin synthesis, allowing the establishment of psychological symptoms typical of menopause. In consequence, the use of Selective Serotonin Reuptake Inhibitors (SSRI) can control the symptoms of anxiety and depression in menopausal women [50].

The use of SSRI to control symptoms of anxiety and depression in menopausal women includes mainly paroxetine, fluoxetine, sertraline, citalopram, and venlafaxine, which are also used to control vascular symptoms, and mainly hot flushes. Usage of these drugs has an appropriate tolerance and security window, with the exception of some adverse effects including the reduction of libido, insomnia, headache, and nausea [51, 52].

Venlafaxine is used for treatment of anxiety disorders most common in menopause, such as generalized anxiety, panic attacks, and social phobia. Very few studies evaluate the effects of antidepressants in women experiencing menopause and diagnosed with some anxiety disorder, due to the fact that frequently symptoms of anxiety can be confused with emotional disturbances characteristic of menopause, such as palpitations, irritability, and sweating [53].

One study by Iglesias et al. (2009) [54] including women between 45 to 55 years old experiencing natural menopause, showed the anxiolytic effect of venlafaxine (450 mg/day/six months). Despite the use of relatively high doses compared to the standard dose (150 mg/day), no potentially dangerous secondary effects were reported, with the exceptions of mouth dryness, appetite changes, abdominal discomfort, headaches, and, in some cases, sexual dysfunction.

7. Alternative therapies

The collateral effects produced by hormone replacement therapy and the lack of controlled studies evaluating the therapeutic effect of antidepressants in women suffering menopause have encouraged research into new alternative therapies that control the symptoms characteristic of menopause but which few or no undesirable side-effects. At the time of writing, the use of chemical compounds obtained from plants (i.e., phyto-oestrogens) has been evaluated as a potential therapeutic option due to the oestrogenic activity over β-oestrogen receptors in the osseous system, reproductive system, and central nervous system [55, 56]. Although phyto-oestrogens seem to be less potent than conventional oestrogens [57] some preclinical and clinical studies support its potential use in therapeutic treatment of osteoporosis, vascular disorders, and the symptoms of anxiety and depression [38].

Some clinical studies have reported that isoflavones are effective in improving classical menopause symptoms, including those related to anxiety and mood swings. The phyto-oestrogens from magnolia bark extract significantly reduces the relevant psycho-affective symptoms, particularly anxiety, irritability, and insomnia in menopausal women, with a scarcity of side-effects [58].

In women experiencing natural menopause, the therapeutic effect of isoflavones synthetized from extracts of red clover (*Trifolium pratense*) was studied. The administration of 80 mg/day of isoflavones during three months (MF11RCE capsule with 40 mg of isoflavones biochanin A, formonometin, genistein, and daidzein) in women experiencing natural menopause reduced the symptoms of generalized anxiety 76% measured by the Hospital Anxiety and Depression Scale (HADS) and compared with basal measures, while with the Zung's Self Rating Depression Scale there was a reduction of 80.6% of symptoms with respect to basal [38]. It is noteworthy to point out that women who received a placebo also significantly reduced the symptoms of anxiety, but only 21.7% with respect to basal. These authors suggest that isoflavones isolated from red clover are efficient in treating the symptoms of anxiety and depression in women experiencing menopause.

On the other hand, Albert et al. (2001) [59], in a multicentric, open, prospective, observational, and nonrandomized clinical trial involving 190 post-menopausal women, tested the effect of a preparation rich in isoflavones (PHYTO SOYA, capsules containing 17.5 mg isoflavones) on symptomatology derived from the lack of oestrogens (i.e., hot flushes, sleep disorder, anxiety, depression, vaginal dryness, loss of libido, and bone pain). Each patient received 35 mg of isoflavones per day in two doses, during four months of treatment. In this study, most of the women reported a statistically significant decrease in all evaluated parameters, including a significant reduction of symptomatology of anxiety and depression, without severe side-effects and with excellent tolerance. Nonetheless, more data from a double-blind, randomized study performed with 50 women (with an average age of 53.3 ± 3.1 years) with menopausal symptoms, the administration of the phyto-oestrogens genistein and daidzein during three months produced significant reductions in hot flushes only, but not in anxiety, insomnia, or vaginal dryness [60]. In this way, diverse studies of menopausal women have reported a particular effectiveness of phyto-oestrogens in the control of vasomotor symptoms, principally in the control of hot flushes [61–63], but few have demonstrated effectiveness in the control of anxiety and depressive symptoms [38, 58, 59]. There are in fact few studies that explore the clinical relevance of phyto-oestrogens in the control of emotional and affective disorders in menopausal women, which limit the wide use of these substances in the treatment of anxiety and depressive disorders. Considering the controversy of the effectiveness of phyto-oestrogens in the management of physiological and psychiatric disorders associated with the menopause, additional studies are needed to further address the complex array of factors that may affect efficacy, such as dose, isoflavone structure, baseline of typical symptoms in the menopause, and treatment duration [61]. Only then will it be possible to consider phyto-oestrogens as a safe and efficacious alternative for treating symptoms associated with menopause and to remove the present barrier to recommending its use for treatment.

8. Ovariectomized rats as an animal model for surgical menopause

Surgical menopause in women is produced by ablation of the ovaries (oophorectomy) with or without the uterus, which produces a similar symptomatology to that observed in natural menopause, but with an increase in intensity. In this way, bilateral ovariectomy in rats has been proposed as a tool to reproduce physiological and emotional alterations related with the reduction of ovarian hormones (Table 3), as occurring in women subjected to surgical menopause; in other words, that surgical manipulation of rats is proposed as an experimental model to study emotional and physiological changes that occur in women [8].

Some experimental studies of ovariectomized rats show a body-weight gain [64] and reduction of bone density as in osteoporosis [65], similar to that identified in menopausal women as a consequence of the long-term absence of ovarian hormones, in particular oestradiol, progesterone, and their reduced metabolites [65]. In this state, other physiological alterations that produce atrophy of the skin and mucosa also occur [66], such as hair loss, deterioration of attention and concentration capacity, reduced memory capacity, and loss of libido [67, 68]. The absence of oestrogens disrupts the immune, motor [69], and cardiovascular systems [70]; in

http://dx.doi.org/10.5772/60621

Weeks post ovariectomy	Effects	References
1	Reduced activation of glutamatergic receptors in the basolateral amygdala.	[75]
1-2	Reduced density of dendritic spines and synaptophysin in pyramidal neurons in the CA1 layer of the hippocampus.	[90]
3	Reduced density of dendritic spines in the CA1 layer of the hippocampus.	[67]
4	Reduced expression of mRNA of $\alpha 2$ and $\alpha 3$ subunits in the amygdala $GABA_A$ receptors.	[75]
4	Reduced expression of mRNA of the tryptophan hydroxylase enzyme and the serotonergic transporter (SERT) in the dorsal raphe nucleus.	[79]
4	Reduced concentration of serotonin in the hippocampus and nucleus accumbens.	[76]
5	Reduced thickness of the CA1 layer in the hippocampus and the cerebral prefrontal cortex.	[91]
6	Reduced concentration of dopamine in the central nucleus of the amygdala.	[92]
8	Reduced expression of mRNA of estrogen receptors (ERα y ERβ) in the hippocampus and cerebral cortex.	[74]
9	Reduced density of dendritic spines in the cerebral prefrontal cortex.	[93]
12	Anxiety-like behavior was higher in 12-weeks postovariectomized rats than 3-weeks postovariectomized rats in the burying behavioral test	[8]
12	Higher anxiety-like behavior in the elevated plus maze, which was reduced by phytoestrogen genistein treatment.	[6]
1-15	Anxiety-like behavior increase progressively after ovariectomy, it was higher from nine weeks post ovariectomy.	[9]
18	Reduced activity of the tryptophan-2-hydroxylase enzyme in the brain.	[78]

Table 3. Cerebral and anxiety-like behavior changes associated with ovariectomy in the rat.

addition, an increase in emotional (i.e., anxiety) and affective (i.e., depression) alterations that negatively impact on women's quality of life also occurs. It has been suggested that these alterations are related to the long-term absence of ovarian hormones, which play an important role in the regulation of diverse physiological processes in gastrointestinal [71], metabolic, and bone [64, 65] systems, as well as in the regulation of emotional and affective states. All those alterations of the different systems are produced at the experimental level through the ablation of the ovaries in the rat; therefore this surgical manipulation has been considered as an appropriate model to study medical alterations occurring in women undergoing surgical menopause [6, 8, 58, 62].

In rats, the long-term absence of ovarian hormones produced by ovariectomy reduces GABAergic neurotransmission in diverse brain structures [72]. It also produces a reduced sensitivity of the $GABA_A$, possibly associated with a reduced expression of mRNA of $\alpha 2$ and $\alpha 3$ subunits of this receptor [73]. As mentioned above, this is important because the $GABA_A$ receptor is the action site of clinically effective anxiolytic drugs such as benzodiazepines; those molecular modifications in the $GABA_A$ receptor could explain the reduced effectiveness of anxiolytic pharmacological therapies in menopausal women.

On the other hand, ovariectomies performed on rats reduce the density of oestrogen receptor α and β in the hippocampus [74]; in addition, reduced activity of glutamate receptors in the basolateral amygdala also occurs [75], and these neurochemical changes are accompanied by an increase in anxiety-like behaviour. While administration of an agonist of the glutamate receptors produces an anxiolytic-like effect in the ovariectomized rats, it is dependent on the availability of oestrogens in the basolateral amygdala [75].

Likewise, the ovariectomy of rats reduces the monoaminergic neurotransmission affecting the production and release of norepinephrine, dopamine, and serotonin in the brain [76]. It has been proposed that reduced monoaminergic neurotransmission in the hippocampus and accumbens nucleus could be related to the presence of anxiety-like behaviour, while administration of oestrogenic compounds in ovariectomized rats produces anxiolytic-like effects [77], possibly associated with the reactivation of brain neurotransmission. Some investigations indicate that the lower concentration of oestrogens in the brain associated with ovariectomy reduces the activity of the enzyme tryptophan hydroxylase-2, which reduces the availability of serotonin and their transportation in the dorsal raphe nucleus [78]. Administration of oestrogenic compounds in ovariectomized rats, on the other hand, produces anxiolytic-like effects [79].

The rats with a long-term absence of ovarian hormones produced by ovariectomy are more vulnerable to environmental stressors. In this case, rats with long-term ovariectomies subjected to chronic mild stress show more anxiety-like behaviour than rats with short-term ovariectomy in the elevated plus-maze, indicating that the frame time in the absence of ovarian hormones plays an important role in response to stress. Vulnerability to stress in ovariectomized rats is associated with a reduced cellular proliferation in the dentate gyrus [79], and reduced density of dendritic spines in CA1 pyramidal neurons [80]. These neuroanatomical changes at brain level are proposed as part of the neurobiological substrate of the altered stress response and higher predisposition to develop emotional (i.e., anxiety) and affective (i.e., depression) disorders [67] in women experiencing both a natural or a surgical menopause.

In rats with the long-term absence of ovarian hormones induced by ovariectomy, it has been possible to study the same emotional and affective changes as occur in women as a result of surgical menopause. Rats with 12 post-ovariectomy weeks show higher anxiety-like behaviour than rats with three post-ovariectomy weeks [8]. Interestingly, this anxiety-like behaviour is reduced with anxiolytic drugs (i.e., diazepam), some natural chemical compounds (i.e., isoflavones), or some extract of plant (*Montanoa tomentosa*). In rats with long-term absence of ovarian hormones produced by ovariectomy, the effect of several doses of isoflavone genistein (0.25, 0.5, and 1.0 mg/kg) during four consecutive days was explored. This treatment schedule produces an increase in the time spent in exploration of an illuminated compartment and the number of explorations towards this compartment in the light/dark test: a validated model to screen drugs with a potential anxiolytic effect. These changes in rat behaviour are an indicator of a reduced anxiety-like behaviour, such as occur in this experimental model when anxiolytic drugs like diazepam are evaluated [6]. Interestingly, the anxiolytic-like effect produced by the isoflavone genistein is antagonized by tamoxifen, a non-selective antagonist of the β-oestradiol receptors [7]. The aforementioned facts support the idea that isoflavones activate the β-oestrogen receptor which play a important role in the anxiolytic effects produced by natural oestradiol and other oestrogenic synthetic compounds [81]. In this way, these data support the hypothesis that phyto-oestrogen could be a possible therapeutic alternative in the natural management of anxiety disorders in menopausal women. In support, clinical studies have shown that administration of 34–100 mg/day of isoflavones from soya reduces the typical symptomatology of menopausal women: principally, vasomotor problems [82]. In other studies, the administration of isoflavones to menopausal women also reduces symptoms of anxiety and depression disorders [38, 58, 83].

In an early study, the effect of an aqueous extract of *Montanoa tomentosa* in rats with a long-term absence of ovarian hormones was evaluated [84]. In this study, the acute administration of the extract produced a significant reduction of anxiety-like behaviour when rats were evaluated in the elevated plus maze. These findings are interesting because the traditional use of this plant extract had been recommended in the ancient traditional medicine from México, as it was described in the *Badianus Codex* or *Libellus de Medicinalibus Indorum Herbis* (1552). It supports the potential use of this extract in the future as a natural alternative to ameliorate anxiety symptoms related with changes in ovarian hormones [84, 85].

In short, the aforementioned data indicate that ovariectomy in rats produces long-term behavioural and physiological changes that mimic the symptoms that occur in women who have undergone surgical menopause, and permit the exploration of possible therapeutic alternatives at an experimental level to ameliorate emotional and affective disorders associated with the long-term absence of ovarian hormones.

9. Conclusion

Anxiety disorders are strongly associated with natural and surgical menopause, principally due to the prolonged absence of oestrogen concentration levels in plasma and the brain. Anxiety is related to hot flashes in most of clinical studies. Finally, preclinical and clinical research suggested that the long-term absence of ovarian hormones associated with natural or surgical menopause is the principal cause of physiological and psychiatric disorder in the women; therefore, oestrogenic compounds seem to play a important role in the maintenance of the brain structures that regulate anxiety, mood, memory, and cognitive functions in menopausal women. Despite advances in the development of diverse therapeutic schedules to ameliorate typical physiological and psychiatric symptoms associated with natural or surgical menopause, we still lack of an efficient treatment to ameliorate symptoms of menopause. The actual therapeutic schedules are partially effective, but they produce some side-effects that limit their use in sensitive women. In consequence, alternative therapies based on the use of natural products, such as isoflavones, are in an experimental phase, but the data suggest that they could be used in the future as alternative therapies to ameliorate symptoms of natural and surgical menopause.

Acknowledgements

The present chapter was realized with partial sources coming from Programa de Fortalecimiento Académico del Posgrado de Alta Calidad, number: I010/458/2013, C-703/2013, and I010/152/2014, C-133/2014. The second and third authors received fellowships from the Consejo Nacional de Ciencia and Tecnología (CONACyT) for postgraduate studies in neuroethology (numbers 297410 and 297560, Respectively). The fourth author received financial support from CONACyT for Posdoctoral position at Universitary Center of Los Lagos, Universidad de Guadalajara.

Author details

Juan Francisco Rodríguez-Landa[1*], Abraham Puga-Olguín[2], León Jesús Germán-Ponciano[2], Rosa-Isela García-Ríos[2] and Cesar Soria-Fregozo[3]

*Address all correspondence to: juarodriguez@uv.mx

1 Neuroethology Institute, Universidad Veracruzana. Xalapa, Veracruz, México.

2 Postgraduate Studies in Neuroethology, Institute of Neuroethology, Universidad Veracruzana. Xalapa, Veracruz, México

3 Laboratory of Psychobiology, University Center of Los Lagos, Universidad de Guadalajara. Lagos de Moreno, Jalisco, México

References

[1] American-Psychiatric-Association, Diagnostic and statistical manual of mental disorders. Washington: American Psychiatric Press; 2000.

[2] Yang SG, Mlcek M, Kittnar O. Estrogen can modulate menopausal women´s heart rate variability. Physiology Research 2013; 62: 165–171.

[3] Erekson EA, Martin DK, Ratner ES. Oophorectomy: the debate between ovarian conservation and elective oophorectomy. Menopause 2013; 20(1);110–114.

[4] Agosta C, Atlante M, Benvenuti C. Randomized controlled study on clinical efficacy of isoflavones plus Lactobacillus sporogenes, associated or not with a natural anxiolytic agent in menopause. Minerva Ginecologica 2011; 63(1):11–17.

[5] Genazzani AR, Komm BS, Pickar JH. Emerging hormonal treatments for menopausal symptoms. Expert Opinion on Emerging Drugs 2015; 5:1–16.

[6] Rodríguez-Landa JF, Hernández-Figueroa JD, Hernández-Calderón BC, Saavedra M. Anxiolytic-like effect of phytoestrogen genistein in rats with long-term absence of ovarian hormones in the black and white model. Progress in Neuro-Psychopharmacology and Biological Psychiatry 2009; 33(2): 367–372.

[7] Rodríguez-Landa JF, Hernández-López F, Saavedra M. Involvement of estrogen receptors in the anxiolytic-like effect of phytoestrogen genistein in rats with 12-weeks postovariectomy. Pharmacology and Pharmacy 2012; 3(4):439–446.

[8] Picazo O, Estrada-Camarena E, Hernandez-Aragon A. Influence of the post-ovariectomy time frame on the experimental anxiety and the behavioural actions of some anxiolytic agents. European Journal of Pharmacology 2006; 530:88–94.

[9] Puga-Olguín A, Germán-Ponciano LJ, Rodríguez-Landa JF, Rovirosa-Hernández MJ, Rivadeneyra-Domínguez E, Bernal-Morales B. Efecto de la ovariectomía sobre los indicadores de ansiedad en la rata Wistar. In: Vázquez GV, Martínez-García A, Solano-Sosa CE, Sánchez ME (eds.). XI Encuentro Participación de la Mujer en la Ciencia. León, Guanajuato: Centro de Investigaciones en Óptica A.C. 2014:1–5.

[10] Minkin MJ, Wright CV What Every Woman Needs to Know about Menopause. New Haven: Yale University Press; 1997.

[11] Do KA, Treloar SA, Pandeya N, Purdie D, Green AC, Heath AC, Martin NG. Predictive factors of age at menopause in a large Australian twin study. Human Biology 1998; 70(6):1073–1091.

[12] Kato I, Toniolo P, Akhmedkhanov A, Koenig KL, Shore R, Zeleniuch-Jacquotte A. Prospective study of factors influencing the onset of natural menopause. Journal of Clinical Epidemiology 1998;51(12):1271–1276.

[13] Ringa, V. Menopause and treatments. Quality of Life Research 2000; 9(6):695–707.

[14] Bosse R, DiPaolo T. Dopamine and $GABA_A$ receptor imbalance after ovariectomy in rats: model of menopause. Journal of Psychiatry Neuroscience 1995; 20:364–371.

[15] Thornton MJ. Estrogens and aging skin. Dermato-Endocrinology 2013; 5(2):264–270.

[16] Salvador J. Climacteric and menopause: epidemiology and pathophysiology. Revista Peruana de Ginecología y Obstetricia 2008; 54:61–78.

[17] Morrie M, Gelfand MD. Role of androgens in surgical menopause. Obstetric and Gynecology 1999; 180(3):325–328.

[18] Baram D. Physiology and symptoms of menopause. In: Steward DE, Robinson GE (eds.) A Clinician's Guide to Menopause. Washington: Health Press International; 1997:9–28.

[19] Bromberger JT, Assmann SF, Avis NE, Schocken M, Kravitz HM, Cordal A. Persistent mood symptoms in a multiethnic community cohort of pre- and perimenopausal women. American Journal of Epidemiology. 2003; 158(4):347–356.

[20] Wittchen H-U, Kessler RC, Beesdo K, Krause P, Höfler M, Hoyer J. Generalized anxiety and depression in primary care: prevalence, recognition, and management. The Journal Clinical Psychiatry 2002; 63(8):24–34.

[21] Taylor M. Psychological consequences of surgical menopause. Journal of Reproductive Medicine. 2001; 46(3):317–324.

[22] Bromberger JT, Kravitz HM, Chang Y, Randolph JF Jr, Avis NE, Gold EB, Matthews KA. Does risk for anxiety increase during the menopausal transition? Study of women's health across the nation. Menopause. 2013; 20(5):488–495

[23] Jafari F, Hadizadeh MH, Zabihi R, Ganji K. Comparison of depression, anxiety, quality of life, vitality and mental health between premenopausal and postmenopausal women. Climacteric 2014; 17(6):660–665.

[24] Von Muhlen D, Kritz-Silverstein D, Barrett-Connor E. A community-based study of menopause symptoms and estrogen replacement in older women. Maturitas 1995; 22:71–78.

[25] Avis N, Stellato R, Crawford S, Bromberger J, Ganz P, Cain V, Kagawa-Singer M. Is there a menopausal syndrome? Menopausal status and symptoms across racial/ethnic groups. Social Science Medicine 2001; 52:345–356.

[26] Hanisch L, Hantsoo L, Freeman E, Sullivan G, Coyne J. Hot flashes and panic attacks: a comparison of symptomatology, neurobiology, treatment and a role for cognition. Psychological Bulletin, 2008; 134:247–269.

[27] Lambrinoudaki I, Bouziou G, Armeni E, Spyropoulou A, Koundi K, Rizos D, Augoulea A, Alexandrou A, Creatsa M, Panoulis C, Dendrinos S, Leonadrou AA, Zervas IM. Circulating androgens are associated with mood disturbances in young postmenopausal women. Climacteric 2015; 7:1–9.

[28] Smoller JW, Pollack MH, Wassertheil-Smoller S, Barton B, Hendrix SL, Jackson RD, Dicken T, Oberman A, Sheps DS. Prevalence and correlates of panic attacks in postmenopausal women. Archives of Internal Medicine 2003; 163:2041–2047.

[29] Smoller J, Pollack M, Wassertheil-Smoller S, Jackson R, Oberman A, Wong N, Sheps D. Panic attacks and risk of incident cardiovascular events among postmenopausal women in the Women's Health Initiative Observational Study. Archives of General Psychiatry 2007; 64:1153–1160.

[30] Vulink NC, Denys D, Bus L, Westenberg HG. Female hormones affect symptom severity in obsessive-compulsive disorder. International Clinical Psychopharmacology 2006; 21:171–117.

[31] Uguz F, Sahingoz M, Gezginc K, Karatayli R. Obsessive-compulsive disorder in postmenopausal women: prevalence, clinical features, and comorbidity. Australian and New Zealand Journal Psychiatry 2010; 44(2):183–187.

[32] Pacchierotti C, Castrogiovanni A, Cavicchioli C, Luisi S, Morgante G, De Leo V, Petraglia F, Castrogiovanni P. Panic disorder in menopause: a case control study. Maturitas 2004; 48:147–154.

[33] Chung-Park M. Anxiety attacks following surgical menopause: a case report. Holistic Nursing Practice 2005; 5:236–240.

[34] Rocca WA, Grossardt BR, Geda YE, Gostout BS, Bower JH, Maraganore DM, de Andrade M, Melton LJ 3rd. Long-term risk of depressive and anxiety symptoms after early bilateral oophorectomy. Menopause 2008;156:1050–1059.

[35] Tangen T, Mykletun A. Depression and anxiety through the climacteric period: an epidemiological study (HUNT II) Journal of Psychosomatic Obstetrics Gynaecology. 2008; 29:125–131.

[36] Moilanen J, Aalto A, Hemminki E, Aro A, Raitanen J, Luoto R. Prevalence of menopause symptoms and their association with lifestyle among Finnish middle-aged women. Maturitas 2010; 67:358–374.

[37] Freeman EW, Sammel MD, Lin H, Gracia CR, Kapoor S, Ferdousi T. The role of anxiety and hormonal changes in menopausal hot flashes. Menopause. 2005; 3:258–266.

[38] Lipovac M, Chedraui P, Gruenhut C, Gocan A, Stammler M, Imhof M. Improvement of postmenopausal depressive and anxiety symptoms after treatment with isoflavones derived from red clover extracts. Maturitas 2010;65(3):258–261.

[39] Toffol E, Heikinheimo O, Partonen T. Hormone therapy and mood in perimenopausal and postmenopausal women: a narrative review. Menopause. 2014; Sep 8: doi: 10.1097/GME.0000000000000323

[40] Dennerstein L, Burrows GD, Hyman GJ, Sharpe K. Hormone therapy and affect. Maturitas 1979; 1(4):247–259.

[41] Baksu A, Ayas B, Citak S, Kalan A, Baksu B, Goker N. Efficacy of tibolone and transdermal estrogen therapy on psychological symptoms in women following surgical menopause. International Journal of Gynecology and Obstetrics 2005; 91(1):58–62.

[42] Yazici K, Pata O, Yazihi A, Aklas A, Tot S, Kanik A. The effects of hormone replacement therapy in menopause on symptoms of anxiety and depression. Turk Psikiyatri Dergisi 2003; 14 (2):101–105.

[43] Somunkiran A, Erel CT, Demirci F, Senturk ML. The effect of tibolone versus 17beta-estradiol on climacteric symptoms in women with surgical menopause: a randomized, cross-over study. Maturitas 2007; 56(1):61–68.

[44] Canonico M, Oger E, Plu-Bureau G, Conard J, Meyer G, Lévesque H, Trillot N, Barrellier MT, Wahl D, Emmerich J, Scarabin PY, Estrogen and Thromboembolism Risk (ESTHER) Study Group. Hormone therapy and venous thromboembolism among postmenopausal women: impact of the route of estrogen administration and progestogens: the ESTHER study. Circulation 2007; 115(7):840–845.

[45] Welty FK. Alternative hormone replacement regimens: is there a need for further clinical trials? Current Opinion in Lipidology 2003; 14(6):585–591.

[46] Gupta B, Mittal P, Khuteta R, Bhargava A. A comparative study of cee, tibolone, and dhea as hormone replacement therapy for surgical menopause. Journal of Obstetrics and Gynaecology of India 2013; 63(3):194–198.

[47] Genazzani AR, Petralgia F, Facchinetti F, Grasso A, Alessandrini G, Volpe A. Steroid replacement treatment increases β endorphin and β lipoprotein levels in postmenopausal women. Gynaecologic and Obstetric Investigation 1988; 26:153–159.

[48] Formoso G, Perrone E, Maltoni S, Balduzzi S, D'Amico R, Bassi C, Basevi V, Marata AM, Magrini N, Maestri E. Short and long term effects of tibolone in postmenopausal women. Cochrane Database System Review 2012; 2:CD008536.

[49] Cummings SR, Ettinger B, Delmas PD, Kenemans P, Stathopoulos V, Verweij P, Mol-Arts M, Kloosterboer L, Mosca L, Christiansen C, Bilizikian J, Kerberg EM, Johnson S, Zanchetta J, Grobbe DE, Seifer W, Eastell R; LIFT Trial Investigators. The effects of tibolone in older postmenopausal women. New England Journal of Medicine 2008; 359(7):697–708.

[50] Carretti N, Florio P, Reis FM, Comai S, Petraglia F, Costa CV. Menopause alters the metabolism of serum serotonin precursors and their correlation with gonadotropins and estradiol. Climacteric 2007;10(5):393–399.

[51] Hickey M, Davis SR, Sturdee DW. Treatment of menopausal symptoms: what shall we do now? Lancet 2005;366: 409–421

[52] Handley AP, Williams M. The efficacy and tolerability of SSRI/SNRIs in the treatment of vasomotor symptoms in menopausal women: A systematic review. Journal of the American Society of Nurse Practitioners 2015; 27(1):54–61.

[53] Bryant C, Judd FK, Hickey M. Anxiety during the menopausal transition: A systematic review. Journal of Affective Disorders 2012; 139:141–148.

[54] Iglesias C, Pato E, Ocio S, Ortigosa JC, Santamarina S, Merino MJ, Alonso MJ, Fernández L, Alonso JL, Rodríguez L. Treatment with venlafaxine extended release for climacteric women with depression or anxiety diagnosis. An open-label study. Actas Españolas de Psiquiatria 2009; 37(3):137–142.

[55] Miksicek RJ. Commonly occurring plant flavonoids have estrogenic activity. Molecular Pharmacology 1993; 44:37–43.

[56] Miksicek RJ. Interaction of naturally occurring nonsteroidal estrogens with expressed recombinant human estrogen receptor. Journal of Steroid Biochemistry and Molecular Biology 1994; 49:153–160.

[57] Dornstauder E, Jisa E, Unterrieder I, Krenn L, Kubelka W, Jungbauer A. Estrogenic activity of two standardized red clover extracts (Menoflavon) intended for large scale use in hormone replacement therapy. Journal of Steroid Biochemistry and Molecular Biology 2001; 78:67–75.

[58] Glickman-Simon R, Lindsay T. Yoga for back pain, cranberry for cystitis prevention, soy isoflavones for hot flashes, curcumin for pre-diabetes, and breathing retraining for asthma. Explore (NY) 2013; 9(4):251–254.

[59] Albert A, Altabre C, Baró F, Buendía E, Cabero A, Cancelo MJ, Castelo-Branco C, Chantre P, Duran M, Haya J, Imbert P, Julía D, Lanchares JL, Llaneza P, Manubens M, Miñano A, Quereda F, Ribes C, Vázquez F. Efficacy and safety of a phytoestrogen preparation derived from *Glycine max* (L.) Merr in climacteric symptomatology: a multicentric, open, prospective and non-randomized trial. Phytomedicine 2002; 9(2): 85–92.

[60] Russo R, Corosu R. The clinical use of a preparation based on phyto-oestrogens in the treatment of menopausal disorders. Acta Biomedica 2003; 74(3):137–143.

[61] Taku K, Melby MK, Kronenberg F, Kurzer MS, Messina M. Extracted or synthesized soybean isoflavones reduce menopausal hot flash frequency and severity: systematic review and meta-analysis of randomized controlled trials. Menopause 2012; 19(7): 776–790.

[62] Chen MN, Lin CC, Liu CF. Efficacy of phytoestrogens for menopausal symptoms: a meta-analysis and systematic review. Climacteric 2014; 1:1–10.

[63] Depypere HT, Comhaire FH. Herbal preparations for the menopause: Beyond isoflavones and black cohosh. Maturitas 2014; 77(2):191–194.

[64] Diz-Chaves Y, Kwiatkowska-Naqvi A, Von Hülst, Pernía O, Carrero P, Garcia-Segura LM. Behavioral effects of estradiol therapy in ovariectomized rats depend on the age when the treatment is initiated. Experimental Gerontology 2012; 47:93–99.

[65] Li F, Yang X, Yang Y, Guo C, Zhang C, Zhonglin Y, Li P. Antiosteoporotic activity of echinacoside in ovariectomized rats. Phytomedicine 2013; 20:549–557.

[66] Thornton MJ. Estrogens and aging skin. Dermato-Endocrinology 2013; 5(2):264–270.

[67] McLaughlin KJ, Bimonte-Nelson H, Neisewander JL, Conrad CD. Assessment of estradiol influence on spatial tasks and hippocampal CA1 spines: Evidence that the du-

ration of hormone deprivation after ovariectomy compromises 17β-estradiol effectiveness in altering CA1 spines. Hormones and Behavior 2008; 54:386–395.

[68] Leiblum SR, Koochaki PE, Rodenberg CA, Barton IP, Rosen RC. Hypoactive sexual desire disorder in postmenopausal women: US results from the Women′s International Study of Health and Sexuality (WISHeS). Menopausia 2006; 13:46–56.

[69] Baeza I, De Castro NM, Giménez-Llort L, De la Fuente M. Ovariectomy, a model of menopause in rodents, causes a premature aging of the nervous and immune systems. Journal of Neuroimmunology 2010; 219:90–99.

[70] McGregor C, Sau A, Ruddy SC, Leung D, Webb M, Durst T, Wright JS, Lagace D, Pratt C. Novel ligands balance estrogen receptor β and α agonism for safe and effective suppression of vasomotor response in the ovariectomized female rat of menopause. Endocrinology 2014; 155:2480–2491.

[71] Eckel L. The ovarian hormone estradiol plays a crucial role in the control of food intake in female. Physiology and Behavior 201; 105:517–524.

[72] Tominaga K, Yamauchi A, Shuto H, Niizeki M, Makino K, Oishi R, Kataoka Y. Ovariectomy aggravates convulsions and hippocampal gamma-aminobutyric acid inhibition induced by cyclosporin A in rats. European Journal of Pharmacology 2001; 430:243–249.

[73] Daendee S, Thongsong B, Kalandakanond-Thongsong S. Effects of time of estrogen deprivation on anxiety-like behavior and GABAA receptor plasticity in ovariectomized rats. Behavioral Brain Research 2013; 246:86–93.

[74] Jin M, Jin F, Zhang L, Chen Z, Huang H. Two estrogen replacement therapies differentially regulate expression of estrogen receptors alpha and beta in the hippocampus and cortex of ovariectomized rat. Molecular Brain Research 2005; 142:107–114.

[75] De Jesús-Burgos M, Torres-Llenza V, Pérez-Acevedo NL. Activation of amygdalar metabotropic glutamate receptors modulates anxiety, and risk assessment behaviors in ovariectomized estradiol-treated female rats. Pharmacology, Biochemistry and Behavior 2012;101(3):369–378

[76] Pandaranandaka J, Poonyachoti S, Kalandakanond-Thongsong S. Differential effects of the exogenous and endogenous estrogen on anxiety as measured by elevated T-maze in relation to the serotonergic system. Behavioural Brain Research 2009; 198:142–148.

[77] Pandaranandaka J, Poonyachoti S, Kalandakanond-Thongsong S. Anxiolytic property of estrogen related to the changes of the monoamine levels in various brain regions of ovariectomized rats. Physiology and Behavior 2006; 87:828–835.

[78] Espinosa J, Neri T, Orozco S, Campos M, Guerra C. Chronic administration of tibolone modulates anxiety-like behavior and enhances cognitive performance in ovariectomized rats. Hormones and Behavior 2012; 61:76–83.

[79] Charoenphandhu J, Teerapornpuntakit J, Nuntapornsak A, Krishnamra N, Charoenphandhu N. Anxiety-like behaviors and expression of SERT and TPH in the dorsal raphe of estrogen- and fluoxetine-treated ovariectomized rats. Pharmacology, Biochemistry and Behavior 2011; 98:503–510.

[80] Nissen I, Estrada FS, Nava-Kopp AT, Irles C, de-la-Peña-Díaz A, Fernández-G JM, Govezensky T, Zhang L. Prolame ameliorates anxiety and spatial learning and memory impairment induced by ovariectomy in rats. Physiology and Behavior 2012; 106(2):278–284.

[81] Gong P, Madak-Erdogan Z, Li J, Cheng J, Greenlief CM, Helferich W, Katzenellenbogen JA, Katzenellenbogen BS. Transcriptomic analysis identifies gene networks regulated by estrogen receptor α (ERα) and ERβ that control distinct effects of different botanical estrogens. Nuclear Receptor Signaling 2014; 12:e001. doi: 10.1621/nrs.12001

[82] González-Jiménez E, Cañadas de la Fuente GA, Fernández-Castillo R, Álvarez-Ferre J, González-Antón C. Phytoestrogens and their effects on osteoporosis in postmenopausal women. Revista Clinica de Medicina Familiar 2010; 3(3): 201–205.

[83] Ishiwata N, Melby MK, Mizuno S, Watanabe S. New equol supplement for relieving menopausal symptoms: randomized, placebo-controlled trial of Japanese women. Menopause 2009; 16(1):141–148.

[84] Rodríguez-Landa JF, Vicente-Serna J, Rodríguez-Blanco LA, Rovirosa-Hernández MJ, García-Orduña F, Carro-Juárez M. *Montanoa frutescens* and *Montanoa grandiflora* extracts reduces anxiety-like behavior during the metestrus-diestrus phase of the ovarian cycle in Wistar rats. BioMed Research International 2014; ID 938060. http://dx.doi.org/10.1155/2014/938060.

[85] Rodríguez-Landa JF, Rodríguez-Santiago MG, Rovirosa-Hernández MJ, García-Orduña F, Carro-Juárez M. Aqueous crude extract of *Montanoa tomentosa* exerts anxiolytic-like effects in female rats with long-term absence of ovarian hormones. Journal of Chemical, Biological and Physical Sciences 2014; 4(5):37–46.

[86] Đoković DD, Jović JJ, Đoković JD, Knežević MŽ, Djukić-Dejanović S, Ristić-Ignjatović DI. Effects of hormone replacement therapy on depressive and anxiety symptoms after oophorectomy. Medicinski Glasnik (Zenica) 2015; 12(1):79–85.

[87] Mendoza N, Suárez AM, Álamo F, Bartual E, Vergara F, Herruzo A. Lipid effects, effectiveness and acceptability of tibolone versus transdermic 17b-estradiol for hormonal replacement therapy in women with surgical menopause. Maturitas 2000; 37: 37–43.

[88] Nathorst-Böös J, Flöter A, Jarkander-Rolff M, Carlström K, Schoultz Bv. Treatment with percutanous testosterone gel in postmenopausal women with decreased libido: effects on sexuality and psychological general well-being. Maturitas 2006; 53(1):11–18.

[89] Zhou B, Xie S, Hu J, Sun X, Guan H, Deng Y. Paroxetine increased the serum estrogen in postmenopausal women with depressive and anxiety symptoms. Open Journal of Depression 2014; 3:184–194.

[90] Velázquez-Zamora DA, González-Tapia D, González-Ramírez MM, Flores-Soto ME, Vázquez-Valls E, Cervantes M, González-Burgos I. Plastic changes in dendritic spines of hippocampal CA1 pyramidal neurons from ovariectomized rats after estradiol treatment. Brain Research, 2012; 1470:1–10.

[91] Xu X, Zhang Z. Effects of estradiol benzoate on learning-memory behavior and synaptic structure in ovariectomized mice. Life Sciences 2006; 79:1553–1560.

[92] Izumo N, Ishibashi Y, Ohba M, Morikawa T, Manabe T. Decreased voluntary activity and amygdala levels of serotonin and dopamine in ovariectomized rats. Brain Research 2012; 227(1):1–6.

[93] Wallacea M, Luine V, Arellanos A, Frankfurt A. Ovariectomized rats show decreased recognition memory and spine density in the hippocampus and prefrontal cortex. Brain Research 2006; 1126:176–182.

Chapter 10

A Systematic Review of Anxiety Disorders following Mild, Moderate and Severe TBI in Children and Adolescents

Michelle Albicini and Audrey McKinlay

Additional information is available at the end of the chapter

http://dx.doi.org/10.5772/60426

Abstract

The aim of this chapter is to systematically review the research exploring the relationship between TBI and anxiety disorders in children and adolescents. A literature search was conducted using Google Scholar, Ovid Medline (1946 - Dec 2013), PsycINFO (1806 - Dec 2013), CINAHL plus (1937 - Dec 2013), Cochrane database (2005 – Dec 2013) and Embase (1946 – Dec 2013). The search returned 346 articles, and 11 of these met the inclusion criteria. Anxiety disorders were often found to be a negative outcome following childhood TBI, with a higher incidence of disorders including GAD, ASD, PTSD, PD, OCD, simple/specific phobia, social phobia and SAD found in children following their injury. In most cases, this relationship was strongest for children with severe TBI who sustained their injury at a younger age. Psychosocial adversity was found to be a consistently significant predictor for the likelihood of children developing anxiety following TBI. It is concluded that children who have suffered from a TBI (mild, moderate or severe), are at a higher risk of developing subsequent anxiety disorders, even 1 year following the injury event, and children with more severe injuries, greater psychosocial adversity, and younger age at injury are considered to be the most vulnerable.

Keywords: traumatic brain injury, children, adolescents, anxiety disorders, risk factors

1. Introduction

Traumatic brain injury (TBI) is a common cause of morbidity and mortality worldwide, with prevalence estimates of 235 per 100,000 individuals in European countries having some form of TBI [1] and for children in particular, rates vary between 280-1373 per 100,000 across the world [2]. Considering the high rates of injury in children and young people, any accompanying long-term negative effects associated with such an injury are likely to represent a significant health concern and burden. Indeed, it is now well-documented that children with TBI may be at an increased risk of long-term, self-reported externalising behavioural problems including increased hyperactivity, aggression and conduct problems [3-8]. In addition to externalising behaviours, a higher incidence of diagnosed psychiatric disorders in children and adolescents following a TBI event has also been established, including Attention Deficit/ Hyperactivity Disorder (ADHD), Oppositional Defiant Disorder (ODD), Conduct Disorder (CD), drug abuse, and personality change disorders [9-10], compared to healthy controls and children with orthopedic injury (OI; an injury, such as fracture or break, to the bones excluding the head, neck or spinal cord [11]). In light of these ongoing problems children and young people may face following their TBI, a review and investigation is required to better understand the need for rehabilitation and recovery, and to understand the children at risk of these long-term effects.

2. Defining traumatic brain injury

Traumatic brain injury (TBI) is defined as an injury to the head as a result of a blow or movement to the head and/or neck, following acceleration/deceleration impact, which causes neurological changes that affect normal brain functioning [12]. Severity of TBI therefore refers to the extent of neurological disruption that has occurred, and is classified as mild, moderate and severe [13]. The assessment of TBI severity is measured by the Glasgow Coma Scale (GCS), length of post-traumatic amnesia (PTA) and duration of loss of consciousness (LOC) [14-16]. The GCS is considered the best indicator of TBI severity, and evaluates three areas, including best motor and verbal responses, and eye opening [17]. Table 1 outlines the levels of severity for TBI and the respective definitions.

Mild TBI	Moderate TBI	Severe TBI
GCS = > 13 after 30 minutes	GCS = 9-13	GCS = ≤8
LOC = < 30 minutes	LOC = 30 minutes to 24 hours	LOC = > 24 hours
PTA = < 1 day	PTA = between 1 and 7 days	PTA = > 7 days

Note: Information in [13-14, 18]; GCS = Glasgow Coma Scale, LOC = loss of consciousness, PTA = post-traumatic amnesia.

Table 1. Defining severity levels of TBI

2.1. Research findings

While it has been established that TBI is associated with an increased rate of externalising behavioural problems, there is a lack in the research exploring the incidence of internalising disorders, and in particular anxiety, following TBI in children. A couple of case studies report on individuals who developed new-onset anxiety symptomatology following TBI, which highlight the need for research in the area. For instance, an 11 year-old girl sustained a severe TBI following a fall from her bicycle, resulting in a coma for 16 days, and following resolution of PTA symptoms, the patient had developed new-onset compulsive behaviours including hand-washing, ordering, arranging and counting rituals [19]. Moreover, the symptoms appeared to worsen at a 6 month follow-up, which was subsequently treated with antidepressant medication [19]. Similarly, another case study reports on a patient who suffered from TBI requiring surgery at the age of 17 years, who reported the onset of social anxiety disorder (SAD) following their injury [20]. The male was previously characterised as extroverted and displayed no evidence of social anxiety. However, following the injury he became socially anxious which worsened until he sought treatment at 21 years, reporting difficulties with authority figures, unknown persons and people of the opposite sex [20]. Both of these aforementioned studies above highlight the important role of the frontal regions of the brain in that their damage following injury may precipitate anxiety symptomatology that is ongoing and requiring treatment or intervention [19-20].

Research exploring the incidence of novel post-injury psychiatric disorders and behavioural problems following TBI in children suggests a greater need for information about the onset of anxiety disorders in the TBI population. There have been reports of rates of novel anxiety disorders in 15% of children with TBI compared to 7.5% of an OI control group [10]. Further, anxiety has been found to occur in higher rates than ADHD and ODD [10]. In children with mild TBI, up to 36% of individuals have been found to exhibit specific anxiety disorders 6-months post-injury [9]. This finding is also evident in other samples for children with mild-TBI, with increased rates on anxious/depressed self-report items on a behavioural rating scale as compared to children with no injury [4]. Others however have reported on different findings. For instance, in an assessment of long-term psychiatric outcomes following preschool mild TBI, no significant difference in the incidence of anxiety disorders were found between individuals with and without TBI when they reached adolescence [7]. Further, while parent reports of behaviour following severe TBI in children has indicated elevated rates of anxiety, the relationship was weak compared to that of ADHD and other externalising problems [21]. Differences in reported outcomes may be due to the length of time that assessments took place post-injury, or in differences in the tools used to evaluate problems. Despite the mixed results, there have been reports of heightened anxiety symptoms following TBI in children and adolescent samples [9-10, 21].

Brain imaging studies further support the potential relationship between an increased incidence of anxiety disorders following TBI in children and adolescents, however again the literature is sparse. While it has been stated that frontal and temporal regions are the most susceptible to impact during a TBI [22], it has been found that deep-brain structures such as the amygdala and hippocampus are also highly vulnerable to such an injury [22]. Indeed, the amygdala has been targeted as an important region in children for processing fearful facial expressions and producing rapid protective responses [23]. Further, right and left amygdala volumes have been found to be significantly larger in children with anxiety [24]. These findings have potential implications for literature involving anxiety and TBI in children and adolescents. Considering the discrepancies in the research mentioned above, and the fact that specific anxiety disorders are rarely the focus of interest in studies exploring the long-term and acute effects of TBI, it is important to review the literature and examine avenues for future research.

2.2. Rationale and aims

It is clear that anxiety negatively affects all areas of function, which is particularly important in the case of children, who are in a rapid state of developmental change. As outlined above, a TBI event can disrupt the developing systems in the brain. Further, research has shown that exposure to events that produce chronic anxiety can have long-term consequences by disrupting the developing architecture of the brain [25-26]. It is therefore important that we understand the impact of anxiety on outcomes following TBI in childhood as this will provide a platform for appropriate intervention to promote a more positive result.

As stated above, the incidence, rate and profile of internalising disorders following TBI in children has been relatively overlooked in the literature when compared to that of externalising disorders. Internalising behaviours represent internal states of distress, whereas externalising behaviours are directed outwardly and therefore tend to be more visibly distressing [27]. This difference in presentation of difficulties may contribute to the lack of research in internalising disorders, given that externalising problems experienced by children following TBI may be more readily reported by parents. The fact that males present with higher rates of TBI than females [28-29] may contribute to this difference, considering that externalising disorders tend to be more common in males than females [27, 30], while females are more likely to report internalising problems [30]. It is evident therefore that there may be a bias in the literature with regards to female oriented behavioural outcomes following TBI, with internalising problems (particularly anxiety) being significantly overlooked.

Based on the literature, this chapter will systematically review original research studies up until 2013 that have explored the relationship between TBI and anxiety disorders in children and adolescents. A comprehensive review investigated the cognitive, behavioural and academic outcomes of mild TBI in children and adolescents, and the merit of each study was strategically analysed according to specified criteria [31]. The rationale behind this procedure was due to the wide variability in methodology for past studies involving mild TBI.

The key criteria set out as essential for studies in this area were as follows:

a. Use of control group,

b. longitudinal design with follow-up assessments,

c. clear definition of mild TBI,

d. inclusion of at least 20 participants with TBI,

e. outcome measures involved standardised tests, and

f. control for pre-injury factors [31].

A study was concluded to have methodological merit if it met at least four of the previously listed criteria [31]. For this review, the methodology of the selected papers was examined according to these criteria, with the inclusion of moderate and severe injuries. When considering anxiety disorders, this refers to disorders including Generalised Anxiety Disorder (GAD), Post-Traumatic Stress Disorder (PTSD), Social Anxiety Disorder (SAD), Obsessive-Compulsive Disorder (OCD), Acute Stress Disorder (ASD), simple/specific phobia, social phobia and Panic Disorder (PD). Search methods and results will be outlined, and methodological considerations and future directions will be discussed and explored.

2.3. Comparison of merit of studies with criteria from Satz (2001)

As mentioned above, a prior literature review examined research studies investigating behavioural problems following mild TBI, and set out criteria regarding what constitutes as a study that has 'methdological merit' [31]. This method was utilised here, and each paper generated from the literature search was analysed according to the review's criteria. The results of the analysis can be found in Table 2 below.

	a) Use of control group	b) Longitudinal design with follow-up	c) Clear definition of TBI	d) At least 20 TBI participants	e) Standardised tests used	f) Controlled for pre-injury factors
[11] Hajek et al. (2010)	√	√	√	√	√	√
[32] Max et al. (1998)		√	√	√	√	√
[33] Levi & Drotar (1999)	√	√	√	√	√	√
[34] Gerring et al. (2002)		√	√	√	√	√
[35] Herskovits et al. (2002)		√	√	√	√	√
[36]Mather et al. (2003)	√	√	√		√	
[37] Grados et al. (2008)		√	√	√	√	√
[38] Luis & Mittenberg (2002)	√	√	√	√	√	√
[39] Max et al. (2011)		√	√	√	√	√

	a) Use of control group	b) Longitudinal design with follow-up	c) Clear definition of TBI	d) At least 20 TBI participants	e) Standardised tests used	f) Controlled for pre-injury factors
[40] Vasa et al. (2002)		√	√	√	√	√
[41] Vasa et al. (2004)		√	√	√	√	√

Table 2. Literature search results based on research methodology criteria

As is evident in Table 2, in accordance to the criteria set out by the review [31], all of the studies involving anxiety disorders following TBI in children and adolescents had methodological merit, possessing at least four of the essential criteria. A discussion of this analysis will be provided later in the chapter.

3. Method

A systematised literature search was conducted using the following search engines: Google Scholar, Ovid Medline (1946 - Dec 2013), PsycINFO (1806 - Dec 2013), Comprehensive Journal Index and Additional Resources for Nursing and Allied Health Professionals (CINAHL) plus (1937 - Dec 2013), Cochrane database (2005 – Dec 2013) and Embase (1946 – Dec 2013). A search was conducted in each database using the terms "traumatic brain injury" or "brain injury" or "head injury" and "anxiety disorders" or "anxiety" and "pediatric" or "paediatric" or "children" or "child". Returned articles were screened by title, abstract or full-text accordingly. Manual searching of articles based on the reference lists of relevant manuscripts was also conducted.

Inclusion criteria for studies were as follows:

a. Participants were children aged 0-18 years,

b. the study included a TBI group, and

c. anxiety symptoms or anxiety disorder diagnosis was included as an outcome measure.

Exclusion criteria involved:

a. Adult participants or a mixture of children and adults, and

b. participants with acquired brain injury (ABI).

4. Results

The search returned a total of 346 articles. Of these, 221 were screened by title, and 82 were screened based on abstract. The full text was examined for 43 of the articles. Of the articles examined by full text, 32 of these were excluded for the following reasons: not an original research paper (n=6), case study (n=1), not specifically assessing anxiety as an outcome measure (n=21), not assessing TBI participants (n=3), or couldn't access the article (n=1). Manual searching of additional studies using the reference lists of relevant articles was conducted, however no further studies were found. The final result included 11 research studies fitting the above criteria, for which study characteristics and findings are outlined in Table 3.

4.1. Anxiety disorders following TBI in children and adolescents

As is evident in Table 3, results from the studies generally reveal some relationship between the presence of anxiety disorders following TBI in children and adolescents. The majority of studies focused on correlates of PTSD following childhood TBI [11, 32-36], with generally mixed but similar findings. The focus on PTSD in such a sample is unsurprising given the close link between such an injury and trauma. Main findings indicate that PTSD within 1 year following TBI can occur despite experiencing post-traumatic amnesia (PTA) [32-33], and that PTSD symptomatology is more prominent in children with severe TBI than those with moderate TBI or OI [33]. Analysis of factors that can predict the development of PTSD in children following TBI reveal that levels of PTSD symptoms are related to social disadvantage/ family social status [33-34], anxiety diagnoses and aggregate anxiety scores [34], other psychiatric diagnoses and symptoms [34] and the presence of internalising disorders at time of injury [32]. Furthermore, predicting the diagnosis of PTSD following TBI was significantly related to anxiety diagnoses and scores, depression symptoms and non-anxiety psychiatric diagnoses [34]. When examining gender differences, female gender was a significant predictor of PTSD in one study [34], however was not the case for other investigators [32]. It is interesting to note that gender was unexamined in one study [33] considering anxiety disorders are seen in higher rates in a female population, it would be beneficial to the literature to compare anxiety symptomatology among groups.

Conversely, two studies exploring the relationship between PTSD and TBI report on different findings. One study explored PTSD following road traffic accidents in children with OI and mild TBI [36], and the other assessed the relationship between post-concussion symptoms (PCS) and PTSD in children with mild TBI and OI [11], with both papers reporting no significant difference among the sample groups on levels of PTSD symptomatology. This result may suggest that those with milder TBI are no more likely to develop PTSD following their injury than children who have sustained an OI. However, differences in the presentation of PTSD symptomatology following injury were found among the two papers. In [11], children with mild TBI tended to report a more frequent occurrence of mild PTSD symptoms, whereas severe PTSD occurred at a higher rate in the OI group. Moreover, another found that those in the mild TBI group reported higher levels of hyperarousal at 3 and 12 months, but not when controlling for PCS, whereas OI participants had higher levels of PTSD when controlling for baseline PCS and were more likely to meet PTSD criteria [26]. Therefore, these findings indicate that while there were no differences in the rate of PTSD symptomatology and diagnoses between mild TBI and OI children, the clinical manifestations of such symptomatology may be quite different across groups. Again, neither study examined any influence of gender on the likelihood of developing PTSD following TBI.

Authors	Aims	Participants	Classifying TBI Severity	Inclusion/ Exclusion Criteria	Anxiety Measures	General Results
[32] Max et al. (1998)	Identify PTSD and PTSD symptomatology following TBI Determine predictors of PTSD following TBI	50 consecutively admitted TBI patients aged 6-14 years at TOI - 26 mild TBI, 9 moderate TBI, 15 severe TBI - 64% male	Severe injury = Glasgow Coma Scale (GCS) score ≤ 8 Moderate injury = GCS score 9-12 or 3-15 with positive CT scan Mild injury = GCS score 13-15	Inclusion: admitted to tertiary care centre and 3 regional hospitals, CT scan on admission, English spoken language Exclusion: PTA > 3 months, penetrating TBI, documented history of child abuse and/or TBI involving hospital admission, history of CNS disorders, pre-existing serious illness	Neuropsychiatry Rating Scale (NRS) Baseline: - Schedule for Affective Disorders and Schizophrenia for School-Age Children – Epidemiologic version (K-SADS-E) plus PTSD module Follow-ups: - K-SADS-E plus sections on ADHD, ODD, CD, alcohol and substance abuse and PTSD module	2/50 with PTSD (resolved by 3 months) Increase in PTSD symptoms in first 3 months, then gradual decline 68% experienced ≥ 1 PTSD symptom at any point in first 3 months; 45%, 33%, 16% and 12% at 3, 6, 12 and 24 months Presence of internalising disorders, and severity of injury were main predictors of PTSD
[33] Levi & Drotar (1999)	Explore PTSD symptoms in children who have experienced traumatic injuries Compare PTSD symptoms of children with TBI and OI	Children 6-12 years at TOI 81 TBI children - 44 moderate, 37 severe - 74% males 59 OI children - 61% males	Severe TBI = GCS score ≤ 8 Moderate TBI = GCS score 9-12, or >12 plus positive CT scans or LOC > 15mins	Inclusion: hospitalised ≥1 night, participants from a prospective study on impact of TBI, English as primary language Exclusion: history of child abuse, TBI or brain disease, children with brain injuries other than closed head injury (e.g. anoxic injuries)	Child PTSD Index (CPTSDRI) (child report) Post Traumatic Stress Scale (PTSS) (parent report)	Parent reports for moderate TBI and OI in doubtful range for PTSD; mild levels PTSD reported for severe TBI at 6- and 12-months PTSD symptoms reported as higher for severe TBI group Younger age and higher social disadvantage associated with more PTSD symptoms Children displayed PTSD symptoms for >1 year post-TBI
[34] Gerring et al. (2002)	Examine the presence and rate of PTSD diagnosis and PTSD symptomatology following TBI	95 children aged 4-19 years with severe TBI and PTA - mean age at TOI 10.5 years -54 boys, 41 girls - 90 inpatient; 5 outpatient	GCS score of 3-8 indicated severe TBI classification	Inclusion: children admitted to neurorehabilitation unit of university-affiliated center Exclusion: previous hospitalisations for TBI, premorbid PTSD, premorbid mental retardation or CNS	Baseline: - Diagnostic Interview for Children and Adolescents parent form (DICA-p) - Child Behavior Checklist (CBCL) -- parents reported retrospectively of premorbid behavior	13% sample developed PTSD within 1 year of TBI - 5 according to parent reports, 5 to child reports and 2 to both Premorbid anxiety symptoms predisposed participants to PTSD symptoms 1 year post TBI Risk factors for PTSD and PTSD symptoms: female gender, high psychosocial adversity, greater

http://dx.doi.org/10.5772/60426

Authors	Aims	Participants	Classifying TBI Severity	Inclusion/ Exclusion Criteria	Anxiety Measures	General Results
				pathology, history of child abuse	- DICA child form (DICA-c/a) 1-year follow-up: - DICA-p, DICA-c/a - CBCL	injury severity, psychiatric disorders early after injury
[35] Herskovits et al. (2002)	Explore PTSD symptomatology post-TBI Compare spatial distribution of brain lesions due to TBI among participants with and without PTSD	94 participants aged 4-19 years with severe TBI - 53 boys, 41 girls - mean age TOI 10.5 years	GCS score of 3-8 indicated severe TBI classification	Inclusion: children referred from tertiary trauma centres to a university-affiliated center for neurological disorders Exclusion: previous hospitalisations for TBI, premorbid PTSD, premorbid mental retardation or CNS pathology, history of child abuse	PTSD diagnosis and symptoms ascertained with same procedure as Gerring et al. (2002) (above) MR Imaging: - imaging at 3 months post-TBI - abnormalities included hematoma, contusion, infarct, axonal-shear injury	9 participants met full PTSD criteria; 41 had re-experiencing criteria, 12 had avoidance criteria, and 55 had hyper-arousal criteria Participants with full PTSD criteria at 1 year post-TBI displayed lower lesion fractions in right medial frontal cortex and greater lesion fractions in left middle temporal gyrus High lesion burden was associated with lower probability of having PTSD
[38] Luis & Mitten-berg (2002)	Investigate relationship between TBI and anxiety/ mood disorders Examine factors that predict children who will suffer from anxiety/ mood disorders following TBI	96 children aged 6-15 years - 42 mild (66.7% male), 19 moderate/severe (68.4% male), - 35 OI (74% male)	Reviewed medical charts GCS score on admission - mild TBI – GCS 13-15 and normal CT/ neurological findings - moderate/severe TBI – GCS <13, abnormal CT, and/or skull fracture	Inclusion: children consecutively admitted to general hospital Exclusion: history of neurological disorders, history of abuse/neglect	Diagnostic Interview Schedule for Children (DISC-IV) - Module A: Anxiety Disorders Diagnoses based on DSM-IV criteria Social Readjustment Rating Questionnaire (SRRQ) (stress)	OI groups reported less post-injury stress Anxiety diagnoses: - Social Phobia: 5.7% OI, 10.5% moderate/severe - SAD: 7% mild, 21% moderate/ severe - Specific Phobia: 9.5% mild - Panic Attacks: 4.7% mild - Agoraphobia:7 % mild, 5.3% moderate/severe - GAD: 5.7% OI, 16.7% mild, 15.8% moderate/severe - OCD: 5.7% OI, 7% mild, 10.5% moderate/severe - PTSD: 10% mild, 10.5% moderate/ severe

Authors	Aims	Participants	Classifying TBI Severity	Inclusion/ Exclusion Criteria	Anxiety Measures	General Results
						- ASD: 2.3% mild, 10.5% moderate/ severe - overall Anxiety Disorders: 11.4% OI, 35.7% mild, 63.2% moderate/severe
[40] Vasa et al. (2002)	Compare rate of pre- and post-TBI anxiety disorders and symptoms Examine relationship between risk factors and anxiety outcomes following TBI	97 children aged 4-19 years with severe TBI - 58% male - mean age at TOI 10.56 years	GCS score of ≤8 taken at admission indicated severe TBI	Inclusion: referred from tertiary trauma centres and recruited from consecutive admissions from 1992-1996 to neurorehabilitation unit of university-affiliated center Exclusion: previous hospitalisations or emergency room visits for TBI, history of child abuse, premorbid mental retardation or CNS pathology	DICA-p assessed anxiety disorders at baseline and 1-year follow-up - derived symptoms from each anxiety disorder in addition	Mean aggregate Anxiety score of 1.86 pre-injury and 3.73 post-injury - pre-TBI, 84% reported 0-3 anxiety symptoms, 13% reported 4-9, and 3 reported ≥10 - post-TBI, 66% reported 0-3, 22% reported 4-9 and 12% reported ≥10 - significant increases in amount that had 4-9 and more than 10 symptoms Pre-injury anxiety and younger age at injury risk factors for post-injury anxiety
[36] Mather et al. (2003)	Compare the presence of PTSD in children who have been in a traffic accident with and without mild TBI Compare child and parent reports of PTSD following the accident	43 children from Casualty section of Sydney hospital aged 6-16 years - 20 males, 23 females - 14 mild TBI, 29 no TBI	Mild TBI defined by: - witnessed LOC - GCS 13-15 taken from medical file - return to full GCS score after 24 hours	Inclusion: enrolled in normal stream school, involved in recent traffic accident, sustained an injury other than TBI or a TBI Exclusion: prior TBI history, current TBI of moderate or severe classification, limited English comprehension of families	CPTSDRI – children report of PTSD Revised Children's Manifest Anxiety Scale (RCMAS) – child report of anxiety PTSD module of Anxiety Disorders Interview Schedule-child version (ADIS-c) – parent report or PTSD CBCL	No significant differences between groups for PTSD symptomatology 69% no-TBI and 85.7% TBI group suffered from PTSD Mean scores indicated improvements in PTSD symptoms Presence of PTSD strongly associated with anxiety Child and parent report of PTSD not significantly correlated
[41] Vasa et al. (2004)	Examine whether damage to specific brain regions are associated	97 children aged 4-19 years with severe TBI - 57% males	Initial GCS score on admission of ≤ 8	Inclusion: referred from tertiary trauma centres and recruited from	MR Imaging conducted 3 months post-TBI	12 subjects had 1 post-injury disorder, 1 had 2 disorders: 6 simple

Authors	Aims	Participants	Classifying TBI Severity	Inclusion/ Exclusion Criteria	Anxiety Measures	General Results
	with anxiety in children with severe TBI	- mean age at TOI 10.62 years	indicated presence of severe TBI	consecutive admissions from 1992-1996 to neurorehabilitation unit of university-affiliated center Exclusion: previous hospitalisations or emergency room visits for TBI, history of child abuse, premorbid mental retardation or CNS pathology	DICA was given to parents of children to assess anxiety disorders and symptoms	phobia, 5 overanxious disorder, 1 SAD and 1 OCD 7 subjects had post-injury PTSD; 1 had anxiety disorder and PTSD Mean number of anxiety symptoms: 1/88 pre- and 3.76 post-injury Inverse relationship between OFC damage and post-injury anxiety
[37] Grados et al. (2008)	Identify prevalence of new onset obsessive-compulsive symptoms (OCS) after severe childhood TBI Assess risk factors and comorbidities of OCS post-TBI	72 children aged 6-18 years with severe TBI - mean age at TOI 10.5 years - 54% males	Initial GCS score on admission of ≤ 8 to indicate severe TBI Also monitored duration of coma	Inclusion: referred to neurorehabilitation unit of a university-affiliated hospital between 1992-1997 Exclusion: previous hospitalisations for TBI, premorbid PTSD, premorbid mental retardation or CNS pathology, history of child abuse	DICA-revised was used to determine OCD, OCS, mood, anxiety and behavioural problems MR Imaging 3 months after TBI	21 children had new onset OCS – 12 had obsessions, 13 had compulsions, 4 had both Greater number of females in OCS group (70%) compared to non-OCS (37%) Those with OCS had higher number of psychiatric disorders – SAD, specific phobia, PTSD hyperarousal, mania, dysthymia and depressive symptoms more common in those with OCS Obsessions related to mesial prefrontal and temporal lesions; compulsions related to smaller OFC lesions
[11] Hajek et al. (2010)	Examine the rate and the relationship between PCS and PTSD in children following TBI and OI	251 children aged 8-15 years - 167 mild TBI (71% male), 84 OI (63% male)	Mild TBI – observed LOC ≤30 minutes, GCS of 13-14 or at least 2 symptoms of concussion OI – fracture injury within Abbreviated Injury Scale (AIS) score of ≤3	Inclusion: aged 8-15 years, recruited from emergency departments at selected hospitals, had suffered OI or mild TBI Exclusion: injury-related surgery, hypoxia or shock post-injury,	PTSD Checklist for Children/Parent Report (PCL-C/PR) to assess parent ratings of PTSD in children	PTSD diagnoses for Mild TBI: baseline 8%, 3 months 8% and 12 months 2% - OI: 7%, 7% and 7% respectively Across groups, PCS and PTSD ratings were correlated

Authors	Aims	Participants	Classifying TBI Severity	Inclusion/ Exclusion Criteria	Anxiety Measures	General Results
				previous TBI needing hospitalisation, premorbid neurological disorders, severe psychiatric disorder needing hospitalisation, AIS of greater than 3, injuries that would hinder assessment, child abuse/neglect		After controlling for PCS, OI group reported higher scores on PCL-C/PR than mild TBI group at baseline Symptoms of PTSD and PCS correlated more highly for OI group than mild TBI
[39] Max et al. (2011)	Examine the rate and nature of novel anxiety disorders and novel subclinical anxiety disorders in children following TBI	177 children aged 5-14 years with TBI - 86 mild, 27 moderate, 64 severe - mean age at TOI 10.13 years - 71% male	GCS scores of 3-8 for severe TBI, 9-12 for moderate TBI and 13-15 for mild TBI - also assessed MR scans	Inclusion: Consecutive admissions to 3 academic medical centres for TBI between 1998-2003 Exclusion: pre-existing autism, ADHD or schizophrenia, mental deficiency, injury due to child abuse or penetrating injury	DSM-IV diagnoses derived from KSADS present and lifetime version, and NRS MR Imaging scans at 3 months	8.5% developed novel clinical anxiety disorder and 17% developed novel subclinical anxiety disorder post-TBI - mild TBI: 11% clinical and 20% subclinical anxiety - moderate TBI: 0% clinical and 24% subclinical anxiety - severe TBI: 7% clinical and 11% subclinical anxiety 9 PTSD, 6 SAD, 4 simple phobia, 3 GAD, 3 adjustment disorder with anxious mood, 3 social phobia, 1 panic disorder Younger age at injury associated with novel anxiety disorder

Note. PTSD = Post-Traumatic Stress Disorder; TBI = traumatic brain injury; TOI = time of injury; CT = computed tomography; PTA = post-traumatic amnesia; CNS = central nervous system; ADHD = Attention-Deficit/Hyperactivity Disorder; ODD = Oppositional Defiant Disorder; CD = Conduct Disorder; OI = orthopaedic injury; LOC = loss of consciousness; MR = magnetic resonance; DSM-IV = Diagnostic and Statistical Manual for Mental Disorders fourth edition; SAD = separation anxiety disorder, GAD = Generalised Anxiety Disorder; OCD = Obsessive-Compulsive Disorder; ASD = Acute Stress Disorder; OFC = Orbitofrontal Cortex; PCS = post-concussion symptoms

Table 3. Characteristics of studies from literature search presented in order of study recency

When focusing on the incidence and presentation of anxiety disorders in general, only four studies were found relevant. One study focused on the incidence of OCD and presence of OCD symptomatology following severe TBI in children and adolescents [37], while the remaining studies explored the relationship between TBI and the incidence of disorders including GAD, ASD, PTSD, PD, OCD, simple/specific phobia, social phobia and SAD [38-40]. Only two studies included participants with mild, moderate and severe TBI [38-39], while the rest focused on severe TBI [37, 40]. Generally, the results demonstrate that in children and adolescents who have sustained aTBI of any severity, there is a statistically significant higher risk of developing subsequent anxiety disorders [37-40].

Overanxious (heightened anxiety which is generalised and non-specific) was a commonly reported disorder in children with severe TBI [40], and the presence of OCD symptomatology following severe TBI was significantly more common in females. When comparing children with mild TBI, moderate/severe TBI and OI, results suggest a potential relationship between degree of neurological insult and risk of developing subsequent anxiety disorders [38], in that overall anxiety disorders were most common in children with moderate/severe TBI, followed by mild TBI and OI. However, similarly to research on PTSD after TBI, the pattern of results is often quite different among the sample groups, including differing age ranges, varying use of control groups, and severity of TBI. For instance, a few of the studies [37, 39-40] didn't use any comparison group when examining rates of anxiety symptomatology and diagnoses, and as such the conclusion that such diagnoses are heightened in a TBI sample is relatively weak, as compared to another study [38] which compared incidence of anxiety diagnoses to an OI comparison group. In terms of gender differences, among two of the studies, gender as a predictor was either not considered [38] or not discussed in any detail [39-40]. Only one study found that being female was associated with a higher number of obsessive compulsive symptoms, with a greater number of females reporting obsessive compulsive symptoms following TBI [37].

Predictors/Risk Factors
· Internalising disorders [32, 34, 37]
· Severity of TBI [32, 34, 38]
· Younger age at injury [33, 39, 40]
· Social disadvantage [33-34]
· Family social status [33-34]
· High levels of pre-morbid psychosocial adversity [34-35, 37, 40-41]
· Female gender [34, 37]
· Pre-morbid mood or anxiety disorders [32, 34, 37-38]
· Pre-morbid ADHD [38]
· Pre-morbid learning disabilities [38]
· Parent education [38]
· Post-injury stress scores [38]
· Post-concussive symptoms [11]
· Concurrent depression [39]
· Concurrent personality change [39]

Table 4. Predictors and risk factors for anxiety following TBI

Among the research, common themes exist in reference to the relationship between anxiety disorders and TBI in children and adolescents. A number of the studies presented here assessed for pre-morbid psychosocial adversity, with all studies reporting higher rates of anxiety and PTSD symptomatology and diagnoses in children from families with higher pre-morbid psychosocial adversity [34-35, 37, 40-41]. In addition, when the impact of age was assessed within the methodology, it was found that younger age at injury tended to be associated with a higher number of anxiety symptoms [33, 39-40] in such children. Alternatively however, there have been conflicting results, in that one found no support for age as a significant predictor of PTSD in their sample of children with severe TBI [34]. This is comparative to results found in a sample of children with mild, moderate and severe TBI, whereby younger age was associated with a higher number of PTSD symptoms [33]. This may be accounted for by the fact that in [34], the researchers utilised a large age range of participants (4-19 years), versus the other study which restricted their sample to children aged 6-12 years [33]. The implications of age ranges utilised in the study samples is discussed further below. See Table 4 for the predictors and risk factors for children and adolescents to develop anxiety disorders and symptomology following TBI.

4.2. Neural substrates and brain regions associated with anxiety following TBI

In examining the brain regions associated with a higher risk of anxiety following childhood TBI, it is important to first review the areas of the brain that are commonly injured and implicated in TBI. Damage as a result of TBI can be either focal, whereby forces have caused localised damage, or diffuse, whereby damage has occurred to axonal properties across the brain [42-43]. Due to the fact that TBI can occur under many different, individualised circumstances, damage to the brain is heterogeneous [44]. However, it has been noted that the frontal and temporal regions are highly vulnerable to injury, due to the shape of the skull and the way the head is held [22, 44-46]. The frontotemporal susceptibility to damage from TBI has been noted as the major cause of the cognitive and neurobehavioral consequences of TBI that some go on to experience, including emotional regulation [45]. Further, white matter tracts have been demonstrated to be more susceptible to damage due to the acceleration-deceleration forces and their direct exposure to shear and strain forces [43-44, 47], and this white matter tract damage tends to occur more frequently again within the frontotemporal areas of the brain [44].

Due to the diffuse damage likely to occur following TBI, and the heterogeneity that occurs across individuals, research has sought to explore and highlight the most commonly affected regions within the brain that may be associated with long-term behavioural and emotional problems. Reports from a multicentre study of children with TBI have noted white matter hypersensitivities and focal atrophy distributed across frontotemporal areas of the brain [44]. More specifically, Magnetic Resonance Imaging (MRI) scans highlighted that among children with mild, moderate and severe TBI, there were lesions evident in frontal regions, temporal poles, and right medial temporal lobe, and damage was also evident to the amygdala, hippocampus, thalamus and basal ganglia [44]. MRI procedures were also used in another sample of children with moderate and severe TBI, to evaluate brain volume differences in the whole brain and also prefrontal, temporal and posterior regions [22]. Imaging results indicated that children with TBI had significantly reduced whole brain, prefrontal and temporal regional tissue volumes compared to that of uninjured children. Further, there were also group differences on white matter and grey matter in superior medial and ventromedial prefrontal regions [22]. Additional research has also utilised MRI procedures to locate brain regions more commonly affected following TBI, with one study including individuals with mild to moderate TBI [46]. In terms of number of lesions, results showed that the frontal and temporal areas had significantly more lesions than parietal and occipital areas of the brain. Again, this is supported by the Toronto TBI study, which recruited individuals with chronic TBI across all levels of severity to undergo MRI 1 year following injury [42]. The most reliable effects noted in the results were brain volume changes within the frontal, temporal and cingulate regions, with focal lesions associated with greater volume loss in frontal and temporal regions [42]. Finally, MRI has been used to examine reductions in fractional anisotropy (reflects fibre density, axonal diameter and myelination in white matter) in adults with mild TBI [47]. Results again demonstrated more reductions in frontal and temporal regions, and also parietal regions, and among association bundles, fronto-temporal-occipital fibre bundles were most often involved [48]. Table 5 provides a concise summary of the above findings within the literature.

As is evident, the frontal and temporal regions are highly implicated following TBI of all severities. In looking at the neural regions implicated in those with anxiety disorders following TBI, it may be possible to discover overlapping regions. However, only two studies have specifically attempted to delineate the neural correlates and brain regions involved in the development of anxiety disorders following TBI in children and adolescents [35, 40]. One of these studies focused on lesion burden in children with severe TBI and their relationship with PTSD symptomatology [35]. Data was obtained from a cohort from a pre-existing study [34], which utilised participants with only severe TBI, and did not include any comparison group. Magnetic Resonance Imaging (MRI) at 3 months following the TBI event revealed associations between lesion fractions in the right cingulum, right hippocampus, right medial frontal gyrus and left hippocampus at 3 months post-TBI, and the presence of PTSD re-experiencing symptoms at 1 year [35]. In addition, assignment to the PTSD versus no-PTSD diagnosis group was dependent on lesions in the right medial frontal and left middle temporal gryi [35]. Furthermore, a lower probability of suffering from PTSD hyperarousal correlated with higher lesion fraction in the left subcallosal gyrus, and avoidance symptoms were associated with lower lesion burden in the right medial frontal and left inferior temporal gyri and higher lesion burden in the left middle temporal gyrus [35]. Interestingly, the researchers found no association between the re-experiencing criterion of PTSD and lesions in the right amygdala, despite research which has suggested that the amygdala is an important structure in the processing of fear and emotional signals [23], and in anxiety symptoms [24].

Again utilising the same cohort of participants in [34], the incidence and presence of anxiety disorders in general and their neural correlates in patients with severe TBI was examined, using MRI procedures [41]. The study was unique in that it attempted to correlate specific brain lesions and their location, with different anxiety outcomes among children with severe TBI. In a 1-year prospective study, with a focus on the orbitofrontal cortex (OFC), imaging results

Study	Main results
[46] Levin et al. (1992)	Number of lesions from MRI: · Total = 145 · Frontal = 60 · Temporal = 55 · Parietal = 15 · Occipital = 10
[22] Wilde et al. (2005)	MRI volumetric findings: · Prefrontal regions smaller in those with TBI · Superior medial grey and white matter, lateral frontal white matter, and ventromedial grey matter smaller in TBI group · Lesion volumes from MRI: · Majority lesions in frontal and temporal areas
[42] Levine et al. (2008)	· Volume changes in ventral frontal and temporal regions · Cerebrospinal fluid increases in left medial frontal and posterior temporal regions · Grey matter volume changes in ventral frontal, middle frontal, superior frontal, bilateral posterior temporal, left medial temporal, left occipital and basal ganglia/thalamic regions
[47] Rutgers et al. (2008)	Brain regions with reduced fractional anisotropy from MRI: · Frontal lobe = 42 individuals (22%) · Parietal lobe = 31 individuals (16%) · Temporal lobe = 28 individuals (15%) · Occipital lobe = 4 individuals (2%)
[44] Bigler et al. (2013)	· Distribution of lesions was more frequent in frontal and temporal regions · Mean group volume differences for white matter, grey matter, hippocampus, amygdala, thalamus, basal ganglia · Focal signal abnormalities and white matter hypersensitivities located predominantly in frontal and temporal lobe regions

Table 5. Summary of commonly damaged brain regions following TBI

revealed that the presence of OFC lesions decreased the risk of anxiety disorders when control variables (demographics, psychosocial adversity, preinjury anxiety, injury severity, post-injury PTSD, whole brain volume) were included in the analyses [41]. Therefore, an inverse relationship exists in that children with more lesions to the OFC as a result of TBI are less likely to develop anxiety disorders than those with fewer lesions. This is said to be due to a disruption between the OFC and amygdala, which results in a disrupted ability to modify responses to cues based on processing the emotional valence of a stimulus [41].The OFC is purported to have important reciprocal connections with the amygdala [41], which again further supports the brain region studies which target the amygdala in having some role in anxiety disorders in children [23-24].

In addition, two other studies included MRI procedures in their methodology - however brain lesion analysis was not a major aim of their study [33, 37, 39]. In examining the nature of OCD symptomatology in children and adolescents with a history of severe TBI, some specific areas were located to potentially be associated with the onset of OCD symptomatology following TBI [37]. MRI scans revealed relationships between OCD symptoms and lesions in the OFC and temporal lobe regions, and also thalamic lesions for males [37]. Alternatively, in their study of anxiety disorders in children and adolescents following severe TBI [39], it was reported that a trend association exists between lesions to the superior frontal gyrus and the presence of novel anxiety disorders. Furthermore, a statistically significant association was found between lesions to the superior frontal gyrus and novel subclinical anxiety disorder [39]. However, no other statistically significant relationships between specific brain lesions and anxiety symptomatology were found in the study.

The above studies implicate certain regions in relation to the elevated incidence of anxiety disorders following TBI in children and adolescents, with emphasis on structures such as the OFC, right medial frontal gyri and temporal gyri. Table 3 outlines the specific regions implicated in anxiety following TBI from the literature. Evidently, these findings highlight a link with commonly affected brain regions following TBI, where research has implicated areas associated with the frontal and temporal regions. While these studies provide some compelling initial evidence for the neurobiological basis of anxiety disorders following TBI, it is clear that the literature in this area is still very sparse and lacking.

Brain Regions Implicated
· Right cingulum [35]
· Right hippocampus [35]
· Frontal regions [35, 37, 39]
- Right medial frontal gyrus [35]
- Right medial frontal cortex [35]
- Mesial prefrontal cortex [41]
- Frontal lobes [37]
- Superior frontal gyrus [39]
· Left hippocampus [35]
· Temporal regions [35, 37, 41]
- Left temporal regions [37]
- Left middle temporal gyri [35]
- Temporal lobes [37]
· Right amygdala [35]
· Orbitofrontal cortex [37, 41]

Table 6. Brain regions associated with anxiety in children and adolescents with TBI

5. Discussion

The above literature demonstrates that the presence of mild, moderate and severe TBI in children and adolescents significantly increases the risk of developing subsequent anxiety disorders [37-40], with feeling overanxious being a commonly reported anxiety symptom in children with severe TBI [40]. When comparing children with mild TBI, moderate/

severe TBI and OI, overall results suggests a potential relationship between the degree of neurological insult that has occurred, and the risk of developing new-onset anxiety disorders [38]. In addition, it has been noted that there is a similar link found for those with PTSD following TBI. The research suggests that while there is a rare (yet, noted) occurrence of PTSD following moderate or severe TBI in children, and a statistically significant difference in the frequency of this occurrence between children with moderate or severe TBI to children with OI, this relationship may not exist for children with only mild TBI. Furthermore, the most important predictors for anxiety symptomatology following childhood TBI include social disadvantage/family social status, severity of TBI, psychosocial adversity and younger age of injury [33-35, 37, 40-41].

5.1. Methodological concerns

As indicated above in Table 2, the studies were analysed according to their methodological merit, as determined by set criteria [31]. Three of the studies [11, 33, 38] included all of the listed criteria, and the most commonly missed criteria was a lack of a control group in 7 out of the 11 papers [32, 34-35, 37, 39-41]. All included studies showed evidence of criteria b), c) and e), indicating the use of longitudinal designs, well-defined TBI groups and standardised outcome measures and assessments. Only one study did not include more than 20 TBI participants or control for pre-injury characteristics [36].

Of concern is the number of studies that did not include a non-TBI group. The research being discussed explores the rate of anxiety disorders following TBI in children and adolescents, and although this information can be obtained using only a TBI group, the strength of the results may be enhanced if authors could compare these rates to a non-injured or OI group of participants, particularly when anxiety is already evident in high rates in the general population. It is also interesting to note that of the studies that did include a control group [11, 33, 36, 38], all utilised an OI group with injuries sustained to regions of the body other than the head or neck. There is therefore an absence of studies that have compared the incidence of anxiety disorders in children and adolescents with TBI and healthy control subjects. While it is useful to use an OI comparison group as this eliminates confounding variables associated with the nature of injury and exposure to hospital/rehabilitation services, the literature is in need of research that compares the incidence of anxiety following TBI to what is expected in the general child population.

In addition, while all but one controlled for pre-injury characteristics and risk factors [36], issues pertain to the validity of such measures regarding the timing of testing. In all cases, premorbid functioning such as behavior scores, pre-existing psychiatric disorders and family functioning assessments were conducted at 'baseline' – meaning that they were assessed following the TBI event. This presents a large issue within the TBI literature as it is difficult to ascertain the validity of reports on child variables that were present before the injury when they are considered retrospectively. Psychological stress as a result of the injury, for both the child and the parent, is likely to affect the ability for the parent or child to recall incidents and functioning before the TBI event. Furthermore, the child's current behavior and functioning may change the child or parent's perspective of what occurred before the TBI. However, the authors do attempt to alleviate the effects of this issue in that testing at 'baseline' was always conducted as soon as possible, once major concussion symptoms (such as PTA) had resided.

A major strength among the literature on anxiety disorders following TBI in children and adolescents is the use of a prospective, longitudinal design with follow-up assessments of behavior and anxiety. Several studies conducted follow-ups up to 1 year after TBI [11, 32-35, 37, 40-41], which allowed for the examination of long-term effects of TBI and the persistence and chronicity of anxiety in such participants. Furthermore, in fewer studies [11, 32-33], participants were assessed at multiple time points, which is essential for exploring the pattern of anxiety disorders and symptomatology following TBI across time. Additionally, well-defined severity groups are important when conducting TBI studies, particularly when comparing groups and when assessing the influence of injury severity on outcomes. Evidently, the studies presented in this paper all assessed and defined severity of TBI using the GCS. The GCS is regarded as the most common method of assessing TBI severity [17], and has been proven both useful and valid in multiple studies. In addition, in many cases other markers of TBI severity were also examined, such as positive CT scans [32-33, 38-39] and the duration of LOC [33, 36-37, 39].

Overall, when considering the methodological merit of the studies listed in this paper, the results seem quite positive. While the absence of a control group for over half of the studies poses some concern for the generalizability of findings, their methodology is strengthened by the use of a longitudinal design with timely follow-up assessments post-TBI and well-defined and accurately assessed TBI severity for each injury group. In addition, all but one study [36] had an adequately sized sample of TBI participants. Furthermore, outcome measures for all of the papers were assessed using standardised, common measures and procedures for examining the presence of anxiety disorders in children and adolescents.

5.2. Other concerns

Examining the literature, common methodological concerns arise across the featured studies. An important finding is that there is a lack of research which has included participants with mild TBI, with a large focus on children with severe TBI. Of the studies in this review, five included participants who had suffered mild TBI [11, 32, 36, 38-39], while the majority only included participants with moderate-severe TBI or severe TBI. Considering that studies on externalising disorders have indicated an increased incidence of psychiatric disorders such as ADHD, ODD, CD, drug and alcohol abuse/use and personality disorders in children with even mild TBI [6-7, 9], it surprising that such a sample has been relatively neglected in the literature.

In relation to this, it is often suggested within the PTSD literature that the diagnosis of PTSD following TBI is not valid due to the nature of the psychological events that follow such an injury [32-33, 36]. This argument states that children who suffer from TBI and lose consciousness or experience PTA are unable to suffer the anxiety of PTSD that is associated with re-experiencing a traumatic event, as the event itself cannot be recalled and subsequently emotionally suppressed [32-33]. The authors, however, do not discuss this argument in relation to children who suffer from a TBI mild enough that it does not result in loss of consciousness (LOC) or PTA. However, instead they tended to utilise samples of children with more severe injuries [33-35], thereby contradicting their argument. Furthermore, over half of the research has focused on solely PTSD following TBI [11, 32-36] and excluded other anxiety disorders, due to the close relationship it has with trauma [40]. Moreover, one study [36] applied more focus on PTSD in children following road traffic accidents, and utilised the TBI group as a control for confounds associated with such an injury, rather than exploring long-term anxiety outcomes following TBI.

Also interesting to note in regards to PTSD following TBI is the discrepancy that is often found between reports of PTSD symptomatology from the child versus the parents. For instance, in [32] and [36], both studies utilised both parent and child report questionnaires to assess PTSD. However, correlational analyses indicated a relatively low relationship between reports from children and adults, and of which the relationship was non-significant in both cases. The meaning of this is not well discussed, which poses a challenge to the methodology of papers which utilise only one source of PTSD symptom reporting. In addition, it is not well-known whether this relationship (or lack thereof) also exists for other anxiety measures. Indeed, some have questioned the validity of parent-report methods for assessing anxiety, arguing that these internal states can be reliably reported by the children themselves, without need for parental reports [38]. Internalising disorders in children and adolescents are not as readily observable for parents, and as such, it may be difficult to report their presence or absence in their children. Further, younger children and children who have sustained a TBI and have developed cognitive deficits may not understand or be able to articulate the internalising problems they are experiencing. As such, this discrepancy between parent and child reports of internalising symptoms should be explored further to examine the best possible way to accurately assess difficulties such children and adolescents may exhibit following TBI.

The importance of gender as a predictor of anxiety disorders following TBI has been significantly neglected within this literature. Considering that a higher number of females experience and report internalising and anxiety problems compared to males in both a normal [48] and TBI [30] population, it is surprising that gender differences in these studies hasn't been thoroughly explored. Women are at greater risk of developing anxiety disorders including GAD, PD and PTSD [49], and also some phobias [50]. However, differences in the psychopathology of children following TBI is has rarely been compared across gender groups, as is evident in the above samples. Given that much work has been done exploring externalising behavioural outcomes of children post-TBI, such as attention, hyperactivity and aggressive behaviours [3-6], it is important that behaviours that are more likely to be seen in a female population are also as extensively explored.

Finally, while there have been some advancements towards the study of internalising problems, including anxiety disorders, following TBI in children and adolescents, it is vital to note that of the 11 papers presented here, 5 of these utilised the same cohort of individuals [34-35, 37, 40-41]. While the sample itself was derived from a large database of referrals from tertiary trauma centres over a relatively large period of time (years 1992-1996), the fact that these studies were replicated among the same cohort limits the generalizability of the results to anxiety and TBI literature. Although the studies provided useful information regarding the relationship between TBI and anxiety disorders [34, 37, 40] and also neural correlates associated with anxiety disorders after TBI [35, 41], the literature remains sparse in relation to different cohorts of children and adolescents being examined for such variables.

5.3. Practical implications

Given the findings in the literature, when assessing children who have been admitted for TBI, it may be important to screen for factors associated with family psychiatric history of internalising disorders, the individual's past psychiatric history of internalising disorders, and also to examine levels of psychosocial adversity. Furthermore, the increased vulnerability of children with a younger age at injury to developing subsequent anxiety disorders would be considered in such assessments. Children who are younger at the time of TBI, have greater psychosocial adversity and have some history of psychiatric internalising disorders may be at greater risk of developing anxiety disorders, and so if such children are targeted early, appropriate intervention practices may be put in place.

Intervention programs for children vulnerable to developing anxiety disorders following TBI may include relaxation procedures for the parent and the child, coping strategies, self-esteem building activities, or open communication between the parent and child regarding the child's anxiety symptoms or worries. Furthermore, those at high risk of developing anxiety disorders may benefit from a follow-up screen following their TBI to assess for any anxiety symptoms, and potentially undergo typical anxiety management procedures such as cognitive-behavior therapy, behavioural assessment and psychotherapy. It is important that such poor outcomes following TBI are targeted and managed early, to enhance quality of life and prevent the negative effects anxiety would have on both social and academic learning and development.

5.4. Limitations

One major limitation of this review is that only 11 papers have been reviewed for discussion. In addition, among these papers, 5 utilised the same cohort of participants. However, this fact highlights further the need for more work in the field of anxiety disorders following childhood TBI. As mentioned above, it is likely that there is less of a focus on internalising behaviours because males have been reported to be at greater risk of TBI than females [28-29], and that the more overt and distressing nature of externalising problems [27] are more readily reported by parents, and also more observable to the human eye.

5.5. Future directions and conclusions

It is clear from the small number of studies generated in this literature search that much work needs to be done in examining the incidence and rate of anxiety disorders following TBI in children and adolescents. Studies that have investigated the presence and rate of PTSD diagnoses and symptomatology [34], and the rate of pre- and post-TBI anxiety disorders and symptoms [40], should be replicated in different samples, with the inclusion of children with both mild and moderate TBI. Moreover, future studies should include the use of control groups to compare against children with TBI, and utilise both healthy control participants and children with OI, as the presence and rate of anxiety disorders is expected to be different among each of these groups. Furthermore, the relationship between parent and child reports of anxiety disorders should be examined, considering the low correlation scores found among reports of PTSD in the present literature [33, 36]. Finally, more studies should attempt to explore brain regions and lesion burdens associated with anxiety disorders in such a sample, as such studies are severely lacking.

This chapter examined the current literature assessing the presence of anxiety disorders following TBI in children and adolescents. While the literature to date is sparse, it may be concluded that children who have suffered from a TBI (mild, moderate or severe), are at a higher risk of developing subsequent anxiety disorders, even 1 year following the injury event. Moreover, children with more severe injuries, greater psychosocial adversity, and younger age at injury may be at the greatest risk, and are a group who would benefit from early intervention. Further studies are needed to replicate all the above findings and generate a more comprehensive view of the relationship between TBI and internalising disorders within the literature.

Author details

Michelle Albicini[1*] and Audrey McKinlay[2]

*Address all correspondence to: michelle.albicini@monash.edu

1 Monash University; School of Psychological Sciences, Australia

2 The University of Melbourne, School of Psychological Sciences, Psychology Clinic, Australia

References

[1] Styrke J, Stalnacke B, Sojka P, Bjorstig. Traumatic brain injuries in a well-defined population: epidemiological aspects and severity. Journal of Neurotrauma 2007;24 1425-1436.

[2] McKinlay A, Hawley CA. Incidence rates for traumatic brain injury in children: International Brain Injury Association. http://www.internationalbrain.org/incidence-rates-for-traumatic-brain-injury-in-children/ (accessed 4 December 2014)

[3] Hawley CA. Reported problems and their resolution following mild, moderate and severe traumatic brain injury amongst children and adolescents in the UK. Brain Injury 2003;17(2) 105-129. doi: 10.1080/0269905021000010131

[4] Liu J, Li L. Parent-reported mild head injury history and behavioural performance in children at 6 years. Brain Injury 2013;27(11) 1263-1270. doi: 10.3109/02699052.2013.804205

[5] Massagli TL, Fann JR, Burington BE, Jaffe KM, Katon WJ, Thompson RS. Psychiatric illness after mild traumatic brain injury in children. Archives of Physical Medicine and Rehabilitation 2004;85(9), 1428-1434. doi: 10.1016/j.apmr.2003.12.036

[6] McKinlay A, Dalrymple-Alford J, Horwood J, Fergusson D. Long term psychosocial outcomes after mild head injury in early childhood. Journal of Neurology, Neurosurgery and Psychiatry 2002;73 281-288.

[7] McKinlay A, Grace R, Horwood J, Fergusson D, MacFarlane M. Adolescent psychiatric symptoms following preschool childhood mild traumatic brain injury: Evidence from a birth cohort. Journal of Head Trauma Rehabilitation 2009;24(3) 221-227.

[8] Schwartz L. Long-Term Behavior Problems Following Pediatric Traumatic Brain Injury: Prevalence, Predictors, and Correlates. Journal of Pediatric Psychology 2013;28(4) 251-263. doi: 10.1093/jpepsy/jsg013

[9] Max JE, Schachar R, Landis J, Bigler E, Wilde E, Saunders A... Levin H. Psychiatric disorders in children and adolescents in the first six months after mild traumatic brain injury. Journal of Neuropsychiatry and Clinical Neuroscience 2013;25(3) 187-197.

[10] Max JE, Wilde E, Bigler E, MacLeod M, Vasquez A, Schmidt A... Levin H. Psychiatric disorders after pediatric traumatic brain injury: A prospective, longitudinal, controlled study Journal of Neuropsychiatry and Clinical Neuroscience 2012;24(4) 427-436.

[11] Hajek CA, Yeates KO, Gerry TH, Bangert B, Dietrich A, Nuss KE... Wright M. Relationships among post-concussive symptoms and symptoms of PTSD in children following mild traumatic brain injury. Brain Injury 2010;24(2) 100-109. doi: 10.3109/02699050903508226

[12] Centers for Disease Control and Injury Prevention. CDC: Traumatic Brain Injury. http://www.cdc.gov/TraumaticBrainInjury/ (accessed 13 February 2014)

[13] Corrigan J, Selassie A, Orman J. The epidemiology of traumatic brain injury. Journal of Head Trauma Rehabilitation 2010;25(2) 72-80.

[14] American Congress of Rehabilitation Medicine. Definition of mild traumatic brain injury. Journal of Head Trauma Rehabilitation 1993;8(3) 86-87.

[15] Maas AIR, Stocchetti N, Bullock R. Moderate and severe traumatic brain injury in adults. The Lancet Neurology 2008;7(8) 728-741. doi: 10.1016/s1474-4422(08)70164-9

[16] McKinlay A. Controversies and outcomes associated with mild traumatic brain injury in childhood and adolescences. Child Care and Health Development 2010;36(1) 3-21. doi: 10.1111/j.1365-2214.2009.01006.x

[17] Greenwood R. Head injury for neurologists. Journal of Neurology, Neurosurgery and Psychiatry 2002;73 (Suppl I) i8-i16.

[18] Baalen B, Odding E, Maas AIR, Ribbers G, Bergen M, Stam H. Traumatic brain injury: Classification of initial severity and determination of final outcome. Disability and Rehabilitation 2003;25(1) 9-18.

[19] Max JE, Smith W, Lindgren S, Robin D, Mattheis P, Stierwalt J, Morrisey M. Case study: Obsessive-Compulsive Disorder after severe traumatic brain injury in an adolescent. Journal of the American Academy of Child and Adolescent Psychiatry 1995;34(1) 45-49.

[20] Chaves C, Trzesniak C, Derenusson GN, Araujo D, Wichert-Ana L, Machado-De-Sousa JP....Hallak JEC. Late-onset social anxiety disorder following traumatic brain injury. Brain Injury 2012;26(6) 882-886.

[21] Karver CL, Wade SL, Cassedy A, Taylor HG, Stancin T, Yeates KO, Walz NC. Age at injury and long-term behavior problems after traumatic brain injury in young children. Rehabilitation Psychology 2012;57(3) 256-265. doi: 10.1037/a0029522

[22] Wilde EA, Bigler ED, Hunter JV, Fearing M, Scheibel R, Newsome M... Levin HS. Hippocampus, amygdala and basal ganglia morphometrics in children after moderate-to-severe traumatic brain injury. Developmental Medicine and Child Neurology 2007;49 294-299.

[23] Baird A, Gruber S, Fein D, Maas L, Steingard R, Renshaw P... Yurgelun-Todd D. Functional magnetic resonance imaging of facial affect recognition in children and adolescents. Journal of American Academy of Child and Adolescent Psychiatry 1999;38(2) 195-199.

[24] De Bellis M, Casey B, Dahl R, Birmaher B, Williamson D, Thomas K... Ryan N. A pilot study of amygdala volumes in pediatric Generalised Anxiety Disorder. Society of Biological Psychiatry 2009;48 51-57.

[25] Arnsten AF. Stress signaling pathways that impair prefrontal cortex structure and function. Nature Reviews Neuroscience 2009;10 410–422.

[26] Brinks V, de Kloet ER, Oitzl MS. Strain specific fear behaviour and glucocorticoid response to aversive events: modelling ptsd in mice. Progress in Brain Research 2008;167 257–261.

[27] Bayer JK, Ukoumunne OC, Mathers M, Wake M, Abdi N, Hiscock H. Development of children's internalising and externalising problems from infancy to five years of age. Psychiatry 2012;46(7) 659-668.

[28] Crowe L, Babl F, Anderson V, Catroppa C. The epidemiology of paediatric head injuries: data from a referral centre in Victoria, Australia. Journal of Paediatric and Child Health 2009;45(6) 346-350. doi: 10.1111/j.1440-1754.2009.01499.x

[29] McKinlay A, Grace RC, Horwood LJ, Fergusson DM, Ridder EM, MacFarlane MR. Prevalence of traumatic brain injury among children, adolescents and young adults: prospective evidence from a birth cohort. Brain Injury2008;22(2) 175-181. doi: 10.1080/02699050801888824

[30] Scott C, McKinlay A, McLellan T, Britt E, Grace R, McFarlane M. A comparison of adult outcomes for males compared to females following paediatric traumatic brain injury. Neuropsychology 2014. No Pagination Specified.

[31] Satz P. Mild Head Injury in Children and Adolescents. Current Directions in Psychological Science 2001;10(3) 106-109. doi: 10.1111/1467-8721.00127

[32] Max JE, Castillo C, Robin D, Lindgren S, Smith W, Sato Y, Arndt S. Posttraumatic stress symptomatology after childhood traumatic brain injury. The Journal of Nervous and Mental Disease 1998;186(10) 589-596.

[33] Levi RB, Drotar D, Yeates KO, Taylor HG. Posttraumatic stress symptoms in children following orthopedic or traumatic brain injury. Journal of Clinical Child Psychology 1999;28(2) 232-243. doi: 10.1207/s15374424jccp2802_10

[34] Gerring J, Slomine BS, Vasa RA, Grados MA, Chen A, Rising W... Ernst M. Clinical predictors of Posttraumatic Stress Disorder after closed head injury in children. Journal of the American Academy of Child and Adolescent Psychiatry 2002;41(2) 157-165.

[35] Herskovits EH, Gerring J, Davatzikos C, Bryan R. Is the spatial distribution of brain lesions associated with closed-head injury in children predictive of subsequent development of Posttraumatic Stress Disorder?. Radiology 2002;224 345-351.

[36] Mather FJ, Tate RL, Hannan TJ. Post-traumatic stress disorder in children following road traffic accidents: a comparison of those with and without mild traumatic brain injury. Brain Injury 2003;17(12) 1077-1087. doi: 10.1080/0269905031000114045

[37] Grados MA, Vasa RA, Riddle MA, Slomine BS, SalorioC, Christensen J, Gerring J. New onset obsessive-compulsive symptoms in children and adolescents with severe traumatic brain injury. Depression and Anxiety 2008;25(5) 398-407. doi: 10.1002/da.20398

[38] Luis CA, Mittenberg W. Mood and anxiety disorders following pediatric traumatic brain injury: a prospective study. Journal of Clinical and Experimental Neuropsychology 2002;24(3) 270-279. doi: 10.1076/jcen.24.3.270.982

[39] Max JE, Keatley E, Wilde E, Bigler E, Levin H, Schachar R... Yang T. Anxiety disorders in children and adolescents in the first six months after traumatic brain injury. The Journal of Neuropsychaitry and Clinical Neurosciences 2011;23 29-39.

[40] Vasa R, Gerring JP, Grados M, Slomine B, Christensen J, Rising W... Riddle MA. Anxiety after severe pediatric closed head injury. American Academy of Child and Adolescent Psychitry 2002;41(2) 148-156.

[41] Vasa RA, Grados M, Slomine B, Herskovits EH, Thompson RE, Salorio C... Gerring JP. Neuroimaging correlates of anxiety after pediatric traumatic brain injury. Biological Psychiatry 2004;55(3) 208-216. doi: 10.1016/s0006-3223(03)00708-x

[42] Levine B, Kovacevic N, Nica EI, Cheung G, Gao F, Schwartz ML, Black SE. The Torronto traumatic brain injury study. Neurology 2008;7 771-778.

[43] Povlishock JT, Katz DI. Update of neuropathology and neurological recovery after traumatic brain injury. Journal of Head Trauma Rehabilitation 2008;20(1) 76-94.

[44] Bigler ED, Dennis M, Taylor HG, Vannatta K, Gerhardt CA, Abildskov TJ.... Yeates KO. Heterogeneity of brain lesions in pediatric traumatic brain injury. Neuropsychology 2013;27(4) 438-451.

[45] Bigler ED. Anterior and middle cranial fossa in traumatic brain injury: Relevant neuroanatomy and neuropathology in the study of neuropsychological outcome. Neuropsychology 2007;21(5) 515-531.

[46] Levin HS, Williams DJ, Eisenberg HM, High WM Jr, Guinto FC Jr. Serial MRI and neurobehavioural findings after mild to moderate closed head injury. Journal of Neurology, Neurosurgery and Psychiatry 1992;55 255-262.

[47] Rutgers DR, Toulgoat F, Cazejust J, Fillard P, Lasjaunias P, Ducreux D. White matter abnormalities in mild traumatic brain injury : A diffusion tensor imaging study. American Journal of Neuroradiology 2008;29, 514-519.

[48] McLean CP, Asnaani A, Litz BT, Hofmann SG. Gender differences in anxiety disorders: prevalence, course of illness, comorbidity and burden of illness. Journal of psychiatric research 2011;45(8) 1027-1035.

[49] Carr A, McNulty M., Editors. The handbook of adult clinical psychology: An evidence-based approach. London: Routledge; 2006.

[50] Seeman MV. Psychopathology in women and men: Focus on female hormones. American Journal of Psychiatry 1997;154 1641-1647.

Chapter 11

Impact of Anxiety and Depression Symptoms on Scholar Performance in High School and University Students

Blandina Bernal-Morales,
Juan Francisco Rodríguez-Landa and
Frank Pulido-Criollo

Additional information is available at the end of the chapter

Abstract

Emotional processes are important to survive. The Darwinian adaptive concept of stress refers to natural selection since evolved individuals have acquired effective strategies to adapt to the environment and to unavoidable changes. If demands are abrupt and intense, there might be insufficient time to successful responses. Usually, stress produces a cognitive or perceptual evaluation (emotional memory) which motivates to make a plan, to take a decision and to perform an action to face successfully the demand. Between several kinds of stresses, there are psychosocial and emotional stresses with cultural, social and political influences. The cultural changes have modified the way in which individuals socially interact. Deficits in familiar relationships and social isolation alter physical and mental health in young students, producing reduction of their capacities of facing stressors in school. Adolescence is characterized by significant physiological, anatomical, and psychological changes in boys and girls, who become vulnerable to psychiatric disorders. In particular for young adult students, anxiety and depression symptoms could interfere in their academic performance. In this chapter, we reviewed approaches to the study of anxiety and depression symptoms related with the academic performance in adolescent and graduate students. Results from available published studies in academic journals are reviewed to discuss the importance to detect information about academic performance, which leads to discover in many cases the very commonly subdiagnosed psychiatric disorders in adolescents, that is, anxiety and depression. With the reviewed evidence of how anxiety and depression in young adult students may alter their main activity in life (studying and academic performance), we discussed data in order to show a way in which professionals involved in schools could support students and stablish a routine of intervention in any case.

Keywords: anxiety, depression, scholar performance, students, education, mental health

1. Introduction

Anxiety is a natural emotion characterized by alertness, vegetative autonomous and behavioral responses, accompanied by subjective sensations, all important for surviving. In the long term, an overexposition to adverse stimuli may lead to a depression comorbid to anxiety. Usually, human beings facing a stressor develop a cognitive or perceptual evaluation comparing previous experiences to solve the threat through an action. Consequently to natural anxiety, a state of heightened attention occurs preparing the body to fight or run away from the perceived threat. This fight-or-flight anxiety response follows an inverted U-shape curve; there is an optimum quantity of anxiety that produces the best response to success. A high level of anxiety interferes with concentration and memory, which are critical for academic success. Without any anxiety, however, people would lack the motivation to study for exams, write papers, or do daily homework, among others. In addition, deficits in familiar relationships and social isolation alter physical and mental health in young students, which reduce their capacities at school. Adolescence is characterized by significant physiological, anatomical and psychological changes in boys and girls, who become vulnerable to psychiatric disorders. Disorders such as anxiety and depression affect scholar performance and students might not be appropriately attended. In this chapter we describe anxiety and depression focused on adolescents and reviewed approaches to the study of anxiety and depression symptoms related with the academic performance in adolescents and young guys. The research literature was based on PubMed and Google Advanced Scholar databases. Results from available published studies in academic journals are reviewed to discuss the importance to detect information about anxiety, depression, academic performance and further considerations.

2. Anxiety and depression

2.1. Concept

Anxiety is an adaptive response generated by environmental stressful situations that activate alarm mechanisms in the individual to assure survival. This emotion is a series of biochemical changes in the brain and body, which makes the heart to beat faster due to an increase in adrenaline, and feeling less pain due to a decrease in cerebral dopamine. However, if the state of anxiety is not adequately affronted or it is produced by an inexistent stimulus in the longterm, natural anxiety is now converted in an anxiety disorder. In this way, natural anxiety is beneficial for the individual but if the level of anxiety is exceeded, it deteriorates the habitual activity of the organism; in this case, higher anxiety produces a lower efficiency of the individual [1, 2]. In human beings, anxiety disorders are characterized by excessive fear and distress in the absence of real danger, that is to say, an excessive preoccupation, fatigue, problems of sleeping or concentrating, irritability, muscle tension, aggressive behavior, vulnerability sensation, surveillance exacerbation, and exaggerated emotional reactions to danger [3]. The anxiety symptoms reflect an excessive autonomic activity caused by the over-release of adrenaline, noradrenaline and cortisol, which in consequence produces perspiration, palpitations, rise in blood pressure, loss of sphincters control, development of gastric ulcers, among others. Anxiety and depressive disorders are classified in the Diagnostic and Statistical Manual of Mental Disorders (DSM-IV-TR and recent DSM-5) and International Classification of Diseases (ICD-10), according to the duration, intensity and origin of symptoms. Anxiety is classified in some types of phobia, separation and social anxiety disorders, among others [3].

Anxiety disorders are influenced by environmental stimuli that are stressful for the individual. Antiquely, it was believed that anxiety disorders were learned, and although the familiar and social context influence in the possibility to develop an anxiety disorder, nowadays, it is known that anxiety disorders have a neurobiological substrate that involves neurochemical changes modifying the correct function of diverse brain structures [4]. In fact, they are the same brain structures involved in the etiology of depressive disorders, which explain the comorbidity among anxiety and depressive disorders, as well as the observation that some antidepressant drugs (i.e., selective serotonin reuptake inhibitors) produce also anxiolytic actions at the clinical level [3,5]

On the other hand, depression is an affective disorder identified from antique cultures around the world [6, 7]. Nowadays, it is considered as a psychiatric disorder classified in the DSM-5 [3]. Its prevalence and incidence have a marked sexual dimorphism; it is estimated that in the general population, it is 10–25% in women and 5–12% in men [8]. The morbidity and mortality associated with depressive disorders are higher and increasing continuously. Depression occupies the fourth place among principal causes of major incapacity around the world, occupying the first place before respiratory affections, perinatal problems, and HIV/AIDS (Human Immunodeficiency Virus/Acquired Immunodeficiency Syndrome) [9]. It is estimated that 17% of the population experiment any depressive episode during their lifespan, and those who suffer a chronic illness have a higher predisposition to develop depressive episodes with an incidence of 30-50% [10]. By 2020, it is estimated that major unipolar depression will be the second cause of incapacity of human beings around the world [11]. Depression is characterized by anhedonia (incapacity to experiment pleasure) as a central symptom but also includes episodes of irritability, anxiety and fear, in addition to alterations in appetite, body weight, sleep and motor efficiency—all accompanied by low self-esteem, guilt and the idea of death that predispose to suicide risk [3].

3. Anxiety and depression in adolescents

3.1. Anxiety

Affective disorders in young people may come from early stress exposition. For example, young adulthood with emotional distress disorders is associated with frequent and recurrent physical distress during childhood [12]. Human epidemiological and animal studies indicate that stressful experiences in utero or during early life may increase the risk of neurological and psychiatric disorders, arguably via altered epigenetic regulation [13]. In case of anxiety and depression disorders, the symptomatology could be quite different from adults.

Anxiety has been considered as a psychiatric disorder in childhood since the 1980s, and depression since the 1970s, always associated with the psychopathological concepts of the psychiatric adult. During childhood fear and sadness are developed, but it changes progressively since breastfeeding and childhood until adolescence. Frequently, anxiety and depressive disorders are expressed in the same individual at the same time, probably because fear is frequently accompanied by sadness in these pathologies. Anxiety disorders are the most frequently psychiatric disorders in the pediatric period, but most patients might not receive pharmacological or psychological treatment. The social anxiety, the anxiety by separation and generalized anxiety produce high suffering; interfere in educational performance and social relationships. In addition, anxiety in adolescence increases the risk of psychiatric disorders in the adult stage; increase the risk to develop anxiety disorders, major depression, suicide attempts and clinical hospitalization associated with psychiatric illness [14-16]. The aforementioned may negatively impact the educational performance in students.

Epidemiological studies have reported that anxiety disorders are common in children and adolescents [17] and are comorbid to depressive disorders in 8–17-year-olds [18, 19]. Data of anxiety prevalence from the United States of America reported in DSM-5 showed 0.9% for generalized anxiety in adolescents; prevalence of anxiety separation disorder in children younger than 12 years old is approximately 4% and decreases through adolescence to approximately 1.6%; for specific phobia prevalence rates are approximately 16% in adolescents; social anxiety prevalence of 7% is similar in adolescents and adults decreasing with age; agoraphobia prevalence is 1.7% [20]. Sexual dimorphism is common for anxiety disorders. More female are affected by anxiety disorder than males with 2:1 to 3:1 preponderance in adolescence [21-23] and the age of onset for anxiety symptoms in the United States is 14 years [24].

For adults and adolescents there are challenges in distinguishing "normal" from "pathological" fear and anxiety, and there is some controversy regarding whether anxiety disorders differ from "normal" fears and worries by kind or degree [14]. Practically, transient worries and fears are common in children and adolescents, but are considered pathologic only when associated with significant impairment, distress and persistence. As mentioned, sweating, shaking and blushing are obvious signs of anxiety but some other elusive behavioral signs in young people make it difficult to detect it. For example, somebody may find it difficult to associate increased inflexibility, over-reactivity, emotional intensity, impulsivity, anger, constant arguments, trials to escape or avoid school or exams, for example, to anxiety-related behaviors associated to an underlying cause. In addition, anxiety disorders have a somewhat different age and gender distribution during childhood and adolescence. Excessive worries about past behavior, self-image, competence and socio-sexual acceptance, excessive perfectionism, somatic complaints, onicophagia, nightmares, trichotillomania and internal tension are common in adolescents [25]. Panic disorder and social phobia are more frequent in adolescents [26]. Female adolescents have higher rates of specific phobia, post-traumatic stress disorder and panic disorder [27, 28]. In addition, anxiety disorders in adolescents often co-exist with either another anxiety disorder or another psychiatric disorder [29].

3.2. Depression

Negative cognitive functioning, cognitive distortions, negative attributions, hopelessness and low self-esteem are common in children, adolescents and adults. But the central symptoms of depression such as anhedonia and helplessness could also be a problem for detecting the disorder on time at school. It is important to know that adolescent onset is associated with a more chronic, severe and disabling form of depression, higher rates of family history and more suicide attempts than depression that first emerges in adulthood [30]. Adolescents with major depression disorder have recurrent episodes; and they differ from adults because sadness is not so prominent but they are more likely to present with irritability, anhedonia, suicidality, hypersomnia, cognitive and circadian rest–activity rhythm problems [31-33]. Although the diagnostic criteria are similar for children and adolescents, typical symptomatology differs by age group. Kovacs [34] noted that adolescents report more hypersomnia, fewer appetite and weight changes, and fewer reported delusions than children, and depressed preschool children show typical symptoms of depression, such as mood disturbance and anhedonia, but have less "masked" symptoms (e.g., sleep problems, appetite changes). In severe depression, the incidence of suicide progresses with age in the United States. Rare cases of suicide are observed before 10 years old children and surprisingly expand to 100-fold up to 14 years, being 10 times higher between the ages of 15 and 19. Similar to anxiety disorders, prevalence rates for depression are higher in females than males from adolescence but not before [35]. The age of female depressed adolescents is associated to a hormonal mechanism activated by menarche, in which anxiety, fatigue and sleep/appetite disturbances are observed [36]. For those who experience premenstrual dysphoric disorder in which body image dissatisfaction, feelings of failure, concentration problems and work difficulties are common, there is a hypothesis of withdrawal syndrome of progesterone to explain symptomatology; this observation has been observed in clinical and preclinical studies [37]. In summary, female adolescent are likely to exhibit more cognitive and somatic symptoms and boys experience elevated "boredom" possibly because depressed boys are more anhedonic [38].

Comorbidity of 30–75% of anxiety disorders and depression is reported in adolescents, which is associated with severe anxiety symptoms [39-41] and greater suicidality [42].

4. Diagnosis

There is a concern that many children and adolescent with anxiety and depression may not be receiving appropriate diagnosis and treatment. Diagnosis of affective disorders in adolescents and young adults could be difficult for many reasons, impossibility to reach mental health facilities, lack of professional training and scarcity of child and adolescent psychiatrists. Maybe it takes longer to diagnose an affective disorder in young than adults due to the common symptoms shared by other comorbid disorders [43, 44]. Diagnosis of anxiety and depression in adolescents requires clinical interviews of the adolescent and parent separately, using both open-ended questions and specific symptom review as well as with children. In addition to assessing for symptoms, the evaluation will also include the assessment of comorbid conditions (both general medical conditions and psychiatric illnesses), and the assessment of contextual factors (i.e., peer and family relationships, school/work, stressors). To Arrivillaga and collaborators [45], the family history of affective disorders with conditions, experiences of negative events, such as parental loss in childhood, the absence of a confident, living in a chaotic family environment and physical or psychological abuse are vulnerabilities to suffer depressive symptoms.

The first step in the differential diagnosis of a given symptom or complaint is typically a search for unrecognized physical disease. Although most adolescents with cognitive and physical symptoms consistent with an anxiety disorder will not be found to suffer from causal physical disease, clinicians should entertain the hypothesis that anxiety might be caused, exacerbated or perpetuated by an unrecognized general medical condition. This is important to emphasize because behavioral health professionals, although having little difficulty accepting that mental disorders are commonly underdiagnosed and undertreated in general medical settings, are vulnerable to overlooking the often important relationship between anxiety and physical disease in traditional mental health settings. The onset and duration of specific cognitive and somatic symptoms of anxiety should be examined and an attempt made to identify a temporal relationship between symptoms of anxiety and the course of the comorbid general medical condition. Inquiry should be made regarding recent and past stressors and traumas, including medical traumas as well as academic problems, family issues, maltreatment and difficulties with peers such as bullying. There is no substitute for a comprehensive psychiatric and medical history, as well as review of the medical record, medication list, laboratory and other diagnostic tests and procedures, and a directed physical examination when appropriate. Children with chronic physical illness are at increased risk to develop anxiety disorders. So anxiety can predispose to physical health problems and negatively impact the course of comorbid physical disease [46]. In addition, anxiety and depression must be differentially diagnosed from attention-deficit /hyperactivity disorder (ADHD) because they share some symptoms such as inattention; the difference is that anxiety inattention is due to worry and rumination, and depressive youths present poor concentration only during depressive episodes, which is distinguished from inattention due to the attraction to external stimuli, new and enjoyable activities observed in ADHD disorder [3].

Diagnosis criteria for anxiety and depression are found in the DSM-5 or ICD-10 among other documents for diagnosis. In students a sudden fall in grades may be a sign of lack of concentration associated to mood or anxiety disorder. Underdiagnosis and undertreatment of anxiety and depression in children and adolescents are not only a matter of mental health services; members of the family, friends and teachers can provide useful information to an early detection of these disorders, and the problem, for example, is the lack of acceptance in some families, the lack of awareness to identify depression symptoms because parents are also depressive, the atypical presentation of symptoms that may be confused or unclear for relatives, and the scarce communication of negative emotions and thoughts that may lead to somatization (general aches and pains, headaches or stomachaches) in children and adolescents [3]. Older age must be easier to diagnose because of the capacity of communication between individuals, but it is not so simplistic. Depressive symptoms in adolescence will have continuity to depression in adulthood; this has been observed in homeless adolescent victims of adverse experiences early in life [47]. Monteiros and collaborators [48] explain that traumatic experiences among young men and women can be a predictor of depressive symptoms and moderate the effect on the emotional reactions of gender. The diagnosis of primary depressive mood disorders requires that physicians also rule out depression from physiological effects of other medical conditions, that is, endocrinopathies, malignancies, chronic and infectious diseases, anemia and vitamin deficiency [3], and from medications such as Isotretinoin, which is used for acne problems [49]. The *DSM-IV-TR* and recent DSM-5 criteria for diagnosing major depressive disorder in children and adolescents are similar to those for adults [3, 50-53]. If substance abuse is present, an independent diagnosis of major depression requires the presence of depression before substance abuse or during periods of remission. Concurrent treatment of substance use disorder and depression is needed to improve outcomes for both [54]. Although less common, bipolar disorder is an important differential diagnosis. In 40% of children and adolescents with bipolar disorder, the illness begins with a major depressive episode [55]. Physicians should maintain a higher level of surveillance in patients at greater risk of bipolar disorder.

Other concerns are psychiatric emergencies. In developing countries, staff in schools and hospitals have little knowledge about psychiatric emergencies in young people, which is worsened by the fact that sometimes saturation in primary attention, the lack of mental services, medical insurance or health facilities make difficult the communication with emergency services and vice versa [56] and could interfere with the appropriate diagnosis leading to a subdiagnosis or misdiagnosis in youth.

5. Treatment

Safe and effective treatment for anxiety and depression requires accurate diagnosis, a detailed family history, suicide risk assessment and the use of evidence-based therapies [57]. Despite increasing evidence of effective treatments in the pediatric age group, adolescents with depression (major depressive disorder, dysthymia, depression not otherwise specified or "minor depression," and adjustment disorder with depressed mood) receive inadequate treatment [57]. Furthermore, physicians uncomfortable with prescribing complex therapies should consider referral to a child psychiatrist, especially for patients with multiple comorbidities [58]. Sometimes there is a lack of sufficiently informative comparative studies of different treatments (i.e., for depressive and anxiety disorders in childhood and adolescence) in health-care systems [21, 59].

Cognitive-behavioral combined with interpersonal approaches may help in prevention and mild depression. A mild depressive disorder without comorbidity or significant risk factors can be initially managed with support in coping with everyday tasks and counseling or psychoeducation about the manifestations of the disorder, its causes, the expected course and the options for treatment for six to eight weeks. Psychotherapy interventions of all kinds have been found to lessen depression more effectively over the short term (mean, 12 weeks) in children and adolescents (age 6–18) than various alternative management strategies. Cognitive-behavioral therapy, interpersonal psychotherapy or other kinds of psychological interventions are recommended for depression in adolescents [59]. When needed, pharmacotherapy is applied to young people. Fluoxetine is the only one drug approved for the treatment of depressive disorders in children and adolescents and sometimes fluoxetine can be combined with psychotherapy for better results. However, the adverse effects of selective serotonin reuptake inhibitors (i.e., headache, vomiting, sleep disturbance, fatigue and loss of appetite at the start of treatment) and their controversial tendency to reinforce suicidal ideation make psychotherapy the first choice to start treatment. Afterward, if needed, the fluoxetine or almost any drug should be given at lower doses than for adults increasing them progressively to be near the adult dose [60, 61].

Modern information technologies offer new opportunities to deliver mental health interventions via computer-based or mobile phone-based internet, which include online self-help with therapist support via email, SMS and/or phone call, family support, school-based group support and teacher support. A meta-analysis showed that this kind of treatment was apparently effective in reducing anxiety symptom severity compared to no intervention, and this effect may be equal to that of face-to-face interventions. The meta-analysis found a larger effect size for anxiety than for depression but the interpretation of the findings analysis needs to consider several factors and has methodological limitations. However, given the rapid adoption of mobile devices among children, youth and young adults, it is also important to develop and evaluate mobile device-based interventions [62].

6. Social problems associated with anxiety and depression

Anxiety and depression in youth result in functional impairment, increased difficulties with schoolwork, peer and family relationships. There are a range of predictors of anxiety and depression disorders in children and adolescents. These include various indices of social disadvantage such as increased family size, overcrowding, low socioeconomic status, family disruptions, parental non-employment, father's criminality and school disadvantage [63]. Anxiety and depression and other mental disorders have impact on several aspects of personal and social functioning. Patients may not complete even secondary school because the early onset of a mental disorder prevents attainment of goals at school, and even more, they tend to get married before the age of 18 and divorce later [64]. Depression is considered disabling, even more than physical illness, in a social context in daily activities or otherwise productive task [65]; and sometimes depressed people tend to use more health services than other diseases; therefore health costs are also significant. Wagner and collaborators [65] mention that people with anxiety or depression disorders have higher rates of utilization of health services, with a higher cost of care. Ritakallio and collaborators [66] found that depression and antisocial behavior among adolescents had considerable continuity, and concurrent comorbidity between these disorders was high. In relation to suicide, Aradilla and collaborators [67] found in a sample of nursing students that emotional care, self-esteem and depression are risk factors for suicidal thoughts, in which women were found to have a high significance of correlation. Also depressive symptoms were associated with other risk behaviors such as alcohol and snuff, besides violence. In other study [68], depression showed to be a risk factor of suicidal behavior in adolescents: suicide ideation was present in male (75%) and female (83.2%) adolescents with depressive symptomatology, and 77.3% of male and 64.8% of female depressive adolescents had attempted suicide. In the study by Vázquez and Blanco [69], suicidal ideation also correlates with poor subjective and negative self-judgment, pessimism and low self-esteem, which is compounded by the stress of academic life, the kind of experiences in early life and personality.

7. Academic achievement

Academic achievement has been identified as a high prevalence of anxiety in the population of college students, even above the prevalence of depression, which is dependent on the age and gender of the study population. Anxiety in adolescents depends on the concept of the student about school demands related to comprehension and auto-control. He or she frequently faces academic situations whose demands must compare with his or her own resources. When evaluation of school tasks lead to conclude that they are more than he or she can do then threat and humiliation are experienced and justify rejection to school. Teachers face many challenges mainly when new policies in education indicate the evaluations of teaching and learning in a standardized form without understanding particular needs in each environment. Hence, an intense anxiety in evaluations reduces scholar performance, affecting self-esteem and social relationships [70]. A study with Mexican male and female 21–26 years old at university showed that students with the lowest academic performance had highest levels of negative interference in Stroop paradigm about school failure; also there was a direct relation between the academic auto-concept and performance in exams; students who had been systematically located in the lower levels of the study index showed the highest levels of anxiety [71]. The finding of an inverse relation in anxiety to examinations and grades had also been observed in university students in the United States [72].

Also, there is a negative relationship between adolescent depression and educational achievement, being that depression affects academic achievement and not the other way around [64, 73]. Humensky and collaborators [74] showed an association between the self-perception of depressive symptoms in adolescents and difficulties to concentrate and complete school tasks making a detrimental cycle. Furthermore, adolescent depression and its consequences might be particularly destructive to subsequent higher education in males [75].

Depressive episodes in the education of students affect learning ability, academic performance and adaptation to college life as well as performance of future professionals. Frojd and collaborators [76] also found association between severity of depression with concentration difficulties, social relationships, self-learning, academic performance, and reading and writing in 13–17-year-old youth.

In other study it was found that the prevalence of depressive symptoms in college students affects almost one-third of the population [77]. Other studies have suggested that the incidence of depression in college students decreases if there are positive adjustments to academic life and adequate social support to cushion stressful scholar stimuli. In this sense, it has been found that when increase women education depression decreases compared to men [78]. Perhaps it is because education increases the levels of creativity in women compared to men.

Parent, child and teacher reports of emotional and behavioral problems to recognize the existence of a situation in school might be limited. Mason et al. suggest the need of studying the course of the emotional and violent behavioral problems from childhood to adolescence reported at school, because more readily identifiable symptoms of depression and anxiety may emerge later in adolescence [79].

Depression and anxiety are serious problems for students in both developed and developing countries. In a study with 139 male Mexican adolescents 18 years old who finished high school, it was observed that mild depression evaluated by mean of the Zung Self-Rating Scale was frequent in students with very low grades; a higher score in depression was observed in those guys who fail to approve the college entrance examination [80]. This suggests that depressed students are shown to have problems with academic work and motivation, and report receiving lower grades than non-depressed students. The problem is that in the future depression symptoms are related to work absences and impaired work performance, and results partly confirmed that work stressors add to this impact [81]. A study of 145 university students at Mexico evaluated the score of the Zung Self-Rating Scale for depression in 21-year-old male guys and showed 55% of students with mild depression and 9% with moderate depression. The latter reported to live with dysfunctional family, to have a self-perception of poor mental health and augmented body weight, as well as to fail more subject written exams [82]. Brain alterations in depression affect the affective behavior as well as cognitive and intellectual aspects in university students [83].

Studies about scholar performance vary in sample age and multifactorial aspects of low grades and individual dysfunction; however, there is an agreement in ensuring attention as soon as possible to give an appropriate treatment to young people.

8. Conclusion

To ensure the scholar success of anxious and depressive students is necessary to clinically manage the disorders. Teachers must consider anxiety and depression as illnesses. It is more difficult for adolescent patients to practice the usual methods of studying. The intensity of emotional tension experimented depends on the cognitive auto-concept of examinations and the capacity to face them. Sometimes, the relationship between anxiety and school performance is indirect because of the valuation of auto efficacy, which means that people with low perception of auto efficacy generate high levels of anxiety. For a diagnosed anxiety or depressive disorder in adolescents and university students, school staff should communicate the problem to allow medical attendance on time.

It is notable that both chronic and acute psychosocial stressors are significant predictors of anxiety disorders and depression. Solutions to low school performance related to anxiety and depression in young people are complex but most of the times depend on family commitment and integration of health promotion services into medical care and school settings. Nowadays, adolescence is strongly related to anxiety and depression disorders, more than any other time of life, and both disorders are related to other psychiatric disorders and substance abuse that negatively impact the academic performance. In addition, the environment plays an important role in the formation of personality and psychiatric illness. There are different types of environments, social, natural, built and virtual, each of which has different effects on human behavior, but few studies about the effects of different types of environment on mental health are available. The social environment, comprising the interactions, networks and social support, for example, social crisis, economic, social mobilization and public policy, can be stressors in which adolescent are involved. Similarly, the virtual environment, such as using the Internet or any other media, where ideal bodies are broadcasting or offering beautiful bodies, can also be stressors. The fact is that adolescence is a vulnerable period in development because of physical, biochemical and social changes that are experienced during this time in spite of the differences in culture, gender, socioeconomic status and education level that lead to cope with external demands and stress. The aforementioned show the importance of identity anxiety and depressive symptoms in this particular population of students, to improve the mental health and academic performance in high school and university students.

Acknowledgements

Present chapter was partially supported by Consejo Nacional de Ciencia y Tecnología, México (CONACyT: Proyecto 1840), Cuerpos Académicos UVE-CA-25, UNPA-CA-26 and Programa de Fortalecimiento Académico del Posgrado de Alta Calidad I010/152/2014C-133/2014.

Author details

Blandina Bernal-Morales[1*], Juan Francisco Rodríguez-Landa[1] and Frank Pulido-Criollo[2]

*Address all correspondence to: bbernalm10@hotmail.com

1 Laboratorio de Neurofarmacología, Instituto de Neuroetología, Universidad Veracruzana, Xalapa, Veracruz, México

2 Licenciatura en Enfermería, Universidad del Papaloapan, campus Tuxtepec, Sistema de Universidades Estatales de Oaxaca, Tuxtepec, Oaxaca, México

References

[1] Nieuwenhuys A, Oudejans RR. Anxiety and perceptual-motor performance: toward an integrated model of concepts, mechanisms, and processes. Psychological Research 2012; 76(6):747-759.

[2] Cody MW, Teachman BA. Global and local evaluations of public speaking performance in social anxiety. Behavior Therapy 2011; 42:601-611.

[3] American Psychiatric Association. Diagnostic and Statistical Manual of Mental Disorders: DSM-V. 5th ed. rev. Arlington, VA: American Psychiatric Association; 2013.

[4] Bernal-Morales B, Contreras CM. Ansiedad y depresión, el enfoque de las neurociencias. In: Fabre Platas DA, Del Callejo Canal DD, Garret Sánchez, De Lozada A, (ed.). Comunidades Vulnerables. México: Serie Mano Vuelta; 2009, pp. 209-228.

[5] Neumann ID, Wegener G, Homberg JR, Cohen H, Slattery DA, Zohar J, et al. Animal models of depression and anxiety: what do they tell us about human condition? Progress in Neuropsychopharmacology and Biological Psychiatry 2011; 35:1357-1375.

[6] Marván ML, Alcalá-Herrera V, Chacón L, Contreras CM. El desarrollo de los conceptos biológicos sobre la depresión. Boletín de Estudios Médico Biológicos de México 1988; 36:61-74.

[7] Rodríguez-Landa JF, Pulido-Criollo F, Saavedra M. La depresión en la medicina mesoamericana precolombina. Revista de Neurología 2007; 44:375-380.

[8] Uriarte-Bonilla V. Psicofarmacología. México DF: Trillas; 2009.

[9] World Health Organization Mental Health. New Understanding, New Hope. Geneva: World Health Organization; 2001.

[10] Post RM. Transduction of psychosocial stress into the neurobiology of recurrent affective disorder. American Journal of Psychiatry 1992; 149:999-1010.

[11] Murray CJL, Lopez AD. The Global Burden of Disease: A comprehensive assessment of mortality and disability from diseases, injuries, and risk factors in 1990 and projected to 2020. Cambridge: Harvard University Press; 1996.

[12] Shanahan L, Zucker N, Copeland WE, Bondy CL, Egger HL, Costello EJ. Childhood somatic complaints predict generalized anxiety and depressive disorders during young adulthood in a community sample. Psychological Medicine 2014; 18:1-10.

[13] Babenko O, Kovalchuk I, Metz GA. Stress-induced perinatal and transgenerational epigenetic programming of brain development and mental health. Neuroscience and Biobehavioural Reviews 2015; 48:70-91.

[14] Klein RG. Anxiety disorders. Journal of Child Psychology and Psychiatry 2009; 50(1–2):153-162.

[15] The Research Unit on Pediatric Psychofarmacology Anxiety Study Group. Fluvoxamina for treatment of anxiety disorders in children and adolescent. New England Journal of Medicine 2001; 344(17):1279-1285.

[16] Mardomingo MJ. Trastornos de ansiedad. In: Mardomingo MJ (ed), Psiquiatría del niño y del adolescente. Madrid: Díaz de Santos; 1994.

[17] Rockhill C, Kodish I, DiBattisto C, Macias M, Varley C, Ryan S. Anxiety disorders in children and adolescents. Current Problems in Pediatric and Adolescent Health Care 2010; 40(4):66-99.

[18] Chavira D, Stein M, Bailey K, Stein M. Comorbidity of generalized social anxiety disorder and depression in a pediatric primary care sample. Journal of Affective Disorders 2004; 80:163-171.

[19] Bhatia SK, Bhatia SC. Childhood and adolescent depression. American Family Physician 2007; 75:73-80, 83-4.

[20] American Psychiatric Association. Diagnostic and Statistical Manual of Mental Disorders: DSM-5. 5th ed. rev. Washington, D.C.: American Psychiatric Association; 2013.

[21] Waite P, Creswell C. Children and adolescents referred for treatment of anxiety disorders: differences in clinical characteristics. Journal of Affective Disorders 2014; 167:326-332.

[22] Craske M. Origin of Phobias and Anxiety Disorders: Why More Women than Men? Oxford, United Kingdom: ELSEVIER; 2003.

[23] Costello EJ, Mustillo S, Erkanli A, Keeler G, Angold A. Prevalence and development of psychiatric disorders in childhood and adolescence. Archives of General Psychiatry 2003; 60(8):837-844.

[24] Kessler RC, Berglund P, Demler O, Jin R, Merikangas KR, Walters EE. Lifetime prevalence and age-of-onset distributions of DSM-IV disorders in the national comorbidity survey replication. Archives of General Psychiatry 2005; 62(6):593-602.

[25] Godrid García M, Pérez Jiménez S. Trastornos de ansiedad y fobias. In: Alda Díez JA, Gabaldón Fraile S (ed), Urgencias psiquiátricas en el niño y adolescente. Barcelona: Masson-ELSEVIER; 2006. p. 102.

[26] Beesdo K, Knappe S, Pine DS. Anxiety and anxiety disorders in children and adolescents: developmental issues and implications for DSM-V. The Psychiatric Clinics of North America 2009; 32(3):483-524.

[27] Black B. Anxiety disorders in children and adolescents. Current Opinion in Pediatrics 1995; 7(4):387-391.

[28] Bernstein GA, Borchardt CM, Perwien AR. Anxiety disorders in children and adolescents: a review of the past 10 years. Journal of American Academy of Child and Adolescent Psychiatry 1996; 35(9):1110-1119.

[29] Rapee RM, Schniering CA, Hudson JL. Anxiety disorders during childhood and adolescence: Origins and treatment. Annual Review of Clinical Psychology 2009; 5:311-314.

[30] Zisook S, Rush AJ, Lesser I, Wisniewski SR, Trivedi M, Husain MM, Balasubramani GK, Alpert JE, Fava M. Preadult onset vs. adult onset of major depressive disorder: a replication study. Acta Psychiatrica Scandinava 2007; 115:196-205.

[31] Emslie GJ, Mayes TL, Ruberu M. Continuation and maintenance therapy of early-onset major depressive disorder. Paediatric Drugs 2005; 7:203-217.

[32] Sørensen MJ, Nissen JB, Mors O, Thomsen PH. Age and gender differences in depressive symptomatology and comorbidity: an incident sample of psychiatrically admitted children. Journal of Affective Disorders 2005; 84:85-91.

[33] Teicher MH, Glod CA, Harper D, Magnus E, Brasher C, Wren F, Pahlavan K. Locomotor activity in depressed children and adolescents: I. Circadian dysregulation. Journal of the American Academy of Child and Adolescent Psychiatry 1993; 32:760-769.

[34] Kovacs M. Presentation and course of major depressive disorder during childhood and later years of the life span. Journal of the American Academy of Child and Adolescent Psychiatry 1996; 35(6):705-715.

[35] Wade TJ, Cairney J, Pevalin DJ. Emergence of gender differences in depression during adolescence: national panel results from three countries. Journal of the American Academy of Child and Adolescent Psychiatry 2002; 41:190-198.

[36] Patton GC, Hibbert ME, Carlin J, Shao Q, Rosier M, Caust J, Bowes G. Menarche and the onset of depression and anxiety in Victoria, Australia. Journal of Epidemiology and Community Health 1996; 50:661-666.

[37] Saavedra M, Contreras CM, Azamar-Arizmendi G, Hernández-Lozano M. Differential progesterone effects on defensive burying and forced swimming tests depending upon a gradual decrease or an abrupt suppression schedules. Pharmacology, Biochemistry and Behavior 2006; 83: 130-135.

[38] Bennett DS, Ambrosini PJ, Kudes D, Metz C, Rabinovich H. Gender differences in adolescent depression: do symptoms differ for boys and girls? Journal of Affective Disorders 2005; 89:35-44.

[39] Costello EJ, Egger HL, Angold A. The developmental epidemiology of anxiety disorders: phenomenology, revalence, and comorbidity. Child and Adolescent Psychiatric Clinics of North America 2005; 14(4):631-648.

[40] Sala R, Axelson DA, Castro-Fornieles J, Goldstein TR, Ha W, Liao F, Gill MK, Iyengar S, Strober MA, Goldstein BI, et al: Comorbid anxiety in children and adolescents with bipolar spectrum disorders: prevalence and clinical correlates. Journal of Clinical Psychiatry 2010; 71(10):1344-1350.

[41] Kinyanda E, Kizza R, Abbo C, Ndyanabangi S, Levin J. Prevalence and risk factors of depression in childhood and adolescence as seen in 4 districts of north-eastern Uganda. BMC International Health and Human Rights 2013; 13(19):1-10.

[42] Kinyanda E, Kizza R, Levin J, Ndyanabangi S, Abbo C. Adolescent suicidality as seen in rural northeastern Uganda. Crisis 2011; 32(1):43-51.

[43] Hill J, Pickles A, Burnside E, Byatt M, Rollinson L, Davis R, Harvey K. Child sexual abuse, poor parental care and adult depression: evidence for different mechanisms. British Journal of Psychiatry 2001; 179:104-109.

[44] Gillian JC. Are sleep disturbances risk factors for anxiety, depressive and addictive disorders? Acta Psychiatrica Scandinava Supplementum 1998; 393:39-43.

[45] Arrivillaga M, Córtez C, Goicochea VL, Lozano TM. Caracterización de la depresión en jóvenes universitarios. Universitas Psychologica Bogotá, 2004; 3:17-26.

[46] Gandhi B, Cheek S, Campo JV. Anxiety in the pediatric medical setting. Child and Adolescents Psychiatric Clinics of North America 2012; 21(3):643-653.

[47] Bender K, Brown SM, Thompson SJ, Ferguson KM, Langenderfer L. Multiple victimizations before and after leaving home associated with PTSD, depression, and substance use disorder among homeless youth. Child Maltreatment 2014: 1-10.

[48] Monteiros S, Matos AP, Oliveira S. The moderating effect of gender: Traumatic experiences and depression in adolescence. Procedia-social and Behavioral Sciences 2015; 165:251-259.

[49] Wysowski DK, Pitts M, Beitz J. An analysis of reports of depression and suicide in patients treated with isotretinoin. Journal of the American Academy of Dermatology 2001; 45:515-519.

[50] Birmaher B, Williamson DE, Dahl RE, Axelson DA, Kaufman J, Dorn LD, et al. Clinical presentation and course of depression in youth: does onset in childhood differ from onset in adolescence? Journal of the American Academy of Child and Adolescent Psychiatry 2004; 43:63-70.

[51] Weller EB, Weller RA, Danielyan AK. Mood disorders in prepubertal children. In: Wiener JM, Dulcan MK (ed), Textbook of Child and Adolescent Psychiatry. 3rd ed. Washington, D.C.: American Psychiatric Publishing; 2004a, pp. 411-435.

[52] Weller EB, Weller RA, Danielyan AK. Mood disorders in adolescents. In: Wiener JM, Dulcan MK (eds), Textbook of Child and Adolescent Psychiatry. 3rd ed. Washington, D.C.: American Psychiatric Publishing; 2004b, p. 437-481.

[53] Chambers WJ, Puig-Antich J, Tabrizi MA, Davies M. Psychotic symptoms in prepubertal major depressive disorder. Archives of General Psychiatry 1982; 39:921-927.

[54] Riggs PD, Davies RD. A clinical approach to integrating treatment for adolescent depression and substance abuse. Journal of the American Academy of Child and Adolescent Psychiatry 2002; 41:1253-1255.

[55] Birmaher B, Ryan ND, Williamson DE, Brent DA, Kaufman J, Dahl RE, et al. Childhood and adolescent depression: a review of the past 10 years. Part I. Journal of the American Academy of Child and Adolescent Psychiatry 1996; 35:1427-1439.

[56] Herreros-Rodríguez O, Sánchez-Garcia F. Características generales de las urgencias psiquiátricas infanto-juveniles. Historia clínica psiquiátrica. In: Alda Díez JA, Gabaldón Fraile S (eds), Urgencias psiquiátricas en el niño y adolescente. Barcelona: Masson-ELSEVIER; 2006, pp. 12.

[57] Choe C, Graham E, Taryn M. Depression. Child and Adolescents Psychiatric Clinics of North America 2012; 21:807-829.

[58] Pine D, Helfinstein S, Bar-Haim Y, Nelson E, Fox N. Challenges in developing novel treatments for childhood disorders: lessons from research on anxiety. Neuropsychopharmacology 2009; 34:213-228.

[59] Qin B, Zhou X, Michael KD, Liu Y, Whittington C, Cohen D, Zhang Y, Xie P. Psychotherapy for depression in children and adolescents: study protocol for a systematic review and network meta-analysis. BMJ Open 2015; 5(2):e005918. doi: 10.1136/bmjopen-2014-005918.

[60] Dolle K, Schulte-Körne G. The treatment of depressive disorders in children and adolescents. Dtsch Arztebl Int. 2013 Dec 13; 110(50):854-860.

[61] Mohatt J, Bennett SM, Walkup JT. Treatment of separation, generalized, and social anxiety disorders in youths. American Journal of Psychiatry 2014; 171(7):741-748.

[62] Ye X, Bapuji SB, Winters SE, Struthers A, Raynard M, Metge C, Kreindler SA, Charette CJ, Lemaire JA, Synyshyn M, Sutherland K. Effectiveness of internet-based interventions for children, youth, and young adults with anxiety and/or depression: a systematic review and meta-analysis. BMC Health Services Research 2014; 14:313. doi: 10.1186/1472-6963-14-313.

[63] Thabet AAM, Vostanis P. Social adversities and anxiety disorders in the Gaza Strip. Archives of Disease in Childhood 1998; 78(5):439-442.

[64] Kessler RC. The costs of depression. The Psychiatric Clinics of North America 2012; 35(1):1-14.

[65] Wagner AF, González C, Sánchez S, García C, Gallo J. Enfocando la depresión como un problema de salud pública en México. Salud Mental 2012; 35:3-11.

[66] Ritakallio M, Koivisto AM, Pahlen B, Pelkonen M, Marttunen M, Kaltiala-Heino R. Continuity, comorbidity and longitudinal associations between depression and antisocial behavior in middle adolescence: A 2 years prospective follow-up study. Journal of Adolescence 2008; 31:355-370.

[67] Aradilla A, Tomás J, Gómez J. Association between emotional intelligence, depression and suicide risk in nursing students. Nurse Education Today 2014; 34:520-525.

[68] Cubillas MJ, Román R, Valdez A, Galaviz G. Depresión y comportamiento suicida en estudiantes de educación media superior en Sonora. Salud Mental 2012; 35:45-50.

[69] Vázquez, FL, Blanco V. Symptoms of depression and related factors among Spanish university students. Psychological Reports 2006; 99:583-590.

[70] Jadue G. Some effects of anxiety on the students' school performance. Estudios Pedagógicos 2001; (27):111-118.

[71] Hernández-Pozo MR, Coronado Álvarez O, Araújo Contreras V, Cerezo Reséndiz S. Desempeño académico de universitarios en relación con ansiedad escolar y autoevaluación. Acta Colombiana de Psicología 2008; 11(1):13-23.

[72] Chapell MS, Blanding B, Silverstein ME, Takahashi M, Newman B, Gubi A, McCann N. Test anxiety and academic performance in undergraduate and graduate students. Journal of Educational Psychology 2005; 97(2):268-274.

[73] McArdle J, Hamagami F, Chang JY, Hishinuma ES. Longitudinal dynamic analyses of depression and academic achievement in the Hawaiian High Schools Health Survey using contemporary latent variable change models. Structural and Equation Modeling 2014; 21(4):608-629.

[74] Humensky J, Kuwabara SA, Fogel J, Wells C, Goodwin B, Van Voorhees BW. Adolescents with depressive symptoms and their challenges with learning in school. Journal of Scholar Nurs 2010; 26(5):377-392.

[75] Jonsson U, Bohman H, Hjern A, Von Knorring L, Olsson G, Von Knorring AL. Subsequent higher education after adolescent depression: a 15-year follow-up register study. European Psychiatry 2010; 25(7):396-401.

[76] Fröjd SA, Nissinen ES, Pelkonen MU, Marttunen MJ, Koivisto AM, Kaltiala-Heino R. Depression and school performance in middle adolescent boys and girls. Journal of Adolescence 2008; 31(4):485-498.

[77] Ibrahim AK, Kelly SJ, Adams CE, Glazebrook C. A systematic review of studies of depression prevalence in university students. Journal of Psychiatry Research 2013; 47:391-400.

[78] Ross EC, Mirowsky J. Sex differences in the effect of education on depression: Resource multiplication or resource substitution? Social Science and Medicine 2006; 63:1400-1413.

[79] Mason WA, Kosterman R, Hawkins JD, Herrenkohl TI, Lengua LJ, McCauley E. Predicting depression, social phobia, and violence in early adulthood from childhood behavior problems. Journal of the American Academy of Child and Adolescent Psychiatry 2004; 43(3):307-315.

[80] Bernal-Morales M, Rodríguez-Landa JF, Bernal-Morales G. Depresión en alumnos del nivel medio superior. VIII Congreso Argentino de Salud Mental 20014. Argentina, Panamericano Hotel and Resort: Buenos Aires, Argentina; 27-29 August 2014.

[81] Lerner D, Adler DA, Rogers WH, Chang H, Lapitsky L, McLaughlin T, Reed J. Work performance of employees with depression: the impact of work stressors. American Journal of Health Promotion 2010; 24(3):205-213.

[82] Pulido-Criollo F, Rodríguez-Landa JF, Acosta-Uribe B. Algunos efectos de la sintomatología depresiva en universitarios. In: Damián-Simon J, López-Azamar B, Garza-Vargas F, Peralta-Santiago GE, Tejiendo redes para el conocimiento multidisciplinario en Educación y Emprendurismo. Universidad de Papaloapan-PROMEP; 2014, pp. 97-107.

[83] Rodríguez-Landa JF, Bernal-Morales B, Gutiérrez-García AG. Estrés, miedo, ansiedad y depresión. In: Coria-Ávila GA (ed), Neurofisiología de la conducta. México: Universidad Veracruzana; 2012, pp. 136-150.

Chapter 12

The Role of Expectations in Treatment Outcome and Symptom Development in Anxiety Disorders

Theodora E. Katerelos, Claude Bélanger, Marie-Christine Payette, Ghassan El-Baalbaki, André Marchand and Michel Perreault

Additional information is available at the end of the chapter

http://dx.doi.org/10.5772/60668

Abstract

For more than 60 years, researchers have been interested in determining the impact of expectations on treatment outcome. Earlier studies mostly focused on two types of expectations: prognostic and process expectations. Aims: To review how four different types of expectations (prognostic, process, anxiety expectancy and anxiety sensitivity) contribute to psychotherapy outcome, and to the development of clinical disorders, especially anxiety. Conclusions: First, the role of process and prognostic expectancies in clinical disorders and psychotherapy outcome should be clarified by addressing the methodological flaws of the earlier expectancy studies. Second, studies, especially those on anxiety disorders, may benefit from evaluating the four different types of expectations to determine their relative impact on outcome, and on the development and maintenance of these disorders. Third, possible links with other clinical disorders should be further explored. Finally, expectancies should be assessed prior to treatment and after several sessions to determine the extent to which the treatment's failure in modifying initial low expectancies contribute to a poor outcome.

Keywords: Prognostic expectations, process expectations, anxiety sensitivity, anxiety expectancy, anxiety disorders

1. Introduction

Expectations play an important role in the treatment of mental health issues. For more than 60 years, researchers have been interested in determining the impact of client expectations on treatment outcome. Nevertheless, many of the criticisms regarding the flawed methodology implemented to research the impact of expectations that had already been raised by Wilkins in 1973 [1] have not been addressed to this day. As a matter of fact, a recent meta-analysis on the role of client prognostic expectations on treatment outcome argued that these studies continued to be fraught with methodological limitations [2].

In a review on expectancies in psychiatric services, Noble, Douglas and Newman [3] summarised several studies on prognosis and process expectations. Expectations may be defined as "a person's understanding of the probability that an event will occur"[4]. This understanding may derive from "any belief, hypothesis, theory, assumption or accessible construct"[5]. Since the 1950s, studies have examined the impact of expectations on the outcome of treatment services in mental health or with psychological issues. Prognostic and participant role expectations, as identified by Goldstein [6], are the most frequently researched categories. Prognostic expectations refer to the probability of a therapeutic success. Process expectations include the participants' (i.e., therapist and client) roles referring to anticipations regarding therapist characteristics (i.e., expertness, attractiveness and trustworthiness), therapist and client behaviour and attitudes expected to be displayed throughout therapy (e.g., [7-9]). Process expectations also include anticipations referring to therapeutic process and procedures (i.e., duration, the function and general process of therapy) (e.g., [7, 10, 11]). There have been several reviews on expectations (e.g., [1, 3, 7, 10, 12, 13]) and some appear to indicate that the data is inconclusive. Although expectations appear to play an important role in psychotherapy outcome, there are many reported methodological shortcomings within the studies reviewed.

More recently, there has been a resurgence of studies examining the impact of expectations on the development and maintenance of anxiety disorders. The trademark of anxiety disorders appears to be the presence of excessive fear and anxiety, often associated with problematic behavioural responses, such as avoidance [14]. The current interest in expectancies arose out of research conducted on motivation to avoid feared objects, situations or physical symptoms (see [15]). The focus has not been so much on therapy outcome, but on the development and maintenance of clinical disorders, namely, anxiety disorders (e.g., [15]). Reiss's expectancy theory ([15-20]) posits that human fear is composed of two distinct factors: expectations (what one expects will happen to him/her) and sensitivities (why one is afraid of the expected occurrence).

The first factor (i.e., expectations), can be broken down in three ways. According to Reiss's theory, individuals may hold danger expectancies (e.g., "I expect to get injured by that spider "), expectations of being socially evaluated (e.g., "I expect others to think I'm stupid") and anxiety expectancies (e.g., "I expect to have a panic attack if I go on the airplane"). The second factor (i.e., anxiety sensitivity), refers to the belief that the sensations of anxiety have harmful somatic, psychological or social consequences [15]. Individuals may possess sensitivities regarding injury (e.g., "I expect to die if the spider bites me"), social evaluation (e.g., "I expect to turn red if they think I'm stupid") and anxiety (e.g., "I expect to have a heart attack if I have a panic attack on the airplane"). Expectations and sensitivities vary from one individual to the next. However, elevated sensitivities and negative expectations are more likely to contribute to phobic avoidance behaviour and to the development and maintenance of anxiety disorders.

http://dx.doi.org/10.5772/60668

The purpose of this chapter is to explore the relationship between treatment outcome and four different types of expectancies: prognostic (e.g., "I expect to get better at the end of therapy"), process (e.g., "I expect to do exposure therapy") and anxiety expectancies (e.g., "I expect to panic at the grocery store") and anxiety sensitivity (e.g., "I expect to die from a heart attack if I panic"). Their influence on the development and maintenance of anxiety disorders in adults will also be examined.

Type of expectancy	Definition	Example
Prognostic	Probability of a therapeutic success	"I expect to get better at the end of therapy"
Process	1) Roles: Anticipations regarding therapist characteristics, therapist and client behaviour and attitudes expected to be displayed throughout therapy	1) "I expect the therapist to be warm"
	2) Anticipations regarding therapeutic procedures	2) "I expect to do exposure therapy"
Anxiety expectancy	Probability that a particular fearful response will occur	"I expect to panic at the grocery store"
Anxiety sensitivity	Belief that the sensations of anxiety have harmful somatic, psychological or social consequences	"I expect to die from a heart attack if I panic"

Table 1. Summary of type of expectations

2. Expectations in mental health

2.1. Prognostic expectations

Frank's earlier studies (e.g., [21-23]) produced evidence indicating that clients who expect a successful therapy outcome often benefited more from psychotherapy than those who had poorer expectations. A number of other earlier studies also reproduced the above findings, demonstrating an existing relationship between favourable prognostic expectations and therapeutic improvement (e.g., [24, 25]).

Subsequent studies, however, began to report contradictory findings. Certain researchers were not able to establish a significant relationship between clients' expectancy of improvement and therapeutic gains [26]. Imber and colleagues [27] also obtained non-significant results when they attempted to induce positive expectations for improvement in clients. Goldstein and Shipman [28] discovered that a curvilinear relationship existed; those who had either very high or very low prognostic expectations improved the least. Their study appears to suggest that moderate expectations, which may be more realistic than ones that are very high or very low, are linked to outcome.

Following these inconsistencies in the earlier findings, Wilkins [1] wrote a critical review on the research published on clients' expectations of therapeutic gain and focused his criticisms on the methodology used. Some of the major weaknesses identified included (1) outcome measures that were not validated. (i.e., several studies were based on self-reports that described client perceptions of how they feel instead of validated measures of symptom reduction administered by independent raters); (2) using expectancy measures as outcome measures, rather than administering questionnaires that differentiate the two; and (3) using correlational techniques to determine the effect of expectancies on symptom reduction. Other methodological deficiencies noted by separate authors include the use of a minimally disturbed student population [29] and the common administration of global measures of expectations rather than measures evaluating prognostic expectations that refer to specific symptoms and behaviours [30]. Martin and colleagues [30] attempted to address some of these critical issues by using (a) a homogeneous group of people with chronic schizophrenia rather than a small, minimally disturbed, heterogeneous population such as students; (b) validated outcome measures; and (c) a measure of expectancy that assesses expectations for improvement in symptoms and behaviours. A relationship was found between expectations and post-hospital adjustment.

A recent meta-analysis of 46 correlational studies ($n=8,016$) found a small but significant effect ($d=.24$, $p<.001$) of the role of client prognostic expectations on treatment outcome [31]. Similar to previous findings, Constantino and colleagues [31] reported limitations in the studies and shortcomings with expectancy measures. For example, one-item scales were used, there was confusion among constructs (e.g., treatment expectancy versus treatment credibility; treatment outcome versus treatment expectations) and the same questions were used to measure expected outcome and actual outcome. Finally, the authors argued that expectations appear to change, which emphasises the need for greater caution regarding results derived from single time measurements of expectations (i.e. measuring expectations only once).

2.1.1. Shifts in prognostic expectations

Perotti and Hopewell (1980; cited in [10]) concluded that although expectancy effects are important in various interventions including systematic desensitization with phobic individuals, pre-therapy expectations have little effect on outcome. They suggested that it would be important to measure the prognostic expectations during therapy. After being exposed to several components of therapy, patients may become better at predicting their outcome (see [10, 32]). Prognostic expectations may shift in a positive direction if clients perceive improvement or they may become more negative if no benefits are noticed [33]. Although these studies recommended examining expectations only during therapy, measuring pretreatment expectations may also be useful in determining the specific treatment components that contribute to these cognitive shifts. Moreover, it appears equally important to investigate the outcome of patients who were not capable of changing their initial negative expectancies. A poor outcome in such clients may indicate that the treatment may require an added component aimed at addressing initial negative expectations of improvement. Conversely, it may also be suggested that lower expectations of improvement may be realistic if they also suffer from more severe symptomatology. Factors that both preclude and encourage shifts in expectations should be explored in order to address the specific needs of the clients during therapy.

A study by Safren, Heimberg and Juster [34] examined prognostic expectancies of clients with social phobia who were taking part in a cognitive–behavioural group treatment. An expectancy measure was administered at the end of the first therapy session after clients were presented with the cognitive–behaviour therapy (CBT) model (i.e., information) for social phobia and again at the end of the fourth session after clients had the opportunity to experience the different treatment components. The data revealed that severity and duration of social phobia were related to initial low expectations. Moreover, findings showed that initial expectancies significantly predicted improvement in symptomatology at post-therapy. The design implemented, however, did not measure expectancies prior to the first therapy session. Consequently, it is not possible to conclude that initial expectancies were associated with outcome. It may be more accurate to assume that the beliefs of improvement held following the initial therapy session, whereby patients received important information, were related to CBT results. In addition, no cognitive shifts were apparent since expectancy scores did not differ between sessions one and four. As indicated in the previous paragraph, it seems important to verify whether there is a difference between pre-therapy expectations and expectations following the first information session in order to determine the extent to which patients modify their initial expectations. It may be suggested that patients who modify their initial low expectations have a better outcome than those who do not. If this was the case, the components of CBT influential in modifying patient expectations should be examined. Nevertheless, the above study demonstrated that expectations during therapy are important determinants of therapeutic outcome even when they are measured after the first session.

A recent study by Tsai, Ogrodniczuk, Sochting and Mirmiran [35] attempted to address some of the shortcomings of earlier research. This study involved participants engaging in group CBT for depression. The authors examined the change in clients' prognostic expectations between pretreatment and after the third session, where they had received information regarding the treatment content. No significant change in clients' perceptions were observed; however, 33% of participants reported a positive shift in their expectations, 42% reported a negative shift and the remaining 25% reported no change in their expectations. Although increases in expectations were of small magnitude, they were significantly associated with reduced anxiety symptoms and interpersonal problems, and an increase in quality of life. This suggests that helping clients shift their expectations during sessions may improve outcome.

Ruptures in therapeutic alliance may be linked to shifts in prognostic expectations. Westra, Constantino and Aviram [36] measured the impacts of therapeutic alliance changes on prognostic expectations of clients with a primary diagnosis of generalised anxiety disorder (GAD) who were taking part in CBT. The authors found that, on average, clients who perceived a rupture in therapeutic alliance lowered their prognostic expectations (i.e., expectations for improvement) by as much as 25%. Moreover, those clients had higher levels of worry upon treatment termination. Although this study found that shifts in prognostic expectations may occur and influence therapy outcome, studies addressing these shifts remain scarce.

2.2. Process expectations

Similar to the studies dealing with the effects of prognostic expectations, numerous other studies specifically concentrated on examining the links between process expectations and treatment outcome. Process expectations include (1) participants' (i.e., therapist and client) roles referring to anticipations regarding therapist characteristics, therapist and client behaviour and attitudes expected to be displayed throughout therapy, and (2) anticipations referring to therapeutic process and procedures. The majority of the studies conducted on process expectations may be found in counselling research (e.g., [37-41]). Numerous studies in counselling have examined process expectations and expectations referring to the role of the participant and the counsellor (e.g., [40, 43-44]). Duckro and colleagues [7] critically reviewed the effects of confirming or disconfirming process expectations related to the role of the participant. Based on this review, only moderate support was found regarding the relationship between disconfirmed participant role expectations and poor outcome. A subsequent review by Glass, Arnkoff and Shapiro [12] also concluded that the literature on role expectations is vague. Although most of the studies they reviewed found an association between clients' role expectations and outcome, poor methodology and mixed findings raise questions about the validity of expectations as a predictor of outcome.

A more recent qualitative study [45] examined participants diagnosed with GAD who underwent a 14-hour CBT treatment. Following the treatment, the authors found that the disconfirmation of pretreatment expectations was often experienced positively by clients who had good treatment outcome (i.e., a clinically significant change and a post-therapy score in the normal range on the Penn State Worry Questionnaire). Clients with a favourable outcome were more likely to have been pleasantly surprised by the therapist (e.g., clients indicated that the therapist was collaborative or that they were comfortable with the therapist) or their experience in therapy (e.g., clients indicated that they did not expect to change so much or that they could trust the process). Conversely, those with poor outcome following therapy were more likely to have had their positive expectations disconfirmed (e.g., clients indicated their problems were more chronic than they thought). These results must be interpreted with great caution because clients were asked to talk about their initial expectations retrospectively, and treatment outcome may have influenced the recall of their initial expectations. The number of participants was also limited (i.e., n=9). In conclusion, the reported methodological flaws and the paucity of studies published on process expectations over the last few years further support the need for new research in this area.

2.2.1. Participants' role in therapy

Different aspects of the participants' role expectations may be linked to treatment outcome. A recent study by Patterson, Anderson and Wei [99] examined the effect of different components of the Expectations about Counselling Questionnaire-Brief Form on outcome. They found that clients' expectations regarding counsellor expertise (e.g., expectations that the therapist will be helpful) were significantly related to outcome, while expectations regarding personal commitment (e.g., client responsibility and commitment towards the therapy) and facilitative conditions (e.g., therapist personal characteristics such as warmth) were not related to outcome. However, all three factors were found to be significantly related to the clients' perception of working alliance.

Al-Darmaki and Kivlighan [42] examined the effect of expectation congruence on the client–counsellor relationship and on their working alliance. Counsellors and clients completed the questionnaire on expectancies after the third session. The findings suggested that neither high nor low expectancies predict the therapeutic alliance; increased congruence in their expectations with regards to the therapeutic relationship is a better predictor of alliance. The authors concluded that counsellors and researchers should focus on trying to increase congruence in expectations to form a better therapeutic relationship. Although it appears important to have congruent expectations, it may be difficult to increase congruence after patients have been exposed to several components of therapy and no apparent changes in expectations have taken place. If therapist–patient expectancies continue to be incongruent after several sessions and this has a negative impact on the therapeutic relationship, it may be useful for the therapist and patient to discuss this issue in an attempt to modify expectancies. If the therapist and patient cannot come to an agreement at this stage, redirecting the patient to an alternative therapeutic approach or a different therapist corresponding with their expectancies may be a better solution.

Clients' role expectations may be typical of a particular therapeutic approach (e.g., CBT). Seligman, Wuyek, Geers, Hovey and Motley [46] studied role expectations among university students enrolled in an introductory class of psychology. The authors asked the participants about their expectations regarding the therapist's and the clients' role in therapy (e.g., "What does a therapist do during a typical therapy session?"). The participants were asked to list a maximum of three short answers to each question. The authors then coded the participants' responses as either being typical of CBT or not. They found that the majority of the participants' responses (i.e., 96% for therapist role and 97% for client role) were judged by the authors as being non-specific to CBT. For example, expectations regarding the role of a therapist that were identified as non-specific to CBT were "Asks questions to see if the patient's problems have come from childhood" and "Sits behind something so the patient does not see their facial expressions". Expectations regarding the role of a therapist that were identified as specific to CBT were, for example, "Attempts to change how the brain interprets problems" and "Directs patient's thoughts in the direction they need to be in". As for client role, examples of expectations identified as non-specific to CBT were "Stay positive" and "Dig deep into their emotions". Conversely, expectations identified as specific to CBT regarding client role were "Face their fears" and "Be monitored on their path to their goal". Based on these results, the authors argue that many clients may hold inaccurate expectations before entering CBT. As indicated in the preceding studies, the data examining the influence of client role expectations on therapeutic outcome is unequivocal.

One of the earlier criticisms put forward by authors regarding research on process expectations was the ambiguity attached to its definition. A study by Tracey and Dundon [9] directly addressed this problem by distinguishing the "anticipatory role" and the "preferences" of the clients; two constructs which, according to Duckro and associates [7], were often confounded. Tracey and Dundon [9] measured the following process expectations related to the role of the client: approval, advice, listening and relationship. However, in order to verify the actual meaning of expectations, the measure they administered was modified to examine the difference between client anticipations and preferences. Clients were to complete the questionnaire on two separate occasions: first, they were to report how they anticipated counselling to be, and then, they were to indicate what they preferred counselling to be. They found that anticipations and preferences were significantly different; however, each anticipation subscale was highly correlated with its preference counterpart (i.e., range =.51 to .70). The elevated correlations between the two subscales prompted the authors to conclude that these two measures may not be as separate as initially proposed (e.g., [7]). Regardless, a high correlation between anticipations and preferences does not necessarily imply that they are not separate constructs. Furthermore, this study only examined counselling with a student population. Any interpretations made from correlations must take into account the possible selection bias. For instance, people who expect counselling to provide them with what they prefer are more likely to choose to attend counselling. Conversely, there may be a greater discrepancy between preferences and expectancies in situations where the client has little choice regarding his treatment options. For example, in publicly funded psychiatric or emergency services, there may not be many choices available for the client. His expectations may accurately reflect what is being offered, but his preferences may exceed the service options. To date, in the field of mental health, there is a lack of studies defining the relationship between the therapist and the client. Measuring patient preferences and expectations simultaneously and counsellor satisfaction may help define this relationship. Nevertheless, Tracey and Dundon's study [9] suggests that preferences and anticipations of clients should be measured separately due to the bidirectional discrepancy results that were detected. The bidirectional discrepancy found in this study showed that counsellors were more satisfied when clients with initial low role anticipations behaved in the manner in which they preferred with respect to the therapeutic relationship. They also displayed greater dissatisfaction with clients whose behaviour was inconsistent with their role anticipations and preferences in the therapeutic relationship. However, these findings were only detected with initial counsellor satisfaction as opposed to in-session and they were only related with one out of the four subscales (i.e., relationship).

Tinsley and Westcot [4] conducted a study to determine whether the Expectations about Counseling-Brief form measures expectations about the counselling process or other constructs including perceptions about counselling and counselling preferences. In this study, process expectation was defined as "the person's understanding of the probability that an event will occur"; perception referred to "the person's knowledge of an event"; and preference was considered as "the extent to which the person desires an event". Subjects were asked to read each question out loud and state all of their thoughts as they interpreted the question. The results revealed that subjects, for the most part, made statements that referred to expectations, and these were distinct from preferences and perceptions. The authors suggest that interviewers utilise the stem "I expect" in expectancy studies and repeat it more frequently during the interview to tap into the cognitions required to elicit expectation responses.

Many of the studies on participant role expectations have been descriptive. These descriptive studies allowed researchers to gather important information on the types of role expectations different groups of individuals have. For instance, the research has attempted to describe the different pretreatment expectations (a) in gender [38, 47]; (b) in the type of problem [47]; (c) between clients and the general public [38, 44]; (d) between individual and group therapy [38];

(e) referring to the gender of the counsellor [48]; (f) regarding counsellor race [49]; (g) in personality dimensions [50]; and (h) in terms of client readiness to change [51]. Relevant information may also be discovered by examining the impact of expectations on treatment outcome, especially in terms of adherence and satisfaction. Clients who do not receive what they expect may be dissatisfied with the services provided, adhere less to the treatment and eventually drop out. Such research may shed some light into factors that contribute to client dissatisfaction and discontinuation of treatment.

2.2.2. Therapeutic process and procedures

Studies on expectations have mostly focused on the role of the therapist and the client in counselling rather than on the procedures of a specific therapy. It seems important to assess process expectations related to distinct aspects of services. For example, expectations regarding the duration of treatment may influence dropout. A recent study found that when clients were provided with information regarding the relationship between treatment efficacy and the number of sessions attended (i.e., that, on average, 50% of the clients showed a clinically significant change after 13-18 sessions), they were significantly less likely to drop out [52]. However, a recent study by Callahan et al. [53] found that clients' pretreatment expectations regarding the duration of treatment remained unchanged after an education session. Conversely, clients' previous experiences with therapy were significantly related with the number of sessions attended and treatment outcome.

Other studies have focused on the procedures of treatment services by attempting to counteract process expectations that were inconsistent with the treatment being offered. Webster [54] conducted a study contrasting a group of patients who were sent an information sheet describing the nature of the initial assessment session to a control group who received no information sheet. The informed group was more likely to attend the initial appointment and express greater satisfaction; however, no difference was detected between the two groups in levels of state anxiety and expectations. Deane, Spicer and Leathem [55] used video as a means of communicating information on the objectives and process of therapy (see [56, 57] for more information on the pre-orientation video). Although the pre-therapy orientation video did not have a differential impact on psychotherapy outcome after two months, individuals who viewed the video had more accurate expectations about psychotherapy and were less anxious about undergoing psychotherapy than controls immediately following the presentation. These results suggest that even when initial expectations are not congruent with the process and procedures of therapy, patients are capable of readjusting their expectations and diminishing their anxiety about entering into therapy after they are presented with information.

3. Expectations and anxiety disorders

Patients receiving mental health services also hold expectations regarding their physical symptoms, anxiety, danger and pain to name a few. Negative expectancies (i.e., what one expects will happen to him/her) and elevated sensitivities (i.e., why one is afraid of the expected occurrence) are likely to contribute to avoidance behaviours and to the development of clinical disorders, especially anxiety (e.g., [15, 18, 58, 59, 62]). Anxiety sensitivity and expectancy (or expectancy of a fearful response) have been studied with numerous psychological issues. The following will demonstrate the important role these two variables have on the development and maintenance of anxiety.

3.1. Expectancy of a fearful response

Expectations have been identified as important factors in the onset of psychological difficulties such as anxious and avoidance behaviours (e.g., [15, 58, 60]). These types of expectations represent the probability that a particular fearful response will occur. Individuals may demonstrate different expectations including, danger, social evaluation or anxiety expectancies. Irrational danger expectancies often contribute to the onset and maintenance of clinical phobias and phobic avoidance. For instance, studies have demonstrated that people with arachnophobia (i.e., phobia of spiders) and cynophobia (i.e., phobia of dogs) are more likely to have greater expectations of being bitten and injured as a result of being bitten (e.g., [59, 61]).

Magnified fears of pain can also lead to avoidance behaviours [62]. Cipher and Fernandez [60] found that chronic pain sufferers were more likely to avoid an activity if they expected to be harmed by it despite reassurance from the experimenter that no tissue damage would occur. This study suggests that experience of pain does not need to be present for the onset of avoidance behaviours; anticipation of pain is enough to contribute to avoidance behaviours. Several authors have suggested that anticipation of pain prevents such individuals from participating in physical tasks (e.g., [27]). Similarly, exaggerated fears of being negatively evaluated in social contexts, or expectations of experiencing negative emotions following a criticism, may also lead to social phobia or social/interpersonal difficulties (for greater detail see [15, 63]). In a recent study, Rodebaugh, Heimberg, Schultz and Blackmore [64] evaluated the social performance of individuals with social phobia by asking them to give a short speech in front of a camera. The authors found that after receiving video feedback, those who actually had greater social abilities (as rated by an independent observer) than they believed (i.e., high self-observer discrepancy) had significantly lower levels of anticipatory anxiety when asked to give another speech in front of a camera. Thus, it seems that individuals with high self-observer discrepancy were able to adjust their expectations after receiving additional and more realistic information.

Increased levels of anxiety expectancy (i.e., the extent to which individuals expect to experience anxiety) may also contribute towards the development of psychological problems. Numerous studies have demonstrated that a greater association exists between the anticipation of anxiety and avoidance behaviour, rather than with the occurrence of panic attacks (e.g., [65, 66, 67]). This suggests that as expectation of panic increases, so does avoidance. This finding is also supported by Craske and Barlow's [68] hypothesis, indicating that there is a greater relationship between avoidance behaviour and anxiety expectancy rather than with the occurrence of panic attacks. These results have important implications in the treatment of anxiety disorders. Treatments aimed at diminishing the expectation of anxiety may be effective in reducing the amount of fear actually experienced by the individual (e.g., [69]). For instance, Kirsch and colleagues [69] succeeded in diminishing the amount of fear experienced in snake-phobic patients through a systematic desensitization approach that dealt with their expectations of anxiety. Southworth and Kirsch [70] also found that when anxiety expectancies were reduced, patients experienced less fear. By challenging expectations related to irrational fears through cognitive restructuring techniques and education, patients will not only gain greater insight into their difficulties, behaviours may also gradually be modified and the severity of clinical disorders diminished.

3.2. Anxiety sensitivity

Anxiety sensitivity is the belief that the sensations of anxiety have harmful somatic, psychological or social consequences [15]. Thus, people with high anxiety sensitivity believe that experiencing anxiety will cause them somatic (e.g., "I expect my panic attack to cause a heart attack"), psychological (e.g., "If I get trapped in the elevator, I expect to become anxious and lose control") or social harm (e.g., "I expect to turn red if others notice my fear of public speaking"). Essentially, individuals with high anxiety sensitivity fear the sensations of anxiety because of the expected consequences. As a result, they will try to avoid anxiety-inducing situations (e.g., [15]).

Reiss's expectancy theory implies that a high level of anxiety sensitivity can precede panic attacks and may be a risk factor for the development of anxiety disorders ([15, 18, 71, 72]). For instance, Maller and Reiss [71] conducted a longitudinal study whereby they administered the Anxiety Sensitivity Index (ASI; measure most frequently used to measure anxiety sensitivity; [18]) to college students in 1984 and retested them three years later. Low and high scores on the ASI were contrasted. The results indicated that anxiety sensitivity predicted anxiety disorders and the frequency and intensity of panic attacks. Subjects with high anxiety sensitivity were five times more likely to develop anxiety disorders (i.e., panic disorder, generalised anxiety disorder, simple phobia and social phobia), especially panic disorder. In a separate study, Taylor and colleagues [72] contrasted ASI scores between anxiety disorder patients (i.e., panic disorder, post-traumatic stress disorder, generalised anxiety disorder, obsessive compulsive disorder, social phobia and simple phobia) and normal controls. They found that ASI scores were greater for anxiety disorders (excluding simple phobia) in contrast to normal controls. In the same study, they [72] also compared ASI scores between anxiety disorder (excluding panic disorder) and panic disorder patients. Their results showed that ASI scores were significantly more elevated in panic disorder than the other anxiety disorders, except for post-traumatic stress disorder (PTSD). There were, however, trends for higher ASI scores in the panic disorder group in contrast to the PTSD group.

Schmidt, Lerew and Jackson [73] confirmed the above finding in a prospective study using a larger population (i.e., n = 1401), followed over a brief period of time (i.e., 5 weeks). Retrospective studies also show links between high anxiety sensitivity and anxiety disorders (e.g., [74]). High scores on the ASI are also predictive of panic attacks ([75, 76]) and agoraphobic avoidance in individuals with panic attacks that are not frequent enough to be diagnosed as panic disorder [76]. The authors of these studies suggest that anxiety sensitivity is not only predictive of panic disorder with agoraphobia; other types of anxiety disorders may also be influenced by this factor.

A recent meta-analysis also examined the relationship between anxiety sensitivity and panic disorder, generalised anxiety disorder, specific phobia, social phobia and agoraphobia, obsessive–compulsive disorder, post-traumatic stress disorder and depression [77]. The study revealed that anxiety sensitivity was higher in individuals suffering from post-traumatic stress disorder, generalised anxiety disorder and panic disorder. Moreover, individuals with depression, social phobia and obsessive–compulsive disorder had intermediate levels of anxiety sensitivity, while those with specific phobia had lower levels of sensitivity. Finally, the author found that the average anxiety sensitivity levels associated with each of these disorders was significantly higher than the average level found in the community. Another meta-analysis also found that anxiety sensitivity was significantly higher in individuals with anxiety disorders than in nonclinical control groups [78]. This study also found that individuals with panic disorder and post-traumatic stress disorder had higher levels of anxiety sensitivity than their counterparts suffering from other anxiety disorders. However, this meta-analysis did not replicate Naragon-Gainey's findings, indicating varying levels of anxiety sensitivity among the other anxiety disorders. These results suggest that anxiety sensitivity is a common feature of numerous psychological disorders.

Anxiety sensitivity may also interact with other conditions. For example, a recent study found that among regular smokers with panic disorders, a high level of anxiety sensitivity combined with a high level of smoking rate significantly predicted more agoraphobic avoidance, more anticipatory anxiety (i.e., worry about interoceptive cues) and more symptoms of anxiety (e.g., feeling dizzy) [79].

Findings support a relationship between change in anxiety sensitivity and outcome in panic disorder with agoraphobia [80]. Similarly, increased anxiety sensitivity has been detected as a negative predictor of response to cognitive behaviour therapy (CBT) [81]. In addition, a change in ASI scores, after a 50-minute intervention designed to reduce anxiety sensitivity (i.e., computer-assisted psychoeducation and interoceptive exposure), was found to facilitate change in symptoms of depression, anxiety and worry [82]. Finally, high ASI scores at the end of CBT for panic disorder with agoraphobia predict relapse better than alternative measures (e.g., [81, 83]).

Individuals with high anxiety sensitivity are more likely to develop other problems as well, such as chronic pain [84, 85], alcoholism [86, 87] and depression [88] to name a few. Asmundson and colleagues [84] reported that patients with recurring headaches demonstrated scores on the ASI that approached or even exceeded scores detected in anxiety disorders. Similarly, Taylor and associates [88] detected high levels of anxiety sensitivity in individuals with depression. Scores on the ASI were compared for patients suffering from panic disorder, major depression, or both. A principal components analysis revealed three factors of anxiety sensitivity: fear of publicly observable arousal-related reactions (i.e., belief that anxiety sensations have harmful social consequences), phrenophobia (i.e., belief that anxiety sensations have harmful psychological consequences) and fear of somatic sensations (i.e., belief that anxiety sensations have harmful somatic consequences). The findings revealed that subjects with major depression and no comorbid panic disorder presented with high scores on the ASI. High scores were mainly attributable to the phrenophobia (i.e., fear of concentration difficulties and cognitive dyscontrol; belief that difficulties can lead to insanity or mental incapacitation). The findings further showed that this dimension was depression-specific. This is understandable since individuals suffering from depression may have difficulty concentrating and making decisions [88]. Schmidt, Lerew and Joiner [89] did not arrive at the same conclusions but they found that high scores on the ASI were more likely to exacerbate depressive symptoms in the context of anxiety. Finally, Samoluk and colleagues [86] confirmed previous research (e.g., [87, 90]) by demonstrating the important role anxiety sensitivity has on alcohol consumption. Participants with high anxiety sensitivity were more likely to consume greater amounts of alcohol in solitary situations than those with low anxiety sensitivity or individuals drinking in a social context. It may be suggested that individuals with high anxiety sensitivity drink more in order to prevent physical symptoms of anxiety.

Anxiety sensitivity seems to originate from environmental [91, 92] and biological [91] factors. With regards to environmental factors, expectancy theory postulates that anxiety expectancy stems from learned experiences that a given stimulus will generate anxiety or fear [91]. Nevertheless, a person may have never experienced anxiety in a particular situation, but come to anticipate it after witnessing someone else (e.g., a family member) having a panic attack. In fact, Donnell and McNally [92] found that two-thirds of participants with high anxiety sensitivity had never suffered from a panic attack. However, those with high anxiety sensitivity were more likely to have a personal and family history of panic. In addition, Schmidt and colleagues [73] found that anxiety sensitivity predicts the development of panic and other anxiety symptoms, independently of history of panic and trait anxiety. Anxiety sensitivity may be learned through parental reinforcement of sick-role behaviour related to physical symptoms rather than anxiety-related symptoms, as suggested by the findings of a retrospective study [93]. Parental reinforcement may have led to dramatisation about the occurrence of bodily symptoms. These findings parallel Clark's [94] cognitive model of panic, which posits that the development and maintenance of panic arise from a fear that bodily sensations will lead to harmful consequences. These results suggest that anxiety sensitivity is a predisposing biopsychosocial factor to developing panic.

The above findings demonstrate that although anxiety sensitivity has been mostly studied and linked with anxiety disorders, catastrophic expectations with respect to physical symptoms may also extend to other psychological problems. The relationship between anxiety sensitivity and other disorders should be further studied and examined in relation to anxiety disorders. Moreover, Olatunji and Wolitzky-Taylor [78] suggest that different anxiety sensitivity components may be related to different anxiety disorders. It may be suggested that addressing patients' sensitivities to anxiety may help them gain a better understanding regarding some of the factors that contribute to their clinical disorder. Exposure therapy may function as a reality test for such individuals. Exposing oneself to the feared stimulus will gradually disconfirm previous negative expectations related to the consequences of anxiety sensations since the feared outcome will not occur (e.g., [69]). Cognitive techniques [95] may also influence patients into modifying their expectations or beliefs regarding the sensations of anxiety for these cognitions to become more realistic.

4. Conclusion

In light of this review, four main conclusions may be drawn. First, it appears important to measure the different types of expectations (i.e., prognostic, process, and anxiety expectations; anxiety sensitivity) to determine their level of contribution to the development and/or maintenance, and to the outcome of anxiety disorders. Second, future research could explore the extent to which the treatment's failure in modifying clients' initial low expectancies has an influence on therapeutic gain. Third, methodological flaws (e.g., the use of retrospective measures; confusion among constructs; the use of single time measures) exist in numerous studies on expectancies [2] and should be addressed to clarify the role of process and prognostic expectances in clinical disorders, and more specifically, anxiety. Finally, studies have also suggested possible links with other clinical disorders. It appears equally important to measure these expectancies when treating other psychological difficulties since expectancies may be contributing risk factors in the development and/or maintenance of these other problems as well.

Measuring expectations in patients ready to begin therapy may provide valuable information regarding their beliefs about their prognosis and on the process and procedures of therapy [46]. Such expectations will not only reveal information about patients' perspectives on the therapy and on their outcome; knowledge may also be gained on whether their expectations are realistic or correspond to the therapy they will undergo.

Findings have been reported on prognostic and process expectations that demonstrate important implications for psychotherapy. However, future research should not only focus on identifying and addressing patient expectations prior to therapy; expectancies should also be addressed throughout therapy. Identifying and discussing these expectations and following their evolution may shed some light on why some individuals seek help whereas others do not; who will continue or discontinue therapy; and which clients will improve following therapy. Moreover, since process expectations comprise two major categories (i.e., procedures of therapy and participant roles) that have been traditionally assessed using different measures (see [39]), it would be important to evaluate this type of expectation distinctly in order to gain more information on clients' pre-therapy perceptions. Prognostic expectations may also be assessed by examining both overall and specific expectancies of symptom reduction. Most studies have focused on general expectancies of therapeutic outcome. By identifying patients' beliefs regarding the reduction of specific symptoms, therapists may be in a better position to address these expectations early on in therapy. Finally, few studies have explored the relationship between expectations, and satisfaction and treatment adherence. Future studies should examine these relationships in order to gather information that will facilitate the use of treatments with fewer dropouts, greater in-session and between-session compliance and higher satisfaction during therapy and at the end of treatment.

Several procedures could be used to resolve some of the methodological shortcomings of previous studies. These may involve (a) utilising two distinct measures to assess prognostic and process expectations [10]; (b) administering questionnaires that assess prognostic expectations related to distinct aspects of symptomatology and treatment efficacy; (c) assessing process expectations linked to distinct components of therapy; (d) distinguishing the effects of the different expectancies on therapeutic outcome, as measured by change in symptoms, satisfaction and compliance; (e) examining the impact of cognitive shifts in expectations from pre-therapy to early stages of therapy on outcome and (f) assessing expectations in a homogeneous clinical population (as opposed to a non-clinical population, such as students).

Pretreatment expectations may also act as predictors of clinical syndromes. According to Reiss's expectancy theory [15], elevated sensitivities and negative expectancies are more likely to contribute to phobic avoidance behaviour and to the development of psychopathology. Prior to treating clinical disorders, it would be beneficial to identify expectancies and sensitivities in order to deal with them during therapy.

Overall, when confronting a situation, individuals bring the personal expectations they have acquired from past experiences. Patients entering into the mental health care system may possess numerous expectations with respect to their symptoms and symptom improvement, services being offered, therapy, their own behaviour and attitude, as well as that of the mental health care worker, and the expertness, attractiveness and credibility of the therapist treating them. Seeking mental health services may generate anxiety for most. Some of their anxiety may be fuelled by personal expectations. Unfortunately, patient expectancies are frequently overlooked. Identifying and discussing patient expectancy beliefs during the initial assessment and initial treatment sessions may minimise fears with respect to psychotherapy and increase treatment compliance and satisfaction. A pre-therapy orientation video, similar to that of Zwick and Attkisson [56, 57], may be developed (also refer to [55] and [3]). As demonstrated by Reis and Brown [96], this video may be short (i.e., 12 minutes) and presented in the waiting room. However, the scope of the video may be expanded beyond the goals and process of therapy. Issues related to prognosis and the clinical disorder may also be included. One of the important objectives of the video would be to replicate the Deane et al. [55] finding of alleviating patients' worries about undergoing psychotherapy. However, the video should also address patient expectations with respect to all aspects of the treatment and their problems.

Another recommendation with regards to therapy may be to dedicate the first two sessions at identifying patients' expectations and their treatment objectives, and then engaging in a discussion about them (e.g., [97, 98]). Patients should be encouraged to discuss what they want from the therapy and/or therapist. After having identified the different types of expectations, information may be provided in order to cover the four main types of expectancies: 1) prognostic, 2) process, 3) anxiety expectancy and 4) anxiety sensitivity. Initial negative beliefs on the efficacy of the therapy, incongruent expectations on client/therapist roles and the procedures of therapy and catastrophic beliefs regarding the symptoms should also be addressed. These information sessions may provide patients with an opportunity to modify their initial expectations to correspond with the therapy that would be offered. Additionally, by providing information early on in therapy with respect to treatment success, process and procedures and their symptoms, patients' motivation and compliance may be enhanced. Fears related to their clinical disorder and to therapy may also be diminished. It is the role of the therapist to explain to the clients the impact of expectations on treatment and on their clinical disorder. It is also important that clients understand that their expectancies may shift in a positive direction during therapy. Conversely, if the treatment does not succeed in changing patients' initial negative expectancies, they may come to realise that another therapy would be more suitable for their needs. It is the role of the clinician to suggest or offer, when necessary, alternative treatments that could meet their clients' expectations.

Summary of recommendations	
Methodological recommendations	• Utilize two distinct measures to assess prognostic and process expectations • Administer questionnaires that assess prognostic expectations related to distinct aspects of symptomatology and treatment efficacy • Assess process expectations linked to distinct components of therapy • Distinguish the effects of the different expectancies on therapeutic outcome, as measured by change in symptoms, satisfaction and compliance • Examine the impact of cognitive shifts in expectations from pre-therapy to early stages of therapy on outcome • Assess expectations in a homogeneous clinical population
Clinical recommendations	• Assess expectations before and throughout therapy • Use a short pre-therapy orientation video, which may be presented in the waiting room • Dedicate some in-session time at identifying and discussing patients' expectations and their treatment objectives • Suggest or offer, when necessary, a treatment that would better suit the clients' expectations

Table 2. Summary of recommendations

Author details

Theodora E. Katerelos[1], Claude Bélanger[1,2*], Marie-Christine Payette[1], Ghassan El-Baalbaki[1,3], André Marchand[1] and Michel Perreault[2,4]

*Address all correspondence to: belanger.claude@uqam.ca

1 University of Quebec in Montreal, Department of Psychology, Montreal, Quebec, Canada

2 McGill University, Department of Psychiatry, Montreal, Quebec, Canada

3 McGill University, Department of Oncology, Montreal, Quebec, Canada

4 Douglas Mental Health Institute, Montreal, Quebec, Canada

References

[1] Wilkins, W. Expectancy of therapeutic gain. Journal of Consulting and Clinical Psychology. 1973;40:69–77. DOI: 10.1037/h0034056

[2] Constantino, M.J., Arnkoff, D.B., Glass, C.R., Ametrano, R.M., & Smith, J.Z. Expectations. Journal of Clinical Psychology: In Session. 2011;67(2):184–192. DOI: 10.1002/jclp.20754

[3] Noble, L.M., Douglas, B.C., & Newman, S.P. What do patients expect of psychiatric services? A systematic and critical review of empirical studies. Social Science and Medicine. 2001;52(7):985–998. DOI: 10.1016/S0277-9536(00)00210-0

[4] Tinsley, H.E.A., & Westcot, A.M. Analysis of the cognitions stimulated by the items on the expectations about counseling-brief form: An analysis of construct validity. Journal of Counseling Psychology. 1990;37(2):223–226. DOI: 10.1037/0022-0167.37.2.223

[5] Ditto, P.H., & Hilton, J.L. Expectancy processes in the health care interaction sequence. Journal of Social Issues. 1990;46(2):97–124. DOI: 10.1111/j.1540-4560.1990.tb01925.x

[6] Goldstein, A.P. Therapist-patient expectancies in psychotherapy. Psychiatry: Interpersonal and Biological Processes. 1962;25(1):72–79. DOI: 10.1521/00332747.1962.1102329

[7] Duckro, P., Beal, D., & George, C. Research on the effects of disconfirmed client role expectations in psychotherapy: A critical review. Psychological Bulletin. 1979;86(2):260–275. DOI: 10.1037/0033-2909.86.2.260

[8] Lambert, M.J., & Asay, T.P. Patient characteristics and their relationship to psychotherapy outcome. In: Hersen, M., Michelson, L., Bellack, A.S., editors. Issues in Psychotherapy Research. New York: Springer; 1984. pp. 313–359. DOI: 10.1007/978-1-4899-2283-0_10

[9] Tracey, T.J., & Dundon, M. Role anticipation and preferences over the course of counseling. Journal of Counseling Psychology. 1988;35(1):10.1037/0022-0167.35.1.3. DOI: 3–14

[10] Garfield, S.L. Research on client variables in psychotherapy. In: Garfield, S.L., Bergin, A.E., editors. Handbook of Psychotherapy and Behavior Change, 3rd ed. New York: John Wiley & Sons; 1986. pp. 213–256

[11] Deane, F.P. Pretreatment expectations of New Zealand clients receiving cognitive-behavioural psychotherapy: Comparison with a North American sample. The International Journal of Social Psychiatry. 1992;38(2):138–149. DOI: 10.1177/002076409203800207

[12] Glass, C.R., Arnkoff, D.B., & Shapiro, S.J. Expectations and preferences. Psychotherapy: Theory, Research, Practice, Training. 2001;38(4):455–461. DOI: 10.1037/0033-3204.38.4.455

[13] Greenberg, R.P., Constantino, M.J., & Bruce, N. Are patient expectations still relevant for psychotherapy process and outcome?. Clinical Psychology Review. 2006;26(6): 657–678. DOI: 10.1016/j.cpr.2005.03.002

[14] American Psychiatric Association, editor. Diagnostic and Statistical Manual of Mental Disorders, 5th ed. Arlington, VA: American Psychiatric Publishing; 2013. 970 p

[15] Reiss, S. Expectancy model of fear, anxiety, and panic. Clinical Psychology Review. 1991;11(2):141–153. DOI: 10.1016/0272-7358(91)90092-9

[16] Capron, D.W., Norr, A.M., & Schmidt, N.B. Risk of co-occurring psychopathology: Testing a prediction of expectancy theory. Journal of Anxiety Disorders. 2013;27(1): 79–83. DOI: 10.1016/j.janxdis.2012.10.011

[17] Reiss, S., & Havercamp, S. The sensitivity theory of motivation: Implications for psychopathology. Behaviour Research and Therapy. 1996;34(8):621–632. DOI: 10.1016/0005-7967(96)00041-1

[18] Reiss, S., Peterson, R.A., Gursky, D.M., & McNally, R.J. Anxiety sensitivity, anxiety frequency, and the prediction of fearfulness. Behaviour Research and Therapy. 1986;24(1):1–8. DOI: 10.1016/0005-7967(86)90143-9

[19] Schmidt, N.B., & Mallott, M. Evaluating anxiety sensitivity and other fundamental sensitivities predicting anxiety symptoms and fearful responding to a biological challenge. Behavioral Research and Therapy. 2006;44(11):1681–1688. DOI: 10.1016/j.brat. 2005.12.001

[20] Vujanovic, A.A., Zvolensky, M.J., Bernsetin, A., Feldner, M.T., & McLeish, A.C. A test of the interactive effects of anxiety sensitivity and mindfulness in the prediction of anxious arousal, agoraphobic cognitions, and body vigilance. Behavioral Research and Therapy. 2007;45(6):1393–1400. DOI: 10.1016/j.brat.2006.06.002

[21] Frank, J.D. The dynamics of the psychotherapeutic relationship: Determinants and effects of the therapist's influence. Psychiatry: Interpersonal and Biological Processes. 1959;22(1):17–39. DOI: 10.1521/00332747.1959.11023154

[22] Frank, J.D., & Frank, J.B. Persuasion and Healing: A Comprehensive Study of Psychotherapy. Baltimore: John Hopkins University; 1961

[23] Frank, J.D. The influence of patients' and therapists' expectations on the outcome of psychotherapy. British Journal of Medical Psychology. 1968;41(4):349–356. DOI: 10.1111/j.2044-8341.1968.tb02043.x

[24] Freidman, H.J. Patient-expectancy and symptom reduction. Archives of General Psychiatry. 1963;8(1):61–67. DOI: 10.1001/archpsyc.1963.01720070063007

[25] Goldstein, A.P. Patients' expectancies and nonspecific therapy as a basis for (un)spontaneous remission. Journal of Clinical Psychology. 1960;16(4):399–403. DOI: 10.1002/1097-4679(196010)16:4<399::AID-JCLP2270160416>3.0.CO;2-E

[26] Piper, W.E., & Wogan, M. Placebo effect in psychotherapy: An extension of earlier findings. Journal of Consulting and Clinical Psychology. 1970;34(3):447. DOI: 10.1037/h0029345

[27] Imber, S.D., Pande, S.K., Frank, J.D., Hoehn-Saric, R., Stone, A.R., & Wargo, D.G. Time-focused role induction. Journal of Nervous and Mental Diseases. 1970;150(1): 27–30. DOI: 10.1097/00005053-197001000-00004

[28] Goldstein, A.P., & Shipman, W. Patient expectancies, symptom reduction, and aspects of the initial psychotherapeutic interview. Journal of Clinical Psychology. 1961;17(2):123–133. DOI: 10.1002/1097-4679(196104)17:2<129::AID-JCLP2270170207>3.0.CO;2-T

[29] Lick, J., & Bootzin, R. Expectancy factors in the treatment of fear: Methodological and theoretical issues. Psychological Bulletin. 1975;82(6):917–931. DOI: 10.1037/0033-2909.82.6.917

[30] Martin, P.J., Sterne, A.L., Moore, J.E., & Lindsey, C.J. Patients' expectancies and hospital outcome. Journal of Clinical Psychology. 1977;33(1):254–258. DOI: 10.1002/1097-4679(197701)33:1+<254::AID-JCLP2270330159>3.0.CO;2-B

[31] Constantino, M.J., Arnkoff, D.B., Glass, C.R., Ametrano, R.M., & Smith, J.Z. Expectations. Journal of Clinical Psychology: In Session. 2011;67(2):184–192. DOI: 10.1002/jclp.20754

[32] Bandura, A., Jeffrey, R.W., & Wright, C.L. Efficacy of participant modeling as a function of response induction aids. Journal of Abnormal Psychology. 1974;83(1):56–64. DOI: 10.1037/h0036258

[33] Weiner, B. An attributionally based theory of motivation and emotion: Focus, range and issues. In: Feather, N.T., editor. Expectations and Actions: Expectancy-Value Models in Psychology. Hillsdale, NJ: Lawrence Erlbaum Associates; 1982. pp. 163–204. DOI: 10.1007/978-1-4612-4948-1

[34] Safren, S.A., Heimberg, R.G., & Juster, H.R. Clients' expectancies and their relationship to pretreatment symptomatology and outcome of cognitive-behavioral group treatment for social phobia. Journal of Consulting and Clinical Psychology. 1997;65(4):694–698. DOI: 10.1037/0022-006X.65.4.694

[35] Tsai, M., Ogrodniczuk, J.S., Sochting, I., & Mirmiran, J. Forecasting success: Patients' expectations for improvement and their relations to baseline, process and outcome variables in group cognitive–behavioural therapy for depression. Clinical Psychology & Psychotherapy. 2014;21(2):97–107. DOI: 10.1002/cpp.1831

[36] Westra, H.A., Constantino, M.J., & Aviram, A. The impact of alliance ruptures on client outcome expectations in cognitive behavioral therapy. Psychotherapy Research. 2011;21(4):472–481. DOI: 10.1080/10503307.2011.581708

[37] Kunkel, M.A., Hector, M.A., Gongóra Coronado E., & Castillo Vales, V. Expectations about counseling in Yucatán, Mexico: Toward a "Mexican Psychology". Journal of Counseling Psychology. 1989;36(3):322–330. DOI: 10.1037/0022-0167.36.3.322

[38] Mezydlo Subich, L., & Coursol, D.H. Counseling expectation of clients and nonclients for group and individual treatment modes. Journal of Counseling Psychology. 1985;32(2):245–251. DOI: dx.doi.org/10.1037/0022-0167.32.2.245

[39] Tinsley, H.E.A., Bowman, S.L., & Ray, S.B. Manipulation of expectancies about counseling and psychotherapy: Review and analysis of expectancy manipulation strategies and results. Journal of Counseling Psychology. 1988;35(1):99–108. DOI: 10.1037/0022-0167.35.1.99

[40] Tinsley, H.E.A., Brown, M.T., St. Aubin, T.M., & Lucek, J. Relation between expectancies for a helping relationship and tendency to seek help from a campus help provider. Journal of Counseling Psychology. 1984;31(2):149–160. DOI: 10.1037/0022-0167.31.2.149

[41] Tinsley, H.E.A., Workman, K.R., & Kass, R. Factor analysis of the domain of client expectancies about counseling. Journal of Counseling Psychology. 1980;27(6):561–570. DOI: 10.1037/0022-0167.27.6.561

[42] Al-Darmaki, F., & Kivlighan, D.M. Jr. Congruence in client-counselor expectations for relationship and the working alliance. Journal of Counseling Psychology. 1993;40(4):379–384. DOI: 10.1037/0022-0167.40.4.379

[43] Tinsley, H.E.A., Bowman, S.L., & Westcot Barich, A. Counseling psychologists' perceptions of the occurrence and effects of unrealistic expectations about counseling and psychotherapy among their clients. Journal of Counseling Psychology. 1993;40(1):46–52. DOI: 10.1037/0022-0167.40.1.46

[44] Richmond, J. Comparison of clients and nonclients expectations of counseling. Psychological Reports. 1984;54(2):752–754. DOI: 10.1037/0022-0167.32.2.245

[45] Westra, H.A., Aviram, A., Barnes, M., & Angus, L. Therapy was not what I expected: A preliminary qualitative analysis of concordance between client expectations and experience of cognitive–behavioural therapy. Psychotherapy Research. 2010;20(4): 436–446. DOI: 10.1080/10503301003657395

[46] Seligman, L.D., Wuyek, L.A., Geers, A.L., Hovey, J.D., & Motley, R.L. The effects of inaccurate expectations on experiences with psychotherapy. Cognitive Therapy and Research. 2009;33(2):139–149. DOI: 10.1007/s10608-009-9266-6

[47] Hardin, S.I., & Yanico, B.J. Counselor gender, type of problem, and expectations about counseling. Journal of Counseling Psychology. 1983;30(2):294–297. DOI: 10.1037/0022-0167.30.2.294

[48] Boulware, D.W., & Holmes, D.S. Preferences for therapists and related expectancies. Journal of Consulting and Clinical Psychology. 1970;35(2):269–277. DOI: 10.1037/h0030078

[49] Watkins, Jr., C.E., & Terrell, F. Mistrust level and its effects on counseling expectations in black client-white counselor relationships: An analogue study. Journal of Counseling Psychology. 1988;35(2):194–197. DOI: 10.1037/0022-0167.35.2.194

[50] Craig, S.S., & Hennessy, J.J. Personality differences and expectations about counseling. Journal of Counseling Psychology. 1989;36(4):401–407. DOI: 10.1037/0022-0167.36.4.401

[51] Satterfield, W.A., Buelow, S.A., Lyddon, W.J., & Johnson, J.T. Client stages of change and expectations about counseling. Journal of Counseling Psychology. 1995;42(4): 476–478. DOI: 10.1037/0022-0167.42.4.476

[52] Swift, J.K., & Callahan, J.L. Decreasing treatment dropout by addressing expectations for treatment length. Psychotherapy Research. 2011;21(2):193–200. DOI: 10.1080/10503307.2010.541294

[53] Callahan, J.L., Gustafson, S.A., Misner, J.B., Paprocki, C.M., Sauer, E.M., Saules, K.K., et al. Introducing the association of psychology training clinics' collaborative research network: A study on client expectancies. Training and Education in Professional Psychology. 2014;8(2):95–104. DOI: 10.1037/tep0000047

[54] Webster, A. The effect of pre-assessment information on clients' satisfaction, expectation and attendance at a mental health day centre. British Journal of Medical Psychology. 1992;65(2):89–93. DOI: 10.1111/j.2044-8341.1992.tb01689.x

[55] Deane, F.P., Spicer, J., & Leathem, J. Effects of videotaped preparatory information on expectations, anxiety, and psychotherapy outcome. Journal of Consulting and Clinical Psychology. 1992;6(6):980–984. DOI: 10.1037/0022-006X.60.6.980

[56] Zwick, R., & Attkisson, C.C. The use of reception checks in client pretherapy orientation research. Journal of Clinical Psychology. 1984;40(2):446–452. DOI: 10.1002/1097-4679(198403)40:2<446::AID-JCLP2270400210>3.0.CO;2-1

[57] Zwick, R., & Attkisson, C.C. Effectiveness of a client pretherapy orientation videotape. Journal of Counseling Psychology. 1985;32(4):514–524. DOI: 10.1037/0022-0167.32.4.514

[58] Gursky, D.M., & Reiss, S. Identifying danger and anxiety expectancies as components of common fears. Journal of Behavior Therapy and Experimental Psychiatry. 1987;18(4):317–324. DOI: 10.1016/0005-7916(87)90045-0

[59] Jones, M.K., & Menzies, R.G. Danger expectancies, self-efficacy and insight in spider phobia. Behaviour Research and Therapy. 2000;38(6):585–600. DOI: 10.1016/S0005-7967(99)00076-5

[60] Cipher, D.J., & Fernandez, E. Expectancy variables predicting tolerance and avoidance of pain in chronic pain patients. Behaviour Research and Therapy. 1997;35(5):437–444. DOI: 10.1016/S0005-7967(96)00121-0

[61] DiNardo, P.A., Guzy, L.T., Jenkins, J.A., Bak, R.M., Tomasi, S.F., & Copland, M. Etiology and maintenance of dog fears. Behaviour Research and Therapy. 1988;26:241–244. DOI: 10.1016/0005-7967(88)90005-8

[62] McCracken, L.M., Gross, R.T., Sorg, P.J., & Edmands, T.A. Prediction of pain in patients with chronic low back pain: Effects of inaccurate prediction and pain-related anxiety. Behaviour Research and Therapy. 1993;31(7):647–652. DOI: 10.1016/0005-7967(93)90117-D

[63] Jussim, L. Expectancies and social issues: Introduction. Journal of Social Issues. 1990;46(2):1–8. DOI: 10.1111/j.1540-4560.1990.tb01920.x

[64] Rodebaugh, T.L., Heimberg, R.G., Schultz, L.T., & Blackmore, M. The moderated effects of video feedback for social anxiety disorder. Journal of Anxiety Disorders. 2010;24(7):663–671. DOI: 10.1016/j.janxdis.2010.04.007

[65] Cox, B.J., Endler, N.S., & Swinson, R.P. An examination of levels of agoraphobic severity in panic disorder. Behaviour Research and Therapy. 1995;33(1):57–62. DOI: 10.1016/0005-7967(93)E0029-5

[66] Cox, B.J., Swinson, R.P., Norton, G.R., & Kuch, K. Anticipatory anxiety and avoidance in panic disorder with agoraphobia. Behaviour Research and Therapy. 1991;29(4):363–365. DOI: 10.1016/0005-7967(91)90073-C

[67] Craske, M.G., Rapee, R.M., & Barlow, D.H. The significance of panic-expectancy for individual patterns of avoidance. Behavior Therapy. 1988;19(4):577–592. DOI: 10.1016/S0005-7894(88)80025-X

[68] Craske, M.G., & Barlow, D.H. A review of the relationship between panic and avoidance. Clinical Psychology Review. 1988;8(6):667–685. DOI: 10.1016/0272-7358(88)90086-4

[69] Kirsch, I., Tennen, H., Wickless, C., Saccone, A.J., & Cody, S. The role of expectancy in fear reduction. Behavior Therapy. 1983;14(4):520–533. DOI: 10.1016/S0005-7894(83)80075-6

[70] Southworth, S., & Kirsch, I. The role of expectancy in exposure-generated fear reduction in agoraphobia. Behaviour Research and Therapy. 1988;26(2):113–120. DOI: 10.1016/0005-7967(88)90110-6

[71] Maller, R.G., & Reiss, S. Anxiety sensitivity in 1984 and panic attacks in 1987. Journal of Anxiety Disorders. 1992;6(3):241–247. DOI: 10.1016/0887-6185(92)90036-7

[72] Taylor, S., Koch, W.J., & McNally, R.J. How does anxiety sensitivity vary across the anxiety disorders? Journal of Anxiety Disorders. 1992;7(3):249–259. DOI: 10.1016/0887-6185(92)90037-8

[73] Schmidt, N.B., Lerew, D.R., & Jackson, R.J. The role of anxiety sensitivity in the pathogenesis of panic: Prospective evaluation of spontaneous panic attacks during acute stress. Journal of Abnormal Psychology. 1997;106(3):355–365. DOI: 10.1037/0021-843X.106.3.355

[74] McNally, R.J., & Lorenz, M. Anxiety sensitivity in agoraphobics. Journal of Behaviour Therapy and Experimental Psychiatry. 1987;18(1):3–11. DOI: 10.1016/0005-7916(87)90065-6

[75] Cox, B.J., Endler, N.S., Norton, G.R., & Swinson, R.P. Anxiety sensitivity and nonclinical panic attacks. Behaviour Research and Therapy. 1991;29(4):367–369. DOI: 10.1016/0005-7967(91)90074-D

[76] Norton, G.R., Pidlubny, S.R., & Norton, P.J. Prediction of panic attacks and related variables. Behavior Therapy. 1999;30(2):319–330. DOI: 10.1016/S0005-7894(99)80011-2

[77] Naragon-Gainey, K. Meta-analysis of the relations of anxiety sensitivity to the depressive and anxiety disorders. Psychological bulletin. 2010;136(1):128–150. DOI: 10.1037/a0018055

[78] Olatunji, B.O., & Wolitzky-Taylor, K.B. Anxiety sensitivity and the anxiety disorders: A meta-analytic review and synthesis. Psychological Bulletin. 2009;135(6):974–999. DOI: 10.1037/a0017428

[79] McLeish, A.C., Zvolensky, M.J., Del Ben, K.S., & Burke, R.S. Anxiety sensitivity as a moderator of the association between smoking rate and panic-relevant symptoms among a community sample of middle-aged adult daily smokers. The American Journal on Addictions. 2009;18(1):93–99. DOI: 10.1080/10550490802408985

[80] Hazen, A.L., Walker, J.R., & Eldridge, G.D. Anxiety sensitivity and treatment outcome in panic disorder. Anxiety. 1996;2(1):34–39. DOI: 10.1002/(SICI)1522-7154(1996)2:1<34::AID-ANXI5>3.0.CO;2-D

[81] Clark, D.M., Salkovskis, P.M., Hackmann, A., Middleton, H., Anastasiades, P.A., & Gelder, M. A comparison of cognitive therapy, applied relaxation and imipramine in the treatment of panic disorder. British Journal of Psychiatry. 1994;164(6):759–769. DOI: 10.1192/bjp.164.6.759

[82] Norr, A.M., Allan, N.P., Macatee, R.J., Keough, M.E., & Schmidt, N.B. The effects of an anxiety sensitivity intervention on anxiety, depression, and worry: Mediation through affect tolerances. Behaviour Research and Therapy. 2014;59:12–19. DOI: 10.1016/j.brat.2014.05.011

[83] Brown, T.A., & Barlow, D.H. Long-term outcome in cognitive-behavioral treatment of panic disorder: Clinical predictors and alternative strategies for assessment. Journal of Consulting and Clinical Psychology. 1995;63(5):754–765. DOI: 10.1037/0022-006X.63.5.754

[84] Asmundson, G.J.G., Norton, P.J., & Veloso, F. Anxiety sensitivity and fear of pain in patients with recurring headaches. Behaviour Research and Therapy. 1999;37(8):703–713. DOI: 10.1016/S0005-7967(98)00172-7

[85] Asmundson, G.J.G., & Taylor, S. Role of anxiety sensitivity in pain-related fear and avoidance. Journal of Behavioral Medicine. 1996;19(6):577–586. DOI: 10.1007/BF01904905

[86] Samoluk, S.B., Stewart, S.H., Sweet, S.B., & MacDonald, A.B. Anxiety sensitivity and social affiliation as determinants of alcohol consumption. Behavior Therapy. 1999;30(2):285–303. DOI: 10.1016/S0005-7894(99)80009-4

[87] Stewart, S.H., Knize, K., & Phil, R.O. Anxiety sensitivity and dependency in clinical and non-clinical panickers and controls. Journal of Anxiety Disorders. 1992;6(2):119–131. DOI: 10.1016/0887-6185(92)90011-U

[88] Taylor, S., Koch, W.J., Woody, S., & McLean, P.D. Anxiety sensitivity and depression: How are they related?. Journal of Abnormal Psychology. 1996;105(3):474–479. DOI: 10.1037/0021-843X.105.3.474

[89] Schmidt, N.B., Lerew, D.R., & Joiner, T.E. Jr. Anxiety sensitivity and the pathogenesis of anxiety and depression: Evidence for symptom specificity. Behaviour Research and Therapy. 1998;36(2):165–177. DOI: 10.1016/S0005-7967(98)00011-4

[90] Stewart, S.H., Peterson, J.B., & Phil, R.O. Anxiety sensitivity and self-reported alcohol consumption rates in university women. Journal of Anxiety Disorders. 1995;9(4):283–292. DOI: 10.1016/0887-6185(95)00009-D

[91] Reiss, S., & McNally, R.J. The expectancy model of fear. In: Reiss, S., & Bootzin, R.R., editors. Theoretical Issues in Behavior Therapy. New York: Academic Press; 1985. pp. 107–121

[92] Donnell, C.D., & McNally, R.J. Anxiety sensitivity and panic attacks in a nonclinical population. Behaviour Research and Therapy. 1990;29(1):83–85. DOI: 10.1016/0005-7967(90)90058-Q

[93] Watt, M.C., Stewart, S.H., & Cox, B.J. A retrospective study of the learning history of origins of anxiety sensitivity. Behaviour Research and Therapy. 1998;36(5):505–525. DOI: 10.1016/S0005-7967(97)10029-8

[94] Clark, D.M. A cognitive approach to panic. Behaviour Research and Therapy. 1986;24(4):461–470. DOI: 10.1016/0005-7967(86)90011-2

[95] Beck, A.T. Cognitive approaches to panic disorder: Theory and therapy. In: Rackman, S., & Maser, J.D, editors. Panic: Psychological Perspectives. Hillsdale: Lawrence Erlbaum; 1988. pp. 91–109

[96] Reis, B.F., & Brown, L.G. Preventing therapy dropout in the real world: The clinical utility of videotape preparation and client estimate of treatment duration. Professional Psychology: Research and Practice. 2006;37(3):311–316. DOI: 10.1037/0735-7028.37.3.311

[97] Lazare, A., Cohen, F., Jacobson, A.M., Williams, M.W., Mignone, R.J., & Zisook, S. The walk-in patient as a "customer": A key dimension in evaluation and treatment. American Journal of Orthopsychiatry. 1972;42(5):872–883. DOI: 10.1111/j.1939-0025.1972.tb00774.x

[98] Lazare, A., Eisenthal, S., & Wasserman, L. The customer approach to patienthood: Attending to patient requests in a walk-in clinic. Archives of General Psychiatry. 1975;32(5):553–558. DOI: 10.1001/archpsyc.1975.01760230019001

[99] Patterson, C.L., Anderson, T., & Wei, C. Clients' pretreatment role expectations, the therapeutic alliance, and clinical outcomes in outpatient therapy. Journal of Clinical Psychology. 2014;70(7):673–680. DOI: 10.1002/jclp.22054

Practical Applications of Complementary and Alternative Therapies in Adults and Youth with Anxiety Disorders

Sarosh Khalid-Khan, Faiza Khalid-Khan and
David Gratzer

Additional information is available at the end of the chapter

http://dx.doi.org/10.5772/61046

Abstract

The use of complementary and alternative medicine (CAM) therapies is becoming an increasingly popular treatment option for anxiety disorders in adults and youth. Parents often are reluctant to use antidepressants due to fear of potential side effects. Youth are often unwilling to participate in cognitive behaviour therapy (CBT) or it is not readily available. Practitioners are not always knowledgeable or open to considering CAM therapies for their patients. This chapter will review the definition of CAM, prevalence of CAM use, its safety and effectiveness and finally its practical applications. Four case studies are discussed in which practitioners were open to the use of CAM and collaborated successfully with parents of youth with anxiety disorders. Literature review is presented for use of vitamin D, melatonin, acupuncture, acupressure and craniosacral therapy.

Keywords: Complementary therapies, alternative therapy, youth adults, anxiety disorders

1. Introduction

The use of complementary and alternative medicine (CAM) therapies is becoming an increasingly popular treatment option for anxiety disorders. In this chapter, we will review the emerging evidence in the West for CAM therapies commonly used in adults and children to treat anxiety disorders focusing in particular on acupuncture, naturopathy and body-based therapies. We will also consider how the widespread use and acceptance of CAM therapies will impact conventional psychiatric practice. Patients rarely disclose CAM use to physicians and, although physicians recognize patient's interest in CAM, they often do not feel comfortable asking about, discussing or recommending these treatments, due to a lack of knowledge about their effectiveness and safety [1].

Anxiety disorders are amongst the most common psychiatric disorders for both adults and children and include a number of conditions such as panic disorder, phobias, obsessive-compulsive disorder (OCD), generalized anxiety disorder, post-traumatic stress disorder and anxiety disorder due to a general medical condition. The prevalence of anxiety disorders is 3–18% worldwide [2]. The most prevalent condition according to the Office for National Statistics is mixed anxiety and depression [3]. Conventional treatment of these conditions involves antidepressants and cognitive behavior therapy (CBT). These treatments have limitations: antidepressants have been associated with adverse effects and poor adherence while CBT is not widely available. Consequently, patients are turning to CAM treatments. Anxiety, depression and stress were among the most common reasons for seeking CAM therapies in the United Kingdom [4]. Similar findings were reported in the United States and Canada [5, 12]. In 1997, 42% of American adults reported using CAM with 629 million visits to CAM practitioners, exceeding substantially the total visits (386 million) to primary care physicians that year [6].

Despite the inconclusive data on the efficacy and safety of many CAM treatments, there is enough evidence on certain treatments to be useful for researchers and clinicians. In light of the current literature, "it is perhaps helpful to remember that excessive skepticism as well as excessive enthusiasm can stand in the way of patient care" [7]. The low stigma and low costs of many forms of CAM, especially in comparison to many conventional psychiatric treatments, make them popular options for patients and thus clinicians should educate themselves about these treatments. The challenge to individual physicians is whether and how to participate in the emergence of CAM treatments in psychiatry. With more than a third of their patients already using natural remedies, an important question is: will physicians view CAM therapies as a conflict and dismiss their use or view them as an opportunity to expand their repertoire of these treatments?

2. What Is CAM?

CAM is not simple to define due to the variety of healing approaches and therapies that are included under its umbrella. Many aspects of CAM are rooted in Eastern healing practices such as those of China, India, and Africa and have been practiced for thousands of years. Often, it is difficult to distinguish between CAM and conventional medicine due to some CAM therapies that have become a part of conventional practice. For example, physical exercise as a treatment for many diseases might have been considered unconventional 50 years ago, but exercise is now known to benefit many medical as well as psychological conditions. There are a number of other examples of treatments that were unconventional but converted to standard practice once research confirmed their efficacy. The term Integrative Medicine was introduced to include all treatment options that are safe and effective, regardless of their origin. All safe and effective treatments should be used by practitioners, so it is often difficult to define what lies outside of conventional medicine. Another example includes the established use of CBT and mindfulness to treat anxiety and depression which were considered unconventional 20 years ago. By definition, most CAM treatments are not established. As more research is conducted, some CAM therapies that show promise in preliminary research will become part of established care and therefore will no longer be considered "alternative" [7].

Although the difference between conventional medicine and alternative medicine is not always easy to distinguish, a basic philosophic difference exists. Conventional medicine is used to treat symptoms and traditional medicine to restore the body to its natural balance [1]. Conventional medicine generally defines health as the absence of disease or dysfunction. The main causes of disease and dysfunction are usually considered to be isolated factors, such as bacteria or viruses, biochemical imbalances, and aging and treatment often involves drugs or surgery. In contrast, alternative medicine practices often define health holistically, that is, as a balance of systems – physical, emotional and spiritual involving the whole person. Disharmony among these systems is thought to cause illness. Treatment involves strengthening the body's own defenses and restoring these balances.

The National Center for Complementary and Alternative Medicine defines CAM as "a group of diverse medical and health care systems, practices, and products that are not generally considered part of conventional medicine.....Complementary medicine refers to the use of CAM together with conventional medicine and alternative medicine refers to the use of CAM in place of conventional medicine....." [8].

There are five categories of CAM:

1. Alternative medical systems (Ayurveda, naturopathy, homeopathy, acupuncture Chinese/Oriental medicine),
2. Biologically based therapies (vitamins, herbs, special diets),
3. Mind–body therapies (meditation, biofeedback, hypnosis, imagery, prayer),
4. Energy healing, (Reiki, electromagnetic-based therapies), and manipulative and
5. Body-based therapies (chiropractic, massage, craniosacral therapy) [8].

3. Prevalence of CAM use

The use of CAM has been increasing for decades both worldwide [9] and in the United States, specifically [10], and it currently remains in the 25-50% range [11]. Both Canada and United States are similar with regard to prevalence of CAM use [12]. In 2008, it was reported that 38% of adults over the age of 18 years used some form of CAM, with women being the greater consumers (43%) compared with men (34%) [11]. Those with psychiatric disorders tend to be high users of CAM and this is particularly true for the patients with anxiety. Bystritsky et al. [13] reviewed the evidence of CAM use in populations with anxiety in 2012. The results, consistent with earlier studies, show a 43% use of a variety of CAM treatments in the United States. Users most often had a diagnosis of GAD, were older, more educated and had two or more chronic medical conditions.

The numbers for CAM use for children and adolescents are also significant. A 2012 paper [14] looked at a sample of about 6000 children and adolescents aged 7–17 years, with mental health concerns 29% of whom had used CAM therapy (excluding vitamins and minerals). In contrast, only 12% of those without mental health concerns reported CAM use. CAM use was higher for those with anxiety/depression (34%) than those with ADHD (24%). Children with anxiety alone versus mixed anxiety and depression had similar rates of CAM use (35%). For those with mental health conditions, the most commonly used CAM therapies were mind-body practices (16.3%) and biological therapies (11%), followed by manipulative and body-based therapies (8.5%). Alternative medical systems and energy healing modalities were used by fewer than 3% [14].

These numbers confirm the importance of awareness of CAM use in both adults and children with anxiety and depression. With so many individuals using CAM treatments it is important to consider how these treatments may be interfering with conventional first-line treatments of these disorders. The numbers also highlight the importance of finding the best integrative use for patients who may benefit from other non-traditional treatment modalities, for example, when parents refuse standard medication for their children considering them "too strong" and asking for natural products which they perceive as more safe.

With more patients visiting CAM therapists than primary care physicians, according to one survey [6], it is important to consider the reason for this shift. Among adult patients with mental health concerns, surveys have found that patients choose CAM therapy because of its natural approach and perception of being safe, because CAM treatments align with their own beliefs, because prior experience with conventional medicine had unpleasant side effects or were ineffective and patients wanted to avoid consulting with a health care provider [13]. Moreover, parents are very reluctant to give their children conventional medications thinking that they are potentially addictive and are looking for "natural" treatments that they believe are safer and more effective [1]. In children, CAM use is associated with chronic medical conditions, higher maternal age and education, as well as parental CAM use [15]. As more patients turn to CAM treatments, there is increased awareness: both health professionals and the public are exposed to articles on the subject in professional journals, lay magazines, on the internet (from the comfort of their home) and numerous products are available in various stores.

Conventional medications are more effective in treating anxiety disorders than CAM treatments, but come with increased side effects. In the case of SSRIs, a class of medications commonly used to treat anxiety disorders, some side effects can be perceived as intolerable [16]: the Black Box warnings related to increased suicidal ideation. Effectiveness of conventional treatments is also a concern. Only about 50–65% of patients with anxiety disorders benefit from antidepressants and CBT [16], and many patients continue to suffer significant symptoms despite treatment, emphasizing the need for further options. For example, conventional approaches may not always be effective for patients with severe OCD, motivating them to try CAM approaches. One other potential reason for the increasing popularity of CAM treatments is a mistrust of the pharmaceutical industry. The perceived blurred boundaries between the pharmaceutical industry and physicians have led to the concern that the industry may have undue influence on a physician's decision to prescribe certain medications [7].

In response to the parents' and physicians' interest in CAM therapies, the United States government is now beginning to become active in promoting the development of CAM. There are several professional associations developed to aid in the funding, support and development of this field. These are the National Institute of Health (NIH), the National Center for Complementary and Alternative Medicine (NCCAM) and Office of Dietary Supplements (ODS). The American Academy of Child and Adolescent Psychiatry (AACAP) has also established its Committee on Integrative Medicine [7].

4. Safety

There is a widespread perception that natural products and remedies are safe, although it is often not the case. Because herbal medicines and other dietary supplements are not regulated as drugs by the Food and Drug Administration (FDA), their manufacturers do not have to prove their safety. One of the most important concerns relates to the fidelity of natural products. Due to the less rigorous efficacy and safety criteria than prescription drugs, herbal remedies and dietary supplements lack standardized preparation, and thus are more prone to contamination and substitution. They are also prone to incorrect packaging and storage, wrong dosage and inappropriate labeling and advertising [1]. Consumers cannot be sure they are taking the amount they are supposed to take or that the product has the all the ingredients listed on its package. The public is not necessarily aware that there is no safety testing of health food store products or oversight of quality control [1]. Therefore, it may be difficult to say that a treatment that worked in one instance is the same treatment that would be offered under the same name elsewhere.

Also, although some CAM therapies have risky side effects, the greatest risk occurs when a person is treated with an unproven CAM therapy instead of a proven conventional medicine approach. Using a CAM therapy as first-line treatment when there is only inconclusive evidence to support it is a significant risk to patient care. Many CAM therapies are clearly safe such as such as meditation or Reiki [17], however many CAM products have potentially significant interactions with other conventional medications. St. John's Wort, for example, has the potential for drug interactions with SSRIs, a standard treatment for anxiety. Its other interactions include "reduced efficacy of birth control pills, antivirals, and many cardiovascular medications" [13]. Kava's potential for liver toxicity has limited its recommendation by practitioners especially for children and adolescents. Furthermore, Kava and Valerian Root can enhance the sedative effect of benzodiazepines [13]. In addition, it may be potentially difficult to evaluate the effectiveness of a treatment while another treatment is being covertly taken in varying doses.

It is also important for clinicians to know that the adverse effects of CAM treatments tend to be under-reported in many publications in the medical literature as well as in lay media. In many instances, adverse effects are not systematically assessed or might not even be mentioned [7].

The simultaneous use of additional CAM therapies such as relaxation, prayers, meditation and biofeedback that are not part of a patient's CBT treatment could also be potentially problematic. Patients could be given conflicting messages and explanations of their symptoms and how to handle them [13].

5. Effectiveness

The effectiveness of CAM therapies has been difficult to establish and many systematic literature reviews provide inconclusive evidence [7]. Some therapies such as acupuncture have been shown to be effective for specific conditions, but are currently being used more broadly than the specific conditions for which there is evidence. Many forms of CAM have not undergone rigorous scientific evaluation. However, a lack of scientific studies does not mean that a therapy is ineffective. A large number of alternative therapies have been practiced for thousands of years. These include acupuncture, meditation, yoga, therapeutic diets, massage and herbal medicine. However, scientific research on CAM therapies can be difficult due to unique barriers. These include a lack of interest among medical researchers, limited availability of research funds, and difficulties applying conventional research methods to studying alternative therapies [18]. For example, medical researchers often have little scientific interest in acupuncture because its theory depends on non-scientific concepts such as "vital energy". Commercial research funds are limited because CAM therapies cannot be patented and do not generate large profits to drive research and marketing. Government research funds are limited because the scientific community remains skeptical of CAM theory and the validity of its methods [18].

There are several challenges to applying conventional research methods to CAM therapies. Concepts such as standard treatment for each subject in the study, a placebo control group and the method of double blinding are required for a rigorous study. Each of these concepts is difficult to achieve in many CAM treatments [18]. For example, many CAM therapies treat the unique and particular imbalances of an individual. Acupuncture needles are placed at points on the body according to the individual's unique needs. Also, two people with the same condition may be treated with completely different herbal medications.

Double blinding is a process where the subjects as well as the researchers are kept unaware of the difference between the active treatment group versus the placebo control group. This process is designed to eliminate the bias associated with outcome expectations. Placebo designs are used to blind subjects, which are limited in many CAM treatments. Placebo control groups can be created easily for some CAM treatments such as herbal remedies, but for other practices such as acupuncture and chiropractic treatment it becomes difficult to design a placebo. For therapies such as meditation placebo designs are quite impossible. Researcher blinding may also be limited, for example, a Reiki practitioner would know whether a real energy treatment is being given.

For these abovementioned reasons, it is difficult to draw firm clinical conclusions from much of the research in CAM psychiatry. Among the systematic reviews by the Cochrane Collaboration of CAM treatments throughout pediatrics, "about 70% of the reviews (109 of 163) have been deemed inconclusive, not permitting firm positive or negative conclusions regarding treatment recommendations" [7]. Child and adolescent psychiatrists will nonetheless find a review of these treatments to be clinically useful, because families of patients are often interested in these treatments, and are reluctant to use standard treatments. The use of low-risk, low-cost adjunctive treatments may be defensible even when the level of data supporting their use is not compelling

6. Practical applications

The integration of CAM treatments does not necessarily require clinicians to make major changes in the way they practice. It can be as simple as recommending reliable CAM options to patients who will benefit from a trusted referral to an established CAM therapist. Using some CAM treatments as an adjunct to standard treatment and providing a range of options for patients when they refuse first-line treatments are important first steps. Clinicians should also routinely ask of CAM use in their patient consults. Patients expect disapproval or ignorance from physicians regarding CAM treatments. Parents inform the doctor of their child's use of CAM in only 12–44% of cases in the United States. In contrast, the disclosure of CAM treatments to pediatricians is 79% in Germany, where CAM is more supported by professional societies, the government and the public [7]. Clinicians can also incorporate CAM research into their clinical practice and teach students and colleagues of how to effectively use CAM therapies. Joining an integrative practice or start a partnership with local CAM specialists where each share care for the patient can also be a good place to start. Individuals can choose to incorporate diverse holistic treatments or start with just natural products and dietary supplements. Prescribers who use these natural products and dietary supplements will want to become familiar with specific brands and products so that they can recommend reliable products that are safe. ConsumerLab.com is a helpful resource for obtaining specific information about different companies and their products, and for following general developments in this area. Many of these products are available at health food stores, but prescribers can inform patients that certain online sources offer brand name products.

Four case studies are described below in which the child psychiatrist utilized complementary and alternative treatments while collaborating with the families of youth. These are followed by literature reviews for vitamin D, melatonin, acupuncture, acupressure and craniosacral therapy.

6.1. Case study 1

Heidi, a 12-year-old girl, had suffered from severe social anxiety disorder with some depressive symptoms for the past 3 years. Her depressive symptoms became worse every fall through the winter months when she had persistent sadness, increased sleep, fatigue, more social withdrawal than before, school non-attendance and lack of enjoyment in activities. She had not been attending school consistently in the past 3 months. Heidi lived with her mother and younger brother. Heidi's mother suffered from generalized anxiety disorder, major depressive disorder and borderline traits while growing up and had "bad side effects" from psychiatric medications.

On assessment, due to Heidi's lack of functioning in all aspects of her life, the child psychiatrist recommended combined treatment of antidepressant and cognitive behaviour therapy (CBT). Heidi's mother refused to start medication and Heidi did not want to do CBT. The psychiatrist checked her baseline labs including thyroid stimulating hormone (TSH) and vitamin D levels. Heidi's TSH was normal; however, her vitamin D levels were very low <25 nmol/mL, a level which signifies deficiency. Heidi was started on vitamin D, 1,000 IU daily. In the meantime, she was monitored at least once a month. She was also placed in a classroom which was small and the setting was conducive to learning for students struggling with anxiety disorders. In this setting, the principles of CBT were embedded in the program. Heidi did fairly well for a few months but when the winter came, she became worse. At this time, the psychiatrist broached the discussion of starting an antidepressant once more. This time the mother relented and agreed. Heidi was started on escitalopram 5 mg daily titrated up to 10 mg daily in conjunction with vitamin D therapy. Heidi had a swift response to medication towards both her anxiety and mood symptoms and was functioning very well after a month of starting treatment. Her vitamin D level was 100 nmol/mL.

Vitamin D is a hormone that can be synthesized by the skin through exposure to sunlight or obtained through certain foods including fish, beef, eggs and fortified foods like milk, orange juice, cheese and cereals. Optimal vitamin D levels are defined as serum 25 OH D levels above 75 nmol/L. Vitamin D insufficiency is defined as levels between 50 and 75 nmol/L and deficiency as levels lower than 50 nmol/L [19]. Vitamin D supplementation, if effective, would provide a safe, less intensive and less expensive alternative to current therapies for anxiety disorders in adolescents. To date, no studies have specifically been done with vitamin D in adolescents with anxiety disorders. Evidence does exist demonstrating the correlation between vitamin D levels and depressive symptomology in a variety of age groups, including adolescents [20,21]. It is important to establish if this is an avenue that can be used as a treatment option by studying the efficacy of correcting the underlying deficiency.

A limited number of studies have been done on vitamin D supplementation and its impact on depressive symptoms. The majority of studies carried out have focused on adult populations with an emphasis on geriatric, obese and female populations [22–29]. Hogberg et al. [30] specifically looked at adolescents and found an increase in plasma vitamin D 25 OH levels after vitamin D supplementation, in addition to a significant decrease in scores on the Mood and Feelings Questionnaire short version, moving the group from an average in the depression range to a sub-threshold value [22]. Unfortunately, the study did not include a control group, which decreases the strength of the findings [22].

A number of studies in adults have also shown improvements in measures of depressive symptoms after vitamin D supplementation [24–26,29,30]. Individuals in these studies were given vitamin D in various dosages, and measures of depressive symptoms were compared before and after treatment. The dosing regimens of vitamin D given between studies varied substantially. Some studies gave one-time treatment [26], some gave annual vitamin D injection [26] and others had daily oral regimens of varied dosages [22–25,28,29]. Treatment length also varied between studies; however, many studies analyzed improvements at the 8-week or 3-month marks. Certain limitations were apparent within the existing literature. The first was a lack of control groups in many of the studies. This warrants the question of whether the effects seen are the result of placebo or whether depressive episodes subsided in the given time frame regardless of treatment efficacy. Another limitation was the small sample sizes used in some of the studies (in one study only nine individuals were studied [29].

The primary controversy is whether or not vitamin D supplementation is truly an effective treatment for depression. While some studies have shown significance, some have not. Three studies analyzed demonstrated no significant change in measures of depressive symptoms, regardless of increases in serum vitamin D levels [23,27,28]. Of these studies, two used low doses of vitamin D, one utilized annual dosing, and all three looked at postmenopausal female populations without significant vitamin D deficiency [23,27,28]. These methodological differences could account for differences seen.

The existing literature provides compelling reason to believe that vitamin D supplementation for adolescents with known vitamin D deficiency may provide a new manner by which to safely and effectively treat depression. However, the literature is unable to provide strong evidence of treatment efficacy at this point. As a result, further research is required to study the effects of vitamin D supplementation in this specific age group.

6.2. Case study 2

Eric, a 10-year-old male, was brought to child and adolescent psychiatry outpatient clinic by his parents. Eric has had excessive worrying, insomnia, stomachaches and nausea when going to school for the past 6 months. At bedtime, he has anticipatory anxiety about his school day which causes initial insomnia; he takes about 1–2 hours to fall asleep. He had been late to school a few days in the past month due to feeling tired and cranky in the mornings. Eric has a television in his bedroom and watches movies when he cannot sleep. He also has his iPOD with him at night. Eric's parents have a difficult time dealing with his anxiety at bedtime. His mother, having an untreated anxiety disorder herself, is prone to enable Eric's worries whereas his father is more firm with him. Eric is functioning well academically and socially and is very engaged in sports.

On assessment, because Eric symptoms had not expanded to other areas of his life i.e. school and with peers and were situated in one domain i.e. home, the psychiatrist recommended sleep hygiene and exclusion of excessive sugar and caffeine from his diet. Regarding sleep hygiene, his parents were advised to have a firm bedtime for Eric, a calming bedtime ritual, i.e. relaxing bath and story time. They were advised to remove the TV and all electronics out of his bedroom. The family tried this for 2 weeks and returned to report that although Eric was calmer with these interventions, he still could not fall asleep. A trial of medication was discussed but parents were not comfortable with starting a psychiatric medication. The child psychiatrist recommended a trial of Melatonin, over the counter, 3 mg, at night for insomnia and the parents were agreeable. Family returned after 2 weeks and reported Eric was falling asleep within 15 minutes of lying down and was staying asleep for the night. He was waking up in the morning feeling alert and was at school on time.

Insomnia with difficulty either initiating or maintain sleep affects 15–25% of youth [31]. Insomnia is usually a symptom of an anxiety disorder and is usually accompanied with worry, fatigue, irritability and inattention. Having exposure to electronics and screen light before sleeping may contribute to insomnia. Other contributing factors may be use of caffeine and excessive sugar.

Endogenous **melatonin** is important for synchronizing the circadian rhythm; it is a hormone produced by the pineal gland at nighttime. Chronic sleep onset insomnia is present in about 10% of school-aged children; these children have worries, night awakening, difficulty awakening and daytime tiredness [32]. Exogenous melatonin can adjust the circadian rhythm and advance sleep onset [33,34] and may affect chronic insomnia positively.

A 2001 paper [32] studied the efficacy of melatonin in childhood sleep onset insomnia lasting for more than a year. This was a double-blind placebo-controlled trial in 40 elementary school children 6–12 years of age who were randomly assigned to either 5 mg melatonin or placebo for one month. Melatonin treatment was shown to significantly advance sleep onset, reduce sleep latency and increase mean sleep duration in children with chronic sleep onset insomnia. Measures of health status and sleep improved significantly more in the melatonin than in the placebo group. Very few transient side effects were reported [32].

In another study completed in 1999 [35], melatonin was administrated to 18 females and 12 males with mean ages of 14.8 years who had insomnia and school phobia. These patients were compared to 27 age-matched healthy controls. Melatonin was administered 1–10 mg daily for a mean of 7.8 months. The dose was adjusted weekly as needed. Sleep disturbances improved mildly to markedly in 25 patients with very few side effects [35].

Although there are a few randomized controlled trials in youth for melatonin, most of them are not in youth with anxiety disorders except the trial in school phobia [35]. However, this study has a very small sample size so results cannot be generalized to a clinical setting. Further research is needed in this population to determine the efficacy of melatonin.

6.3. Case study 3

Sydney is a 15-year-old girl who came to the outpatient mood and anxiety clinic with her mother. Sydney is of mixed Chinese and Caucasian descent, her mother is Caucasian and father is Chinese. Sydney has had increased anxiety in the past year which has affected her in a way such that she feels constantly overwhelmed. She has stress headaches, tension in her shoulders, frequent nausea and insomnia. All medical tests are normal. Sydney was quite irritable due to her feeling of stress and was having frequent crying episodes at the slightest provocation. She was attending school regularly, enjoying her activities and socializing with friends. Sydney had a few recent stressors: a breakup with her boyfriend of 6 months, her pet dog had died after being hit by a car and her parents were having marital discord.

Sydney's mother was a successful naturopath and was averse to any psychiatric medication. Her father was also in favour of Eastern medicine; Sydney did not want to pursue CBT. The child psychiatrist informed them of the treatments that could be offered and when encountering resistance and refusal, engaged Sydney and her mother and then her father over the phone in a discussion of their preference for complementary and alternative treatments. Parents and Sydney agreed on doing acupuncture for her symptoms. The child psychiatrist got in touch with Sydney's acupuncturist for continued collaboration and ongoing monitoring.

Acupuncture involves inserting extremely thin needles through skin at strategic points on the body. Acupuncture is a key component of traditional Chinese medicine and is most commonly used to treat pain. Acupuncture, in traditional Chinese medicine, is a technique for balancing the flow of energy or life force known as "qi" or "chi" believed to flow through pathways (meridians) in the body. Needles are inserted into specific points along these meridians such that energy flow will re-balance.

Anxiety disorders are often associated with symptoms that are treated with acupuncture, i.e. pain, nausea and depression. Currently, there are no randomized controlled trials for acupuncture in children and adolescents in anxiety disorders. Liu et al. [36] randomized 240 adult patients with anxiety neurosis to either acupuncture, behavioural de-sensitizations and combined treatment of acupuncture and behavioural desensitization. Treatment was provided over range of 1–10 sessions with standard being 4 sessions. Behavioural desensitization was provided over 2 sessions per week. The combined treatment group had a significantly greater improvement after 10 sessions; however, all groups experienced improvement.

A second randomized controlled study [37] enrolled adult patients with minor depression or generalized anxiety disorder. Randomization was done to receiving either body acupuncture at 5 points or sham acupuncture for 10 sessions. The acupuncture group had a significant improvement over the sham group over 10 sessions; however, no improvement was seen over 5 sessions.

Two studies done in China compared antidepressants with acupuncture in adult patients. Chao-Ying et al. [38] compared acupuncture for 45 minutes for 6 weeks to an antidepressant trazodone. No differences in treatment were seen possibly due to the short duration of the study.

Zheng, Zeng and Deng [39] studied a larger adult sample of 296 patients with anxiety disorders and compared them to acupuncture and the antidepressant doxepin over 5 weeks. Patients received a total of 30 sessions of acupuncture. Although there were no differences between the two groups, there were minimal improvements in both groups.

Acupressure is a non-invasive and safer form of treatment than acupuncture. It involves using parts of the body, i.e. fingers, thumbs, palms, elbows and heels of the hand, to apply pressure to stimulate specific points along energy channels or "meridians". Carotenuto et al. [40] studied 25 adolescents with insomnia and used acupressure using an elastic wristband which applied continuous pressure at points to eliminate insomnia. The study duration was 6 months and polysomnography was used for assessment of sleep alterations. Subjects showed an increase in sleep quality and efficiency at the end of the study.

Effects of acupressure on the levels of physical and emotional stress were studied by Dads et al. (2011) in 47 adolescents in high school in the treatment group and 48 in the control group. The students self-applied acupressure for 15 days for 5 minute sessions each day. There was a significant decrease in the levels of stress of these students at the end of the study. This study signifies the importance of this safe, cost-effective and non-invasive treatment for stress or anxiety in youth. However, none of the trials of acupuncture or acupressure are in youth with anxiety disorders.

6.4. Case study 4

Dan, an 8-year-old boy, was referred to the outpatient clinic after his anxiety symptoms had become worse resulting in anger outbursts. He was experiencing obsessions and compulsions about germs and contamination and was avoiding touching things. He was also having difficulty with sleep due to grinding his teeth at night. Dan and his family had experienced an automobile accident in which Dan had suffered severe whiplash. He did not have any flashbacks or nightmares and was not avoidant in his daily functioning.

Parents were looking to help Dan, but were not ready to consider any psychiatric medications; they did not have time to come in for the parent anxiety CBT groups that the clinic offered. Dan's mother, who also had injuries during the accident, had been successfully treated with craniosacral therapy. She had a lot of trust in her craniosacral practitioner and decided to consult her for her son's treatment.

Craniosacral therapy (CST) involves the craniosacral system starting from the skull, face, mouth and the spine down to the sacrum and coccyx. It is described as "a gentle, hands on approach that releases tensions deep in the body to relieve pain and dysfunction and improve whole-body health and performance" [41]. Practitioners of craniosacral therapy "release restrictions in the soft tissues that surround the central nervous system" by using gentle touch [41]. CST is used for headaches, chronic neck and back pain, stress and tension-related disorders, temporomandibulur joint syndrome, attention-deficit hyperactivity disorder, post-traumatic stress disorder [41]. No CST studies have been done on youth or adults with anxiety disorders. There are a few randomized controlled trials.

Mann and authors [42] recruited 69 adult outpatients with migraines and randomized them to CST or sham treatment of 8 weekly sessions. Headache intensity was reduced in CST patients, but the difference was not statistically significant.

A recent study [43] conducted a randomized controlled trial in 50 adult patients with chronic non-specific neck pain. Patients were randomly assigned to CST or sham treatment for 8 weeks and assessments were done for the credibility of the sham treatment. There were no differences between the groups in symptom improvement; however, patients were convinced about the credibility of the sham treatment.

A study in 2011 [44] looked at 84 adult patients with fibromyalgia and the effects of CST on depression, anxiety and quality of life. Patients were randomly assigned to either CST or placebo or sham group for 25 weeks. Patients in the CST showed significant improvement in overall anxiety measures, quality of life and sleep quality. One year later, there were no differences between the groups in anxiety, depression and quality of life, but there was still improved sleep quality index in the CST group.

In summary, although there is overall inconclusive evidence on efficacy and safety on many CAM treatments, there are enough data in some specific treatments to be used safely and judiciously in conjunction with Western psychiatric treatment. One third of patients are already using complementary and alternative treatments. Regardless of the methodological problems of these studies, it is essential that practitioners look beyond the Western treatments as these are often more appropriate for moderate to severe symptoms. For patients having mild to moderate symptoms of an anxiety disorder, CAM treatments can be utilized if the family is unwilling to try conventional treatment and is already convinced that CAM treatments may be more appropriate.

Author details

Sarosh Khalid-Khan[1*], Faiza Khalid-Khan[2] and David Gratzer[2]

*Address all correspondence to: khalids@hdh.kari.net

1 Hotel Dieu Hospital affiliated with Queen's University, Kingston, ON, Canada

2 The Scarborough Hospital, Birchmount campus, affiliated with University of Toronto, Scarborough, ON, Canada

References

[1] Rey MR, Walter G, Soh N. Complementary and alternative medicine (CAM): treatments in pediatric psychopharmacology. J Am Acad Child Adoles Psychiatr 2008; 47:364–8.

[2] World Health Organization (WHO). The World Health Report 2004 [Internet]. 2004. Available from: http://www.who.int/whr/2004/en/index.html [Accessed 2015-03-14].

[3] Office for National Statistics. Psychiatric morbidity among adults living in private household. Summary Report, HMSO. 2000.

[4] McPherson H, Sinclair-Lian N, Thomas K. Patients seeking care from acupuncture practitioners in the UK: a national survey. Complement Ther Med 2006;14:20–30.

[5] Simon GE, Cherkin DC, Sherman KJ, Eisenber DM, Deyo RA, Davis RB. Mental health visits to complementary and alternative medicine providers. Gen Hosp Psychiatr 2004;26(3):171–7.

[6] Eisenberg DM, Davis RB, Ettner SL, et al. Trends in alternative medicine use in the United States, 1990–1997: results of a follow-up national survey. JAMA 1998; 280:1569–75.

[7] Simkin DR, Popper CW. Overview of integrative medicine in child and adolescent psychiatry. Child Adolesc Pscychiatric Clin N Am 2013;22:375–80.

[8] National Center for Complementary and Alternative Medicine. National Institute of Health. What is Complementary and Alternative Medicine? [Internet]. 2011. Available from: http://nccam.nih.gov/health/whatiscam/#definingcam [Accessed 2015-01-22].

[9] Goldbeck-Wood S, Dorozynski A, Lie L. Complementary medicine is booming worldwide. BMJ 1996;313(7050):131–3.

[10] Nguyen LT, Davis RB, Kaptchuk TJ, Phillips RS. Use of complementary and alternative medicine and self-rated health status: results from a national survey. J Gen Intern Med 2011;26(4):399–404.

[11] Barnes PM, Bloom B, Nahin RL. Complementary and alternative medicine use among adults and children: United States, 2007. Natl Health Stat Rep 2008;1–23.

[12] McFarland B, Bigelow D, Zani B, Newsom J, Kaplan M. Complementary and alternative use in Canada and the United States. Am J Public Health, 2002; 92(10); 1616-18.

[13] Bystritsky A, Hovav S, Sherbourne C, Stein BM, Rose RD, Cambell-Sills L, Golinelli D, Sullivan G, Craske MG, Roy-Byrne P. Use of complementary and alternative medicine in a large sample of anxiety patients. Psychosomatic 2012;3:266–72.

[14] Kemper KJ, Gardiner P, Birdee GS. Use of complementary and alternative therapies among youth with mental health concerns. Acad Pediatr 2013;13:540–45.

[15] Yussman, SM, Ryan AS, Auinger P, Weitzman. Visits to complementary and alternative medicine providers by children and adolescents in the United States. Ambulatory Pediatr 2004;4:429–435.

[16] Sarris J, Moylan S, Camfield DA, Pase MP, Michoulon D, Berk M, Jakca RN, Scheitzer I. Complementary medicine, exercise, meditation, diet, and lifestyle modification for anxiety disorders: a review of current evidence. Evidence-Based Comp Altern Med V. 2012 (2012), Article ID 809653, 20 pages.

[17] Pilkington K. Anxiety, depression and acupuncture: a review of the clinical research. Neurosci Basic Clin 2010;157:91–5.

[18] Lewith GT, Breen A, Filshie J, et al. Complementary medicine: evidence base, competence to practice and regulation. Clin Med 2003; 3(3): 235–40.

[19] Godel JC. Vitamin D supplementation: recommendations for Canadian mothers and infants. J Pediatr Child Health 2007; 12(7):583–9.

[20] Bertone-Johnson ER, Powers SI, Spangler L, Brunner RL, Michael YL, Larson JC, et al. Vitamin D intake from foods and supplements and depressive symptoms in a diverse population of older women. AJCN 2011;94:1104–12.

[21] Tolppanen A, Sayer A, Fraser W, Lewix G, Zammit S, Lawlor D. The association of serum 25-hydroxyvitamin D3 and D3 with depressive symptoms in childhood – a prospective cohort study. J Child Psychol Psych 2012;52(7):757–66.

[22] Bertone-Johnson ER, Powers SI, Spangler L, Larson J, Michael YL, Millen AE, et al. Vitamin D supplementation and depression in the women's health initiative calcium and vitamin D trial. AJE 2012;176:1–13.

[23] Jorde R, Sneve M, Figenschau Y, Svartberg J, Waterloo K. Effects of vitamin D supplementation on symptoms of depression in overweight and obese subjects: Randomized double blind trial. J Intern Med 2008;264:599–609.

[24] Khorminya A, Tehrani-Doost M, Jazayeri S, Hosseini A, Djazayery A. Therapeutic effects of vitamin D as adjunctive therapy to fluoxetine in patients with major depressive disorder. ANZJP 2013;47(3):271–5.

[25] Mozaffari-Khosravi H, Nabizade L, Yassini-Ardakani SM, Hadinedoushan H, Barzegar K. The effect of 2 different single injections of high dose of vitamin D on improving the depression in depressed patients with vitamin D deficiency: a randomized clinical trial. J Clin Psychopharmacol 2013;33:378–89.

[26] Sanders KM, Stuart AL, Williamson EJ, Jacka FN, Dodd S, Nicholson G, et al. Annual high-dose vitamin D3 and mental well-being: randomised controlled trial. BJP 2011;198:357–64.

[27] Shipowick C, Moore C, Corbett C, Bindler R. Vitamin D and depressive symptoms in women during the winter: a pilot study. Appl Nursing Res 2009;22(3):221.

[28] Yalamanchili V, Gallagher JC. Treatment with hormone therapy and calcitriol did not affect depression in older postmenopausal women: no interaction with estrogen and vitamin D receptor genotype polymorphisms. Menopause 2012;19:697–703.

[29] Lax-Vanek J, Kanellos-Sutton M, Booij L, Johal R, Khalid-Khan S. Prevalence of suboptimal vitamin D levels in psychiatric adolescent outpatients and association with fatigue and depressive symptoms. 2014; poster presented at Queen's University Medical School Showcase.

[30] Hogberg G, Gustafsson SA, Hallstrom T, Gustafsson T, Klawitter B, Petersson M. Depressed adolescents in a case-series were low in vitamin D and depression was ameliorated by vitamin D supplementation. ActaPaediatrica 2012;101:779–83.

[31] Shamseer L, Vohra S. Complementary, holistic, and integrative medicine: melatonin. Pediatr Rev 2009;30(6):223–8.

[32] Smits MG, Nagtegaal EE, van der Heijden J, Coenen AM, Kerkof GA. Melatonin for chronic sleep onset insomnia in children: A randomized placebo-controlled trial. J Child Neurol 2001;16(2):86–92.

[33] Sack RL, Auckley D, Auger R, et al. Circadian rhythm sleep disorders: Part II, advanced sleep phase disorder, delayed sleep phase disorder, free-running disorder, and irregular sleep-wake rhythm. Sleep 2007;30:1484–501.

[34] Van Geijlswijk IM, Korzilius HPLM, Smits MG. The use of exogenous melatonin in delayed sleep phase disorder: a meta-analysis. Sleep 2010;33:1605–14.

[35] Tomoda A, Miike T, Iwatani N, Ninomiya T, Mabe H, Kageshita T, Ito S. Effect of long-term melatonin administration on school-phobic children and adolescents with sleep disturbances. Curr Therapeut Res 1999;60(11):609–12.

[36] Liu GZ, Zang YJ, Guo LX, Liu AZ. Comparative study on acupuncture combined with behavioural desensitization for treatment of anxiety neuroses. Am J Acupunct 1998;26(2–3):117–20.

[37] Eich H, Agelink MW, Lehmann E, Lemmer W, Kliesser E. Acupuncture in patients with minor depression or generalized anxiety disorders – results of an experimental study. Fortschr Neurol Psychiatr 2000;68(3):137–44.

[38] Chao-Ying W, et al. The electroacupuncture treatment of 20 cases of anxiety disorder. Hunan J Chinese Med 2003;3:26 (abstracted and translated by Wolfe HL.

[39] Zhang H, Zeng Z, Deng H. Acupuncture treatment for 157 cases of anxiety neurosis. J Tradit Chin Med 1986;23(1):55–6.

[40] Carotenuto M, Gallai B, Parisi L, Roccella M, Esposito M. Acupressure therapy for insomnia in adolescents: a polysomnographic study. Neuropsychiatr Disease Treat 2013;9:157.

[41] Das, R, Nayak, BS. Margaret, B. Acupressure and physical stress among high school students. Holistic Nursing Pract 2011;25(2):97-104.

[42] The Upledger Institute International. Frequently asked questions – craniosacral therapy [Internet]. 2011. Available from http://www.upledger.com/content.asp?id=61 [Accessed: 2015-01-18].

[43] Mann J, Gaylord S, Faurot K, Suchindran K, Coeytaux R, Wilkinson L, Coble R, Curtis P. Craniosacral therapy for migraine: a feasibility study. Biomed Central, Complement Alt Med 2012;12:111.

[44] Haller H, Ostermann T, Lauche R, Cramer H, Dobos G. Credibility of a comparative sham control intervention for craniosacral therapy in patients with chronic neck pain. Complement Therap Med 2014;22:1053–9.

[45] Mataran-Penarrocha GA, Castro-Sanchez AM, Garcia GC, Moreno-Lorenzo C, Carreno TP, Zafra MDO. Influence of craniosacral therapy on anxiety, depression and quality of life in patients with fibromyalgia. eCAM 2011;1–9.

Chapter 14

Yoga for Anxiety Management in the Workplace

S. Doria, F. Irtelli, R. Sanlorenzo and F. Durbano

Additional information is available at the end of the chapter

http://dx.doi.org/10.5772/60633

Abstract

Anxiety is a potential cause of serious influence in a person's daily life. This chapter is focused specifically on the effects of the work environment factors in disease development and progression. Working environments are places of significant sources of stress: they put us in connection with our duties and expectations (often not coincide with reality) and with a "forced socialization." Especially forced socialization is to be considered a main source of stress in work places, inducing negative outcomes in work and social relationships. The psychosocial risks of work places can so be defined according to design, organization and management of work as well as to social and environmental contexts that may lead to damage of physical, social and psychological domains. Stress can then be defined as a pattern of emotional, cognitive, behavioral, and physiological reactions to adverse and noxious aspects perceived as the contents of the working environment. Thanks to the beginning of psychosocial research on the working environment, the impact of some aspects of the work environment on health has become an object of study, as the interventions to mitigate it. Yoga, meditation, and mantra techniques, as described in this work (presenting others' experiences and two of own current projects, used in a hospital workplace to control the condition of occupational stress but also in a clinical sample), showed the potential in considerably reducing anxiety and mood symptoms.

Keywords: anxiety, yoga, work, environmental factors, stress, coping and vulnerability, prevention

1. Introduction

This perspective is deep-rooted in the history of medicine. From this perspective, George Engel introduced the term "biopsychosocial approach" as a privileged model for decoding and comprehending in many ways health and stress as existential processes, and to articulate forms of care and of taking responsibility [1]. The biopsychosocial model is based on the paradigm of complexity, in sharp contrast with classical biomedical reductionism, as well as the hierarchy of the sciences. It adopts the perspective of the General Systems Theory developed by Von Bertalanffy, which considers a set of events interrelated as a system with specific properties and functions depending on the level at which it is located with respect to a larger system. The systems theory in fact claims that all levels of an organization are interrelated to each other, so that changing one affects the other, mitigating the dichotomy between holism and reductionism [1]. The model refers to three basic principles: free dialogue, relationship, and humility. In other words, it aims at looking at the person as a "whole" genetic element (bio), the subject of discussion and decision (psycho), as well as a historical, cultural, and familiar subject (social). The axioms of the model are inclusiveness (understanding of diversity) and nonexclusiveness (putting aside what is regarded as their competence), the answers to which are total and global whatever the point of entry into the system (the biological now, psychological time, social hour). The centrality of this model has been confirmed and validated by almost uncountable literature marking the transition to a person-centered medicine [2] and it is now of widespread knowledge that biopsychosocial screening, rather than a compartmentalized approach, can help plan a more effective treatment and help an early and useful stress management. Human beings tend to form themselves through the development of groupal complex systems affecting the three main areas explored in the biopsychosocial model. Therefore, one must bear in mind that every action must always consider the construction of or refunding the mind–body integration. A person's discomfort cannot be considered only in terms of somatic or psychic discomfort, because any discomfort brings the indissoluble unity of consciousness of the self. This should be emphasized because not everyone knows how to use this knowledge in the care of the person as a whole.

2. Work, a question of balance and psychosocial aspects

Workplace can be assumed as a model of a complex system involving biological, psychological, and social aspects, so we have to rely on a biopsychosocial approach to deal effectively with any issue concerning individuals and teams. These three dimensions are interlinked, in fact effective management of health and safety in the workplace is important and recommended to individuals and society alike. This approach is particularly important and relevant in times of economic uncertainty when it is essential for companies to maintain high productivity levels despite the decreasing number of resources and when mistakes and accidents are most likely to occur [3]. The psychosocial risks should be taken in to account when designing, organizing, managing, and evaluating the social and environmental contexts that may lead to damages of the "physical, social, and psychological health." In the '60s, psychosocial research in the work environment highlighted the impact of some aspects of the workplace on health. Today we have strong evidence of how the work-related stress exposes the individual to danger, inefficiency, and error: stress increases the production of cortisol, damages the hippocampus, and causes damage to memory and cognitive skills (which can be reduced by up to 60%) [4].

But what is stress? In the '50s Selye introduced the term stress in everyday language and such term began to take on the meaning which it still retains, also in the field of psychology. Stress, a term that means "pressure," derives from the field of engineering; it is used to refer to any force that is applied to a body in order to test its durability under stress. Over time, this term was progressively used to refer more specifically to "a state of non-specific stress of living matter, which is manifested by morphological transformations tangible in various organs, particularly in the endocrine glands that are under the control of the pituitary" [5,6]. Originally the syndrome "just being sick" covered the stereotypical response of an organism to a wide range of physical, biological, or chemical agents. Selye was the first to use the term stress to describe a range of physical and psychological responses to adverse conditions or influences [7]. Stress occurs when we have to respond to a stimulus from the external world: this response consists of a behavioral adaptation and the activation of biological systems (psycho-neuro-endocrine) in such a way to prevent potential negative consequences and, where it is not possible to solve the situation, possibly develop forms of adaptation. The first important consideration relates to the fact that stress is the result of a process of human adaptation to the environment. There are some specific mechanisms that underlie the identification of a response to stress: a) a dynamic stimulus-response reaction, b) the required adjustment in order to respond appropriately and effectively to the stimulus, c) the high energy (mental and physical) needed to achieve this adaptation effort. In addition to the "active" and "passive" reaction, characterized by inhibition, recent studies have demonstrated the existence of ways of reacting with a great intersubject variability. We filter the stressor by attributing different and personal meanings and values to it depending on a wide range of constitutional and experiential factors, and also on the context. When exposed to stressful situations, the individual puts in place strategies that modify or attempt to modify his/her environment. These strategies are strictly individual and are linked to the personal characteristics of the subject and their historical experience. The term stress stands for stressful event (or stressor), a term that describes the stimulus factor that causes the reaction. Stressors can be major factors (the loss of work), minor factors (small facts of everyday life, or hassles), acute factors (accidents) and chronic factors (a very competitive business environment) [8]. The stress effect is potentially pathogenic when the conditions from which it is derived are chronic or recur with some frequency. Selye also distinguished between eustress (or good stress) and distress (bad stress); such terms were originally included in the broader definition of stress but were immediately indicated as distinct from one another. Selye stated that stress is an inevitable consequence of living, but that distress appears when the requests to which the person is exposed (both in the psychological and physiological dimensions) overtake the capacity and energy that the person has or believes to have to maintain the homeostasis. The stimulus demand can, therefore, have a more or less acceptable meaning [7,9]. Holmes and Rahe, in the construction of the "Social Readjustment Rating Scale [10]," discovered that each stress can be classified into distress and eustress, where the first is caused by a response considered disproportionate in size, while the eustress is caused by a response considered acceptable, which creates a moderate level of tension enabling to successfully address the perceived challenge. This is, however, only one aspect of Eustress. The concept of an optimal level of stress derives from the studies of Yerkes and Dodson Law that explained how stress is beneficial for increasing the performance until it is moderate, after surpassing a certain level of stress the performance will deteriorate according to a inverted "U" diagram—see Figure 1 [11,12].

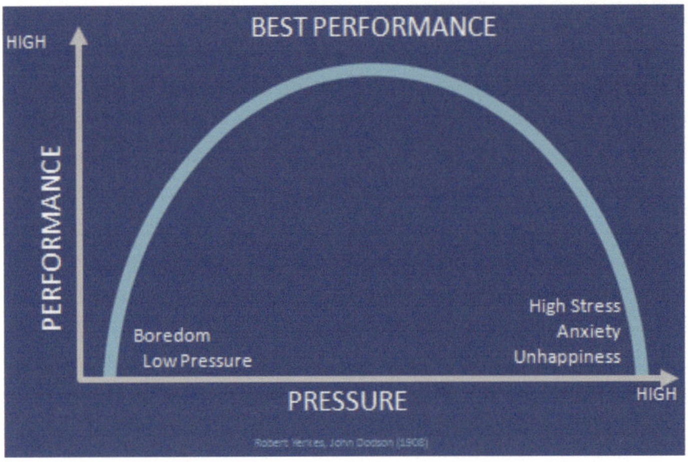

Figure 1. The stress–performance relationship according to Yerkes and Dodson [12] modified.

In order to clarify the connection between the theory of Yerkes and Dodson and Seyle's work, it has to be clear that the effect of any stimulus depends on how each individual interprets it and chooses to react to it. It is the individual that determines whether the stressor will generate eustress or distress. The eustress is the primary result of a positive perception of the stressor, while the distress is the result of a negative perception. The classification depends on how the stressor is perceived by the individual, on which kind of value is assigned to it. Selye suggested that learning how to respond to stressful stimuli with positive emotions, such as hope, maximizes eustress and minimizes the distress, whereas responding with negative emotions, such as despair, greatly increases the distress [9]. In the perception of stressor, and when assigning of its meaning, a key characteristic of the individual is involved: the locus of control (or self-efficacy); people with an internal locus of control (believing they can control and master all external situations) tend to perceive and to respond to stressors quite differently with respect to people with an external locus of control (believing they cannot at all control and master all external situations) [13]. Self-efficacy is the belief of being able to control the environmental challenges by deploying an adaptive action, and, according to the social cognitive theory, strongly influences the effectiveness of self-perceived behaviors being positively associated with adaptation [13]. In fact, it is positively related to an active strategy and negatively to a passive reaction [14]. In the aforementioned works, Selye introduced the notion of "general adaptation syndrome" to describe the way in which the body copes with stressful events; he distinguished three phases that follow this order: 1) alarm phase: it is activated by the autonomic nervous system in the occasion of intense stressful events; 2) resistance stage: the body reacts to stress and, if the stress is intense, there are transient events such as the enlargement of the adrenal glands, gastrointestinal ulcers, etc.; 3) exhaustion stage: if the stressor persists or if the body is not able to put in place appropriate responses, the body undergoes irreversible responses, which can include death. The distress, specifically, is characterized by a stage of alarm, a stage of resistance, and a stage of functional exhaustion. R.S. Lazarus has integrated Selye's model with the purely cognitive aspects related to the subjective perception of specific stressors, creating a more complex model [15,16]. In his model, the same event, as already mentioned, may have different meanings in different subjects, and it is unquestionable that when confronted with stressful factors different people react in different ways with quite different outcomes. The ideal response requires strategies which are active but also multiple, flexible, and tailored to the specific factors or stressful events in action. The stress response is then modulated in two ways by the psychological characteristics of the individual: in the process of perception and processing of the stressors, and in coping with these factors.

3. Workplace and anxiety

Working environments put us in connection with our duties and expectations (which often do not coincide with the reality of the context) and with a "forced socialization." This is a clear model of stress defined as a psychosocial phenomenon; therefore, specific interventions have to be based on the identification of stressors and their original context. Over time, this has led to the identification of two areas of research: 1) study of stress measures, scales, and 2) tools for assessing the effects of stress on individuals. We must remember that the measured stress level may not be strictly related to the work environment and that subjective aspects play a decisive role in the type of reaction. Being subjective, this measure allows us to identify the sources of stress that have occurred in causing discomfort and to certify its effects only [4]. If the stressful events are easily identified, it is much more difficult to predict the subjective reactions to them. In fact, as already stated, the individual response to stress depends on constitutional and experiential factors. There are also particular types of stress and forms of anxiety (i.e., stress response) that could be directly related to the workplace, like "stress in social situations." This is a particular stress that arises from forced participation in social situations perceived as anxiety provoking. People affected by stress in social situations are very upset when forced to interact in social gatherings, tend to avoid public speaking, show anxiety in group settings and invent excuses to avoid encounters with people they do not know; furthermore, those who exceed in this stress often feel uncomfortable when talking with “superior” people of the opposite sex and/or with whom they have never spoken before. Therefore, the resulting stress involves a state that may evolve from an acute condition (where the mind/body is enabled to effectively react to external events that must be addressed and solved) to a chronic condition in which stress remains constant and generates harmful effects on the physiological functions with repercussions on the ability of interpersonal adaptation. Another kind of anxiety that could characterize a person is also “social concern": it is closely related to the activation and the consequent negative emotional condition of tension that occurs in situations in which the subject feels under observation. Individuals with high levels of social concern are very uncomfortable when thinking someone is looking at him, as he often fears negative evaluations by others. Feeling apprehensive about someone becoming aware of their shortcomings, or not approving what they do, is a cause of great anxiety for these individuals, especially when the feared opinion comes from their superiors. People with high social concerns usually see their image as is potentially perceived by others, and believe that physical appearance is very important to establish positive and functional relationships with others. This induces a dysfunctional groping to inspire confidence at all costs, with the negative and unwanted pitfall to behave ridiculously. These elements can originate a condition defined mismatch [17-19]. Concerns about the image perceived by others can lead to the complete avoidance of any potentially stressful situations and, consequently, to a state of interpersonal closure and loss of motivation to affiliate to others [15,20]. In this context, it is very important to prevent negative stress, distress, which occurs when the situation needs an effort to adapt to it that exceeds our perceived ability to achieve it. Since the '60s, there has been a growing awareness on the unavoidable essence of stress as a human condition while coping skills and resources make the difference in the outcomes of the adaptation process [16,21]. The features involved in the modulation of the stress response strategies are called coping skills, and the whole process of reaction and coping of stress is referred to as "coping" [15,16]. Studies on the so-called "good copers" clearly show that these people persistently believe that they will be able to cope with the stress: they are practical and directly address the issues straightforward; on the contrary, "bad copers" are characterized by disappointment and pessimism [22,23]. There are quite recurrent types of coping, which is why we talk about "styles" of coping. They are crucial in the success to achieve personal goals [24-27]. The most common coping styles can be summarized as follows:

1. **Combat**: this style is characterized by the challenge of defeating the stress: the person sees the situation of stress like a challenge, has an optimistic view of the future, and believes that it is possible to exercise control over the stress. This kind of person reveals a coping style aimed at direct confrontation [27]. Therefore, those who adopt this strategy have a so-called internal locus of control, they want to know as much as possible about their own condition, their source of stress and the context and actively change their lifestyle in order to preserve their health; this strategy can be defined as an active, positive coping, because it represents a tendency to actively confront and cope with stress and protects from anxiety. The optimism that characterizes this style of coping has beneficial effects on the health, well-being, and the quality of life of those who adopt it. Recent research confirmed these assumptions [27]. The combative coping mediates these effects positively, while fatalism, anxious worries, and despair mediate these effects negatively. However, it is not enough to be optimistic, if you do not take a combative style of coping. The combative style induces lower levels of anxiety and demoralization, empowers individuals in finding answers for discussion and gives them the feeling they are able to control events, at least partially: "I see this stress as a challenge," "I am determined to overcome it," "I am very optimistic;" combative people adopt more flexible and differentiated cognitive and

behavioral strategies, such as "I am actively trying to improve my health," which promote a more positive view of the events. As a result, and as mentioned above, this style is associated with lower psychological morbidity and a greater sense of personal control [27].

2. **Avoidance-disclaimer**: this strategy is very complex, it is generally characterized by the tendency to not directly address any issues related with stress, and is associated to the use of the refusal defense mechanism (to avoid seeing the unpleasant aspects of reality); it is very common, often plays a really useful role in protecting from anxiety. However, if taken to the extreme and used as the only form of defense, it can cause problems. It has been divided into denial of adaptation and maladaptive avoidance; the first can be defined as a natural method of emotional self-protection, which has positive effects on health, so it was also called "healthy denial" by Druss in 1988 [28]. The maladaptive avoidance, instead, splits up into more extreme forms of denial that can lead to poor cooperation and cause strong anxiety when it is no longer effective as defense mechanism. A high level of avoidance, used as the only coping strategy, can also lead to an unrealistic perception of self-efficacy.

3. **Fatalism**: it is a strategy characterized by an attitude of fatalistic resignation and passive acceptance of the stress. People who adopt this strategy recognize the gravity of the situation and believe they have little control over events. Therefore, they accept what fate ordained with resignation as if that was their destiny. Therefore, we must point out that the tendency to perceive external events as related to fate is typical of those who have an external locus of control, a place of external control, which causes poor adaptation to the stress.

4. **Anxious preoccupation**: it is a strategy characterized by constant feelings, the feelings of danger, stress, and high level of anxiety. Stress assumes a central position in person's existence. It is negatively related to social and emotional functioning. Those who adopt this style of coping are continuously searching for reassurance, demand for visits, or otherwise escape from the context because it is too distressing. It is positively related to coping style despair [27].

5. **Despair**: it is characterized by feelings of loss and the oppression; it is related to high levels of anxiety, poor cognitive strategies, and the belief of having little control over events. In fact, there is a correspondence between despair and demoralization, which leads to affective symptoms of existential distress, cognitive tendency to pessimism, sense of personal failure, lack of motivation to deal with the event, feelings of social isolation and alienation [24-27].

3.1. Burn out, source of stress in workplaces

The '**burn out**' syndrome is a stress-related phenomenon, even if distinct from it. It happens particularly to people working in the social sector and in the helping professions. Burn out consists in a progressive loss of motivation, idealism, objectives and the meaning associated with them, a decreased perception of social utility of one's own work. The "burn out" condition does not coincide with stress but it induces stress in a work environment when the balance between the following three important factors is lost: a) required level of performance, b) control over one's own work, c) reward and gratification. In order not to get into a condition of stress, the worker has to perceive these three factors as balanced. With regard to the analysis of occupational stress the cognitive aspects are very highlighted, assuming that an event can have very different effects on each individual. To better understand the development of burn out it is useful to introduce also the concepts of "work stress" and "work strain." "Work stress" is an objectively measurable occupational stress (an acceptable level of overtime); "work strain" is defined as the particular emotional and mental reverb of the same condition or activity on different people (e.g., the effects of demotivation on a single person in relation to his/her actual potential professionalism or his/her culture) [4]. Only in certain circumstances can an experience of stress turn into a real illness. Since the autonomic nervous system and the neuroendocrine system mediate the body's response to stress, as a result of prolonged and repeated stress a normal physiological response can turn into a meaningful damage to health, especially affecting the cardiovascular, endocrine, gastrointestinal, and immune systems [4]. When the need to tackle stress is over, the chemical responses previously activated should terminate. But when the physiological reaction to stress is not able to recover, the areas assigned to the production of adrenaline and cortisol continue their secretion, creating chronic stress, this in turn leads in particular to systemic alterations that in turn cause physical and psychological problems, such as behavioral and emotional symptoms like recurring irritability, poor concentration, decreased performance, tearfulness, changes in appetite, loss of self-esteem, sleep disorders, cardiovascular disorders, tendency to hyperglycemia, headache, and poor functioning of the immune system [4].

3.2. The importance of stress prevention in working organization

The high psychological and social costs that a person has to pay as a result of negative experiences (stress) at the workplace is becoming an increasing problem not only for the workers or the management, but also for organizations. For this reason, organizations are gearing up (e.g., by promoting yoga courses for employees). In the past, it was noted that the reduction in efficiency due to work stress probably has comparable effects to those caused by the strikes on the economic front [4].

Potentially stressful factors at work involve the relationship with work environment and work content (material factors), the role people play in the organization (organizational factors), and interpersonal relationships (psychosocial factors). Referring to the role that a person plays in the organization we can talk about role-stress when there is a discrepancy between the actual role and the role to that the worker wishes to reach in the organization (this phenomenon is called inconsistency of position).

The classical three levels of prevention are:

1. **Primary prevention**, the purpose of which is to decrease the incidence of the arising of the negative phenomenon, it consists in an attempt to prevent the development of a discomfort in a population at risk.

2. **Secondary prevention**, which tends to reduce the prevalence of morbidity through the curtailment of the period, the spread of the stress.

3. **Tertiary prevention**, which tends to mitigate the effects of negative factors on those affected.

The timing of the intervention with the onset of pathological symptoms is, therefore, the discriminating factor between these three levels. The earlier the preventive intervention takes place, the more efficacy it has in preventing potential damages generated by work processes and environment. Developing trainings aimed at improving stress management can help to reduce stress through greater mastery of the work process, strengthening self-esteem, and developing a higher sense of self-efficacy, but also improving motivation and mood. In the process of designing the work flow it is essential to take in to account not only ergonomic principles, but also the need to develop proper systems of performance evaluation, based on known criteria (preferably shared), on a transparent communication and on constructive feedback from the management. Such evaluation system will concretely reduce stress and increase the sense of control and involvement, facilitating the employees in the assignment of meaning to their activities and contribute to self-esteem [4].

3.3. Mental disorders in the EU, the importance of an early intervention

It is estimated that a third of the European population suffers from mental disorders [29]. Psychiatric disorders are the prominent cost of disability-adjusted life years worldwide [30]. Anxiety is one of the most common psychiatric disorders affecting adults and young adults [29,31-36]. Anxiety disorders have the potential to cause serious interference with a person's daily life, work, and career [29,37]. It is also known that all pharmacological treatments with benzodiazepines can cause troublesome side effects, including anterograde memory impairment, sedation, and the risk of dependence; therefore, they are not recommended for long-term use [38]. Furthermore, response to these treatments tends to be highly variable, ranging from 40% to 70% [39-42]. These limits in terms of efficacy and tolerability often result in poor patient adherence to medication and, thus, long-term remission is often difficult to achieve [43]. On average, only a third of patients achieve remission within a year of follow-up, while patients who do achieve an initial response often relapse [44].

Can we, therefore, intervene before the appearance of a psychiatric disorder? Here stands the importance of primary prevention, which is finalized to prevent pathogenesis preserving the subject from the risk of taking pathogenic behaviors. The literature has largely emphasized that improving "coping style" to stress, and all the problems related to it, may prevent and decrease anxiety and its consequences on working processes (and on social functioning as a whole). In this perspective yoga can be a very effective and promising approach.

3.4. Yoga: A biopsychosocial approach to health

Why should organizations promote yoga and not a generic physical activity for their employees? What is the difference between generic physical activity benefits and yoga benefits? The difference in benefits has been shown in a fairly recent study made by Bonura: both fitness and yoga lead to an improvement of psychological health, although the changes obtained with yoga were generally higher and more durable [45].

Yoga has shown greater enhancement in psychological health than the simple physical exercise, substantiated by the decrease of anger, anxiety, and depression, and increased global wellness, positive overall effects, and feeling of an increase of self-efficacy. Clance and coworkers (1980) concluded that yoga is an effective method to improve the image of the body and, consequently, the self-image [46].

We need to point out that yoga is a time-tested, *ante litteram*, biopsychosocial approach to life: it includes health in the body, peace in the mind, and helps to develop good relationships and harmony in the society; moreover, the body-mind-spirit unity is a key feature of the yogic approach to health and happiness. Yoga techniques range from yoga postures (asanas) and purification techniques (kriyas), more focused on body health, to breathing techniques, cognitive strategies, and meditation for clarity of mind and emotional balance (pranayama, gyana, and dyana), to ethical codes of conduct aimed to establish harmony in the society (yama and nyama). The yoga approach to life is very reliable with the general system theory and to the work of Nicolis and Prigogyne [47] on dissipative systems: life is seen as a flow of energy where the individual (subsystems) is part of the whole (the bigger system) and is striving to keep its harmony (sattva) utilizing energy from nature to implement proper actions and assuming a proactive attitude toward events. The imbalances of the system can be of two types: excess of tamas (inertia) like in depression and misunderstandings or excess of rajas (activity) like in anxiety, and all yoga techniques are aimed at recreating balance (sattva) at physical, psychological and social level. Often yoga is seen as an intangible and philosophical practice that is not suitable for the modern world of competitions and the fast pace that characterizes the work environment. This misunderstanding is due to a lack of knowledge and a cultural bias; in fact Patanjali (a prominent character in the yogic tradition that systematized the discipline in his "yoga sutras" (400 BC)) defines yoga as "skill in action" [48] The usefulness of yoga postures and breathing techniques for general health, stress management and anxiety is easy to understand and to demonstrate and there is a growing body of studies showing evidences in this direction [49,50]. But yoga can also provide cognitive tools to approach stressors in a healthy way. In fact yoga promotes a proactive approach to events and challenges, encouraging the apprentice to develop a keen self-awareness and to take responsibility for how he perceives events and people and for how he responds to events and people's behavior. When properly understood and followed this "practice" leads to a balanced and constructive combative attitude toward stressors. Yoga can be helpful for the development of an effective strategy for reducing tension, through short and simple exercises that are easy to replicate autonomously. In particular, for the constant attention paid to the body–mind relationship, yoga seems to be particularly influential on the activities related to the sympathetic system and, therefore, on the typical symptoms of anxiety: accelerated heartbeat, palpitations, tremors, sweating, increased blood pressure, dry mouth, avoidance behaviors, restlessness, etc. [51]. Yoga can also stabilize mental activity and enhance brain function and resilience to stress [52-54]. Yoga and breathing techniques can also favor a regular nasal breathing, with better lung expandability. Some yogic exercises of relaxation and cleansing of the nasal passages are also very effective in the prevention of sinusitis and rhinitis, and the resulting pharyngitis, laryngitis, and tracheitis [55]. Specific exercises can procure greater elasticity in the muscles needed for breathing, which is important because respiratory deficits are due in large part to the lack of movement secondary to a sedentary lifestyle. Yoga breathing techniques can also prevent excessive tachycardia and hypertensive crises related to anxiety, because of their help in regularizing breathing. Finally, it is also known that stress and sleep disorders, such as insomnia and frequent interruption of sleep, can be fought with specific breathing techniques associated with sequences of dynamic yogic exercises [56]. Yoga can be also considered one of the strategies to cope with pathological conditions that have already taken place (secondary prevention), like Generalized Anxiety Disorder. Today there is enough evidence to consider yoga to be a beneficial, low-risk, low-cost integration to the treatment of stress and anxiety [57-60]. The antidepressant efficacy is also important as demonstrated by quite numerous studies [61-66]. Yoga could be considered a complementary therapy to classical psychological and psychiatric approaches, because many traditional yogic exercises have a therapeutic value. For these reasons today more and more doctors and psychologists recommend yoga as a relaxation technique.

3.5. Yoga and work organization

There are many evidences supporting the hypothesis that the introduction of yoga and meditation in the workplace at a large scale will benefit both the single workers and the performance of teams and organizations. We think that can be useful to analyze the "access barriers" that yoga shows for organizations and also to highlight cases where these barriers have been surpassed:

1. **Language and cultural bias**: yoga is perceived by many managers and decision takers in the corporate and institutional world as unpractical, philosophical, esoteric, religious, and anyway as something that concerns personal life and personal choices. To overcome such preconceptions the yoga teachers need to develop the skill to present yoga and conduct yoga classes with a secular language, introducing scientific evidences of the benefits of yoga. It is a huge cultural experiment that offers very interesting horizons of integration of eastern and western culture.

2. **Budget allocation**: in the middle of the shrinking of budgets, HR departments struggle to give priority to initiative that do not seem very concrete and with short term results. Again to overcome this problem it is necessary to show scientific results both in terms of health prevention and health strategies (and also the reduction of lost working hours) but also in terms of increased personal and team performance.

Some successful initiatives highlighted the potential of introducing yoga and meditation in working organizations, suggesting how to overcome the aforementioned barriers.

The Project Response has been supported and funded by the EU Commission's Directorate General (DG) Research to develop knowledge and understanding on the degree of alignment between companies and their stakeholders about what Corporate Social Responsibility (CSR) entails. The main objective was to study CSR at the level of individual manager's behavior, assessing the relative effectiveness of diverse training interventions on the development of social consciousness in managers. It was conducted from 2004 to 2007 by a multidisciplinary team of academic researchers from a consortium of leading business schools in Europe (INSEAD, France; Copenhagen Business School, Denmark; Università Commerciale Luigi Bocconi, Italy; Leon Kozminski Academy of Entrepreneurship and Management, Poland) and a training consultancy (Impact, Austria). Part of the study was aimed to evaluate, on 93 managers, the impact on their CSR behaviors after following stress management and meditation programs. In the words of Maurizio Zollo, leading the research team, "meditation and relaxation techniques seem to enable managers to break free from patterns of decision making driven by short term outcomes, self interest and reliance on safe solutions to embrace more proactive and innovative approaches to social and environmental challenges" [67]. One might even posit that the strain placed on managers in the workplace leads to short-term time horizons, narrow self-interests and familiar approaches to problem solving. This would, thus, prevent sound decision-making based on search for creative solutions to unstructured problems, on caring and trusting attitudes and on long-term views of the implications of one's decisions on broader audiences internal and external to the company [67].

Mindfulness Based Stress Reduction: the roots of this method are in the Tibetan Buddhist tradition. Mindfulness Based Training was conceived in a hospital setting and developed by Jon Kabat-Zinn at the University of Massachusetts Medical Center, it uses a combination of mindfulness meditation, body awareness, and yoga to help people become more mindful. His specific secular and scientific approach to yoga and meditation coupled with the effectiveness are the base of the wide success of the program in corporations and organizations worldwide [68-70].

TLEX Program: TLEX program is another positive example of how to overcome the barriers expressed in points 1 and 2. The origin of this set of programs is the Sudarshan Kriya Yoga (SKY), a complete yoga method created by Sri Sri Ravi Shankar in 1982. The TLEX program started form the personal experience of some entrepreneurs and managers that experienced SKY and, seeing the potential of introducing such techniques and cognitive strategies in their working environment, requested Sri Sri Ravi Shankar to tailor specific programs for their employees and managers. Starting as a very innovative service, TLEX is now offered in corporations and organizations worldwide [71,72].

4. Two studies focused on yoga and health — The Milan "Fatebenefratelli e Oftalmico" Hospital experience

The promising results of the scientific research, embracing both the neurophysiologic approach and the management approach, the "commercial" success of programs based on yoga and meditation, and positive case histories (like the program conducted at Fatebenefratelli Hospital in Milan, Italy) show the important impact that yoga training has on individual workers and organizations in general. We are still in the initial phase; much more has to be done.

Here we describe two studies regarding yoga and health.

http://dx.doi.org/10.5772/60633

In the first study we applied a particular yogic protocol called SKY (which stands for Sudarshan Kriya Yoga) as a treatment for patients affected by Generalized Anxiety Disorder and depression.

In the second study that we present, yoga, meditation and mantras have been used to deal with work-related stress for employees of a hospital.

4.1. SKY for anxiety disorders

A sample of patients (n=69) diagnosed and treated for anxiety and depression disorders was included in an experimental treatment with SKY techniques [73]. The adult participants (from 25 to 64 years old) were consenting persons with primary diagnosis of DSM-IV-TR Mood (n=18), anxiety disorders (n=39), or mixed condition (n=12) [74]. All patients signed informed consent for participation in the study. The sample was divided in two groups:

Group 1 undergoing pharmacological treatment, SKY treatment and participating to self-help group weekly; Group 1 subjects had a minimum of six months of stable condition due to standard pharmacological treatment with appropriate dose of antidepressant and/or anxiolytic.

Group 2 was not treated with psychiatric medication for at least six months prior to the study. This group received only SKY treatment and participated to self-help group weekly. These subjects were characterized by poor response and/or inadequate adherence to pharmacological treatment, had at least six months of participation to self-help groups and stable conditions.

The procedure of SKY was documented previously [62,63,74,75]. SKY was taught by trained, certified facilitators. The experimental group participated in an intense SKY workshop consisting of 10 sessions in two weeks followed by weekly SKY follow-up classes for six months. Each session lasted approximately two hours.

Assessments were done by a psychologist, uninvolved in treatment, in a quiet ambulatory environment. The severity of anxiety was assessed using Hamilton Rating Scale for Anxiety (HRSA) [76] and Zung Self-Rating Anxiety Scale Inventory (ZASI) [77]. The severity of depression was assessed using Hamilton Rating Scale for Depression (HRSD) [78] and Zung Self-Rating Depression Scale Inventory (ZDSI) [79]. The global symptom situation of patients was also assessed using Symptom Checklist-90 Revised (SCL-90-R) [80].

One of the aims of the study was to verify if SKY was an efficacious adjunctive treatment in pharmacological resistant, anxious-depressive subjects. Other objectives are related to neurophysiological evidences of the effects of SKY on the autonomic nervous system; the data are currently in evaluation for a specific publication.

Table 1 shows the results on anxiety severity assessment both with a subjective and an objective measure (ZASI and HRSA, respectively). Statistical analysis is in press [73], but some results are summarized in Table 1. All the tests measuring anxiety showed a significant improvement, which reaches statistical significance. The Global Score Index of SCL–90–R also showed a marked improvement from the baseline onward, the main effect of medication consumption over GSI scores being not significant.

Statistical analyses have shown that SKY therapy significantly reduces the levels of anxiety as measured by different scales.

SKY seemed to promote a meaningful remission of anxiety symptoms in the outpatients but the study should be replicated on a larger clinical sample for a more in-depth analysis of the efficacy of SKY Protocol and a longer follow-up is needed to evaluate the response maintenance.

Scale	Group	T0	T1	T2	T3	P
Hamilton	Medicine n=30	16,9	12,9	8,8	11,4	P <0.001
	No Medicine n=25	16,6	8,9	8,5	7,6	P <0.001
Zung	Medicine n=30	44,4	36,7	36,6	35,3	p <0.001
	No Medicine n=25	43,3	34,2	32,6	31,8	p <0.001
Scl-90	Medicine n=30	1,27	0,86	0,79	0,78	p <0.001
General Symptoms Index	No Medicine n=25	1,21	0,75	0,71	0,56	p <0.001

In the table the mean scores are reported. Statistical analysis was conducted by ANOVA (see text for details)

T0 (before SKY treatment), T1 (after 15 days of SKY training), T2 (after 3 months), T3 (after 6 months).

Table 1. The improvement of Anxiety level

4.2. Yoga, meditation, and mantras to deal with work-related stress for employees of a hospital

This project took place at the Fatebenefratelli and Ophthalmic Hospital in Milan since 2012, and it is currently ongoing as a quality project of the hospital.

This intervention includes five lessons, two hours weekly; every lesson is structured as follows: 30 minutes for relaxation, breathing, and full asanas (yoga postures to promote lengthening of column and muscles); 60 minutes for asana specifications; and 30 minutes for meditation with mantra listening.

The experimental sample is composed mainly by females (n=90) and to a lesser extent by males (n=10), the mean age being 47.51 yrs (sd=8.3).

The work-related stress measure utilized was the Perceived Stress Scale (PSS) [81]; this self-assessed questionnaire measures the perception of stress (degree to which situations in the life of the subject are evaluated as stressful). This is one of the tools most frequently used for evaluating work-related stress. To evaluate the stress response, the GHQ-12 - General Health Questionnaire [82] was chosen: the questionnaire consists of 12 items, it assesses the degree to which a person experiences the presence of stress symptoms. It can signal a situation of distress and in particular depression, anxiety, somatic symptoms and dysfunction at the social level. It can also discriminate between well-being conditions (scores below 5) and the presence of symptoms of psychological distress (scores greater than or equal to 5). Finally, Profile of Mood

States (POMS) [83] was utilized. This questionnaire evaluates six factors, each of which identifies a particular state of mood: tension-anxiety, depression, aggressiveness-anger, vigor-activity, tiredness-indolence, and confusion-bewilderment.

The results of the pilot study on 100 workers attending the treatment program are summarized by the following Tables 2, 3, and 4.

PSS (N=100)	**Mean (sd)**
before	18.55 (5.089)
after	14.87 (4.923)
Anova: F(1,99) = 63.990, p=.000	

Table 2. Descriptive statistics for Perceived Stress Scale (PSS). Average score of the sample before and after the treatment.

GHQ (N=100)	**Mean (sd)**
before	2.55 (2.749)
after	1.01 (1.664)
Anova: F(1,99) = 46.615, p=.000	

Table 3. Descriptive statistics for General Health Questionnaire Scale (GHQ): Average score of the sample before and after the treatment

POMS-T (N=100)	**Mean (sd)**
before	11.33 (5.853)
after	6.77 (5.272)
Anova: F(1,99) = 76.112, p=.000	

Table 4. Descriptive statistics for POMS-Tension and Anxiety Scale: Average score of the sample before and after the treatment.

For the Scale for the Perceived Stress (PPS) there is a significant decrease in the average score of the sample, from 18.55 to 14.87; for General Health Questionnaire (GHQ) there is a significant decrease in the average score of the sample, from 2,55 to 1,01; and for POMS, in particular, in the subscale tension and anxiety, there is also a significant improvement; finally, there is a clear and significant reduction in the percentage of subjects who experience a condition of distress (from 21% to 8%).

5. Conclusion

In the light of the benefits and the effectiveness showed in preventing and treating anxiety symptoms, yoga and meditation protocols would reasonably be helpful if proposed in organizations and to the general public health system. This person-centred approach generates a prevention culture and a significant costs reduction among all three levels of prevention mentioned earlier.

Workplace being a main place of high level and high intensity interactions, the intervention models presented could be positive examples of an institutional response to stress issue. Another positive outcome is the creation of a widespread culture of efficacious prevention of stress responses without the induction of secondary costs due to medication side effects, medication costs, lost days of work (as the traditional approaches induce instead) and with evident benefits on work efficacy and work–life balance. Moreover, these interventions do not generate a stigmatizing response in the whole system, being "not psychiatric" even if deeply rooted in psychic life and equilibrium. Yoga is focused on empowerment and self-efficacy, acting on body level to effect mind–body system, and it promotes a central role of the worker/ patient in pursuing health and balance in daily life.

Probably it will be necessary to tailor the interventions to the different settings, target groups, and patients. The experience of programs like Mindfulness Based Stress Reduction Program, the project at Hospital Fatebenefratelli, and the TLEX Program can be examples to follow confirming that when yoga and meditation programs are presented in a proper way and adequately sponsored by an organization's leaders, not only is the participation of employees and managers assured, but they also show encouraging results.

More work has to be done in this direction to identify the most effective approaches and to differentiate the interventions based on the target population and the nature of the challenges that the context proposes. Yoga is, however, a new low-risk, without side effects, way to improve health and quality of life [84].

Author details

S. Doria, F. Irtelli*, R. Sanlorenzo and F. Durbano

*Address all correspondence to: dott.ssaflorianairtelli@gmail.com

Department of Psychiatry and Neuroscience, "Fatebenefratelli e Oftalmico" Hospital, Milano, Italy

References

[1] Engel G. The Need for a New Medical Model: A Challenge for Biomedicine. Science; 1977, 196:129-136.

[2] Engel G. How Much Longer Must Medicine's Science Be Bound by a Seventeenth Century World View? Psychother Psychosom. 1992; 57:3-16.

[3] EU-OSHA European Agency for Safety and Health at Work [internet]; 2014. Available from: http://osha.europa.eu; or https://www.healthy-workplaces.eu/en

[4] Ferrari G. Manuale di valutazione dello stress e dei rischi psicosociali [Manual for evaluation of stress and psychosocial risks]. Edizioni Ferrari Sinibaldi, Italy, 2010.

[5] Selye H. A Syndrome Produced by Different Nocuous Agents. Nature, 1936; 138: 32.

[6] Selye H. History of the Stress Concept. In: Goldberger L and Bretznitz S (Eds.), Handbook of Stress: Theoretical and Clinical Aspects. 2nd Ed. New York: The Free Press, 1993.

[7] Selye H. From Dream to Discovery: On Being a Scientist. Ayer Co Pub; New edition, 1975.

[8] Sanavio E, Cornoldi C. Psicologia Clinica [Clinical Psychology] Il Mulino, Bologna, Italy, 2001.

[9] Selye H. Stress without Distress. New York: Harper & Row, 1974.

[10] Holmes T.H, Rahe R.H. The Social Readjustment Rating Scale. J Psychosom Res. 1967; 11: 213-218.

[11] Benson H, Allen RL. How Much Stress is Too Much. Harvard Business Review, 1980; 58(5): 86-92. Available from: https://hbr.org/1980/09/how-much-stress-is-too-much

[12] Yerkes RM, Dodson JD. The Relation of Strength of Stimulus to Rapidity of Habit-Formation. J. Comp. Neurol. Psychol. 1908; 18: 459-482. doi: 10.1002/cne.920180503.

[13] Bandura A. Self-efficacy: The Exercise of Control. New York: Freeman, 1997.

[14] Luszczynska A, Scholz U, Swarzer R. The General Self-efficacy Scale: Multicultural Validation Studies. J Psychol, 2005; 139(5): 439-457.

[15] Lazarus RS. Psychological Stress and the Coping Process. New York: Mc Graw-Hill, 1966.

[16] Lazarus RS, Folkman S. Stress Appraisal and Coping. New York: Springer,1984.

[17] Clarck JV, Arkowitz H. Social Anxiety and Self-evaluation of Interpersonal Performance. Psychological Reports, 1975; 36: 211-221.

[18] Buss AH. Self Consciousness and Social Anxiety. San Francisco: Freeman, 1980.

[19] Villone Betocchi G, Asprea AM. Ansia, Ansia Sociale e Ansia da Esame nella Prospettiva Cognitiva. Arch psicol Neurol psichiatr. 1994; LV(1-2): 326-338.

[20] Bellack M, Hersen AS. (Eds.) Research and Practice in Social Skills Training. New York: Plenum Press, 1979.

[21] Lazarus RS. Coping Theory and Research: Past, Present and Future. Psychosom Med. 1993; 55: 234-247.

[22] Weisman A. Worden JW. Coping and Vulnerability: A Research Report. Boston. MA: Massachusetts General Hospital, 1977.

[23] Folkman S. Positive Psychological States and Coping with Severe Stress. Soc Sci Med. 1997; 45(8): 1207-1221.

[24] Scheirer MF, Carver CS. Optimism, Coping and Health: Assessment and mplications of eneralized Outcome Expectancies on Health. Health Psychology. 1985; 4(3): 219-247.

[25] Scheirer IH, Carver CS. Distinguishing Optimism From Neuroticism (and trait Anxiety, self-mastery, and self-esteem): A Reevaluation of the Life Orientation Test. J Pers Soc Psychol. 1994; 67(6): 1063-1078.

[26] Grassi L, Buda P, Cavana L, Annunziata M, Torta R, Varetto A. Styles of Coping with Cancer: The Italian version of the MINI-MAC Scale. Psycho-Oncol. 2005; 14: 115–124.

[27] Schou I, Ekberg O, Ruland CM. The Mediating Role of Appraisal and Coping in the Relationship between Optimism-Pessimism and Quality of Life. Psycho-Oncol. 2005; 14: 718-727.

[28] Druss RG, Douglas CJ. Adaptive Responses to Illness and Disability. Healthy Denial. Gen Hosp Psychiat. 1988; 10: 163-168.

[29] Wittchen HU, Jacobi F. Size and Burden of Mental Disorders in Europe: A Critical Review and Appraisal of 27 Studies. Eur. Neuropsychopharmacol. 2005; 15: 357–367.

[30] Balasubramaniam M, Telles S, Doraiswamy M. Yoga on Our Minds: A Systematic Review of Yoga for Neuropsychiatric Disorders. 2012; 3: 117.

[31] Da Silva TL, Ravindran LN, Ravindran AV. Yoga in the Treatment of Mood and Anxiety Disorders: A Review. Asian J Psychiat. 2009; 2(1): 6-16.

[32] Alonso J, Angermeyer MC, Bernert S, Bruffaerts R, Brugha TS, Bryson H, et al. Prevalence of Mental Disorders in Europe: Results from the European Study of the Epidemiology of Mental Disorders (ESEMeD) Project. Acta Psychiat Scand. 2004; 109(420): 21–27.

[33] Cassano P, Fava M. Depression and Public Health: An Overview. J Psychosom Res. 2002; 53: 849-857.

[34] Wittchen HU, Lieb R, Schuster P, Oldehinkel AJ. When Is Onset? Investigations into Early Developmental Stages of Anxiety and Depressive Disorders. In: Rapaport JL

(Ed.), Childhood Onset of ''adult'' Psychopathology, Clinical and Research Advances. American Psychiatric Press, Washington, pp 259–302, 1999.

[35] Wittchen HU, Kessler RC, Beesdo K, Krause P, Höfler M, Hoyer J. Generalized Anxiety and Depression in Primary Care: Prevalence, Recognition and Management. J Clin Psychiatry. 2002; 63 Suppl 8: 24-34.

[36] Wittchen HU, Jacobi F, Rehm J, Gustavsson A, Svensson M, Jönsson B. et al. The Size and Burden of Mental Disorders and Other Disorders of the Brain in Europe. Eur Neuropsychopharmacol. 2010; l21(9): 655–679.

[37] Wittchen HU. Generalized Anxiety Disorder: Prevalence Burden and Cost to Society. Depress Anxiety. 2002; 16(4): 162-171.

[38] Michelini S, Cassano GB, Frare F, Perugi G. Long-term Use of Benzodiazepines: Tolerance, Dependence and Clinical Problems in Anxiety and Mood Disorders. Pharmacopsychiatry. 1996; 29: 127-134.

[39] Rickels K, Downing R, Schweizer E, Hassman H. Antidepressants for the Treatment of Generalized Anxiety Disorder. A Placebo-controlled Comparison of Imipramine, Trazodone, and Diazepam. Arch Gen Psychiatry. 1993; 50: 884-895.

[40] Gelenberg AJ, Lydiard RB, Rudolph RL, Aguiar L, Haskins JT, Salinas E. Efficacy of Venlafaxine Extended-release Capsules in Non-depressed Outpatients with Generalized Anxiety Disorder: A 6-month Randomized Controlled Trial. JAMA. 2000; 283: 3082-3088.

[41] Pollack MH, Zaninelli R, Goddard A, McCafferty JP, Bellew KM, Burnham DB, et al. Paroxetine in the Treatment of Generalized Anxiety Disorder: Results of a Placebo-Controlled, Flexible-Dosage Trial. J Clin Psychiatry. 2001; 62: 350-357.

[42] Baldwin DS, Nair RV. Escitalopram in the Treatment of Generalized Anxiety Disorder. Expert Rev Neurother. 2005; 5: 443-449.

[43] Katzman MA, Vermani M, Jacobs L, Marcus M, Kong B, Lessard S, et al. Quetiapine as an Adjunctive Pharmacotherapy for the Treatment of Non-remitting Generalized Anxiety Disorder: A Flexible-Dose, Open-label Pilot Trial. J Anxiety Disord. 2008; 22: 1480-1486.

[44] Andrews G, Slade TC, Issakidis SC. Deconstructing Current Comorbidity: Data from the Australian National Survey of Mental Health and Well-being. Br J Psychiat. 2002; 181(4): 306-314.

[45] Bonura KB. The Impact of Yoga on Psychological Health in Older Adults. Florida State University. Electronic Theses, Treatises and Dissertations. Paper 3549, 2007. Available from: http://diginole.lib.fsu.edu/cgi/viewcontent.cgi?article=2537&context=etd

[46] Clance P, Mitchel M, Engelman S. Body Cathexis in Children as a Function of Awareness Training and Yoga. J Clin Child Psychol. 1980; 9: 82-85.

[47] Nicolis G, Prigogine I. Self-Organization in Nonequilibrium Systems: From Dissipative Structures to Order through Fluctuations. NY: Wiley, 1977.

[48] Woods JH. The Yoga-System of Patañjali. Cambridge, MA: Harvard University Press, 1914.

[49] Brown RP, Gerbarg PL. Sudarshan Kriya Yogic Breathing in the Treatment of Stress, Anxiety, and Depression. Part II-Clinical Applications and Guidelines. J Altern Complement Med. 2005; 11(4): 711-717.

[50] Ravindran AV, Lam RW, Filteau MJ, Lespérance F, Kennedy SH, Parikh SV, Patten SB. Canadian Network for Mood and Anxiety Treatments (CANMAT) Clinical Guidelines for the Management of Major Depressive Disorder in Adults. V. Complementary and Alternative Medicine Treatments. 1. J Affect Disord. 2009; 117 Suppl 1: S54-64.

[51] Michalsen A. Die Komplementärmedizin und der «menschliche Faktor». Forsch Komplementmedizin Innere Medizin V und Integrative Medizin, Kliniken Essen-Mitte, Deutschland 2006; 13(2): 68-69.

[52] Agte VV, Chiplonkar SA. Sudarshan Kriya Yoga for Improving Antioxidant Status and Reducing Anxiety in Adults. Alternative and Complementary Therapies, 2008, 14(2): 96-100. Available from: http://online.liebertpub.com/doi/pdfplus/10.1089/act.2008.14204

[53] Meti BL, Desiraju T. Study of Changes in BEG and Autonomic Parameters After 4 Months of Initiation and Practice of Pranayama. Indian J Physiol Pharmacol. 1984; 28: 34.

[54] Meti BL, Raju TR. Auditory Middle Latency Evoked Potentials in Kriya Yoga. Health Administrator. 1993; 4: 56-58.

[55] Iyengar BKS. Light on Pranayama: The Yogic Art of Breathing. New York: Crossroads Publishing, 1997.

[56] Sarris J, Byrne GJ. A Systematic Review of Insomnia and Complementary Medicine Sleep Medicine Reviews. 2011April; 15(2): 99–106.

[57] Gilbert C. Yoga and Breathing Journal of Bodywork and Movement Therapies, Elsevier, 1999.

[58] Gupta N, Khera S, Vempati RP, Sharma R, Bijlani RL. Effect of Yoga Based Lifestyle Intervention on State and Trait Anxiety. Indian J Physiol Pharmacol. 2006; 50(1): 41-47.

[59] Brown RP, Gerbarg PL. Sudarshan Kriya Yogic Breathing in the Treatment of Stress, Anxiety, and Depression. Part II-Clinical Applications and Guidelines. J. Altern. Complement. Med. 2005b ;11(4): 711-717.

[60] Zope SA, Zope RA. Sudarshan Kriya Yoga: Breathing for Health. Int J Yoga. 2013; 6(1): 4-10.

[61] Naga Venkatesha Murthy PJ, Janakiramaiah N, Gangadhar BN, Subbakrishna DK. P300 Amplitude and Antidepressant Response to Sudarshan Kriya Yoga (SKY). J Affect Disorders. 1998; 50(1): 45-48.

[62] Janakiramaiah N, Gangadhar BN, Naga Venkatesha Murthy PJ, Harish MG, Subbakrishna DK, Vedamurthachar A. Therapeutic Efficacy of Sudarshan Kriya Yoga (SKY) in Dysthymic Disorder. NIMHANS J. 1998; 17: 21–28.

[63] Janakiramaiah N, Gangadhar BN, Naga Venkatesha Murthy PJ, Harish MG, Subbakrishna DK, Vedamurthachar A. Antidepressant Efficacy of Sudarshan Kriya Yoga (SKY) in Melancholia: A Randomized Comparison with Electroconvulsive Therapy (ECT) and Imipramine. J Affect Disord. 2000; 57: 255–259.

[64] Rohini V, Pandey RS, Janakiramaiah N, Gangadhar BN, Vedamarthachar A. Comparative Study of Full and Partial Sudarshana Kriya Yoga (SKY) in Major Depressive Disorder. NIMHANS J. 2000; 18(1-2): 53-57.

[65] Vedamurthachar A, Janakiramaiah N, Hegde JM, Shetty TK, Subbakrishna DK, Sureshbabu SV, Gangadhar BN. Antidepressant Efficacy and Hormonal Effects of Sudarshana Kriya Yoga (SKY) in Alcohol Dependent Individuals. J Affect Disorders. 2006; 94(1-3): 249-253.

[66] Gangadhar BN, Janakiramaiah N, Sudarshan B, Shety KT. Stress-Related Biochemical Effects of Sudarshan Kriya Yoga in Depressed Patients Study #6. Presented at the Conference on Biological Psychiatry. New York: UN NGO Mental Health Committee, 2000.

[67] European Commission's Directorate General [internet]; 2014. Available from: http://www.insead.edu/media_relations/press_release/docs/RESPONSE-Executive-Briefing.pdf

[68] Bazarko D, Rebecca AC, Azocar F, Jo Kreitzer M. The Impact of an Innovative Mindfulness-Based Stress Reduction Program on the Health and Well-Being of Nurses Employed in a Corporate Setting. J Workplace Behav Health. 2013; 28(2):107-133.

[69] University of Massachussetts Medical School; 2014. Available from: http://www.umassmed.edu/cfm/stress-reduction/workplace-programs/

[70] Awareness and Relaxation Training (ART); 2014. Available from: http://www.mindfulnessprograms.com/corporate-program.php

[71] Sri Sri Ravi Shankar, [interneet]; 2014. Available from: http://srisriravishankar.org/entry/tlex-transformational-leadership-for-excellence/

[72] Sri Sri Ravi Shankar; [internet]; 2014. Available from: www.tlexinstitute.com

[73] Doria S, Sanlorenzo R, Irtelli F, Mencacci C. Anti-anxiety Efficacy of Sudarshan Kriya Yoga in General Anxiety Disorder: A multicomponent, Yoga Based, Breath Intervention Program for Patients Suffering from Generalized Anxiety Disorder with or without Comorbidities. J Affect Disorders (2015 in press).

[74] American Psychiatric Association, 1994. Diagnostic and Statistical Manual of Mental Disorders, 4th ed. American Psychiatric Association, Washington, DC.

[75] Yoga Research Group. Treating Depression with Sudarshan Kriya Yoga: A Demonstration Video Cassette. Department of Health Education, National Institute of Mental Health and Neurosciences, Bangalore (1995).

[76] Hamilton M. The Assessment of Anxiety States by Rating. Br J Med Psychol. 1959; 32(1): 50–55.

[77] Zung WWK. A Rating Instrument for Anxiety Disorders. Psychosomatics. 1971; 12(6): 371–379.

[78] Hamilton M. A Rating Scale for Depression. J Neurol Neurosurg Psychiatry. 1960; 23: 56–62.

[79] Zung WWK. A Self-Rating Depression Scale. Arch Gen Psychiatry. 1965; 12(1): 63-70.

[80] Derogatis LR: SCL-90-R, Administration, Scoring and Procedures Manual-II for the R(evised) Version and Other Instruments of the Psychopathology Rating Scale Series. Townson: Clinical Psychometric Research; 1992 [italian version: Emanuele Preti, Antonio Prunas, Irene Sarno e Fabio Madeddu, OS Editions, Florence, Italy, 2011.

[81] Cohen S, Kamarck T, Mermelstein R. A Global Measure of Perceived Stress, J Health Soc Behavior. 1983; 24: 385-396.

[82] Goldberg DP, Gater R, Sartorius N, Ustun TB, Piccinelli M, Gureje O, Rutter C. The Validity of Two Versions of the GHQ in the WHO Study of Mental Illness in General Health Care Psychol Med. 1997; 27(1):191-197.

[83] Spielberger CD. Review of Profile of Mood States. Professional Psychol. 1972; 3(4): 387-388.

[84] Balasubramaniam M, Telles S, Doraiswamy PM. Yoga on Our Minds: A Systematic Review of Yoga for Neuropsychiatric Disorders. Front Psychiatry. 2013; 25(3): 117(1-16). Available from: http://journal.frontiersin.org/Journal/10.3389/fpsyt.2012.00117/full

Mindfulness — New Research and Treatment Directions in Post-traumatic Stress Disorder

Delia M. Podea and Karol J. Wild

Additional information is available at the end of the chapter

http://dx.doi.org/10.5772/60635

Abstract

Combining mindfulness to strengthen emotion regulation with existing empirically supported post-traumatic stress disorder (PTSD) treatments may improve outcomes through increasing (a) engagement, (b) compliance, and (c) decreasing the level of ruminations in PTSD. Several psychotherapeutic interventions incorporating training in mindfulness are clinically relevant to traumatic stress. In order to see how far PTSD treatment could benefit from including mindfulness into the therapeutic process, we analyzed researches regarding: (a) the neuroscience of mindfulness, (b) assessment instruments for mindfulness, (c) mechanism of mindfulness, respective, and (d) the relation between mindfulness and other techniques. Based on this analysis, we can conclude that mindfulness may improve the therapeutic results and the outcome of PTSD patients. Mindfulness can be used in two ways: (a) as an emotion regulation support technique for existing empirically supported PTSD treatments and (b) as a standalone treatment- mindfulness-based cognitive behavior psychotherapies.

Keywords: Mindfulness, Post-Traumatic Stress disorder, PTSD, empirically supported treatments, third-wave CBT

1. Introduction

The "fight-or-flight" response is a natural reaction in order to help the person to react adaptively to harmful events. In post-traumatic stress disorder (PTSD), this reaction is modified or dysfunctional. Persons who develop PTSD may feel a state of stress or frightened even when there is no danger [1]. PTSD develops after experiencing a physical harm or the threat of physical harm in a terrifying way. Persons who develop PTSD may be directly affected or may have witnessed a harmful event that happened to someone significant, or an unknown person [1].

PTSD can cause many symptoms. Symptoms that can be categorized into areas:

1. **Memory and emotional reactivating symptoms**

Repetitive flashbacks that reactivate elements from the traumatic event, including experiencing also the physical symptoms.

Bad dreams

Thoughts with a frightening content.

2. **Behavioral and cognitive avoidance symptoms**

Avoiding places, events, or objects related to the event

Intense emotions (depression, anger, guilt, or anxiety)

Anhedonia

Elective hypoamnesia.

3. **Physiological symptoms**

Being easily startled

Feeling tense or "on edge"

Insomnia,

Irritability or angry outbursts.

The above mentioned symptoms may interfere with daily tasks, circadian rhythm, or concentrating. Sometimes similar symptoms are present after a dangerous event, but there the intensity and quality is not always dysfunctional. Sometimes people present very intense symptoms that disappear after a few weeks; in this case we may speech about acute stress disorder (ASD). So far the symptoms last more than 2–4 weeks there is a possibility that the person present PTSD, in other cases symptoms appear only after weeks or months [1].

These symptoms are well described and presented in [2] The Diagnostic and Statistical Manual of Mental Disorders Fifth Edition DSM 5, [3] The International Classification of Diseases (ICD), and [4] The National Institute for Health and Care Excellence Guidelines for PTSD. Re-experiencing symptoms are the most characteristic symptoms that produce suffering. PTSD patients re-experience aspects of the trauma (flashbacks), very often producing a reactivation of the afferent intense emotions (where the patient acts or feels as if the traumatic experience was reoccurring),

Repetitive and intrusive images, nightmares, or other sensorial impressions of the traumatic event may be also re-experiencing. Stimuli of the traumatic event can produce an increase in

http://dx.doi.org/10.5772/60635

the arousal of the physiological reactions. Children may present some peculiarities in re-experiencing the trauma; their symptoms may include also a form of repetitive play or negative dreams without that the child to be able to recognize the content of the dreams.

Avoidance of various stimuli that are in correlation with the trauma is also a very often present PTSD symptom. Stimuli that can produce a re-experiencing of the trauma can be people, situations, or circumstances that are simulating or associated with the traumatic event. Patients often try to intentionally forget memories related to the event and avoid thinking or talking about what happened. Excessive rumination about: the justice of happening such an event to them, about what could they maybe don different in order to prevent to experience such an event, or scenarios about the way they will revenge what they have experience, are also very often.

Hyperarousal and hypervigilance symptoms include threat, startle, irritability, tension, concentration difficulty, and insomnia. Some PTSD patients present symptoms of emotional numbing which include: lack of ability to feel, detached from others, relinquish implication in previously preferred activities, and selective amnesia of the trauma [4].

Mindfulness mechanism is described as involving intention to direct one's attention to the present moment, in a detached and nonjudgmental way that lead to a state of acceptance [5]. Directing attention to the present moment means observing thoughts, feelings, and sensations that lead to developing awareness of the "here and now" [5]. Though focusing on the present in a nonjudgmental way, mindfulness consequently leads to developing an attitude of acceptance, or willingness to experience negative or discomfortable events [5]. The question is how far Mindfulness has potential to be of benefit to individuals with PTSD?

At this time, the evidence-based treatment interventions presented on the website of The National Institute for Health and Care Excellence and APA Division 12 Society of Clinical Psychology do not include Mindfulness-based psychotherapies. In the following we present how far the evidence-supported therapies could benefit from including Mindfulness.

2. Mindfulness — The *"Third Wave"* in cognitive behavior therapies

Evidence-Based treatments (EBT) for PTSD are Cognitive Processing Therapy [CPT, 6] and Prolonged Exposure [PE, 7]. The efficacy of these techniques in decreasing PTSD symptoms was proven by the many samples of PTSD patients in clinically controlled studies. CPT as well PE encourages the client to recall traumatic events in a controlled setting. Exposure to trauma-related memories, thoughts, and feelings, and cognitive restructuring of the trauma-related dysfunctional beliefs have been considered essential components for an effective treatment of PTSD patients. However, there is an important percentage of population which does not seek help, give up, or refuse the PE treatment because of the expected discomfort during confrontation of the trauma-related stimuli, or because they do not obtain significant results in their cases [5, 8, 9, 10].

Including mindfulness or other emotion regulation techniques in the existing evidence-based treatments protocols for PTSD may improve outcomes in multiple ways such as [5]:

Motivation for the treatment: Mindfulness can be useful for those clients who do not turn to evidence-based treatments or it is hard for them to tolerate the attached discomfort [8, 11, 12]. Mindfulness practice can play a role in decreasing symptoms and may increase the possibility of the clients with low motivation to accept the therapist's recommendations or evidence-based treatments.

Additional or replacing relaxation techniques: Mindfulness can be used prior to exposure or cognitive restructuring. Teaching patients to observe in a nonjudgmental way their internal reactions, feelings, sensations, and thoughts the moment they arise and to accept them can be useful in increasing their tolerance toward unpleasant emotions and discomfort that are associated with the trauma-related stimuli.

Decreasing the level of rumination: In order to increased awareness of trauma-related symptoms, encouraging mindfulness would be useful. Mindfulness may allow patients to decrease the level of rumination by developing detachment and defusion from their intrusive thoughts and feelings. Mindfulness can stimulate acceptance rather than avoidance of the trauma-related situations.

Increasing compliance to EBT: Patients practicing mindfulness during the treatment process may be more willing to follow EBT and accept the attached discomfort.

The *"third-wave"* cognitive behavioral psychotherapies (third-wave CBT) are defined by incorporating mindfulness training as central intervention technique, which can be clinically relevant also for deceasing traumatic stress. In the scientific literature there is a lack of study on the efficacy of these interventions in PTSD patients. Research has supported the efficacy of the third wave CBTs for various mental health problems such as anxiety, depression, or emotion deregulation that are also commonly present in PTSD [5].

2.1.1. Dialectic Behavior Therapy (DBT)

Linehan [13] describes mindfulness practice as an "instance of exposure to naturally arising thoughts, feelings, and sensations" [p. 354] [13]. Mindfulness skills are taught of as the "core" skills of DBT, and emphasize focused attention and awareness through observing, describing, and participating fully in both public and private experience [13, 14]. DBT often has been used prior to the implementation of PTSD-specific treatments such as exposure-based interventions to address difficulties with emotion regulation and distress tolerance [5].

2.1.2. Acceptance and Commitment Therapy (ACT)

ACT is based on relational frame theory [14, 15], which describes how language produces a unique situation in which direct experience is fused with cognition. In such instances, human beings respond to the literal content of thoughts as "truth" rather than responding to the thought as an experience. For example, thoughts such as "I can't do this" or "This will never get better" are responded to as reality. This "cognitive fusion" can then lead to efforts to avoid situations or emotions that give rise to these thoughts, or to escape such thoughts at the time they occur. While some avoidance of private experience may be necessary for healthy functioning and may in fact serve as effective coping [e.g., taking a walk to distract from work-related stress], routine avoidance of unpleasant private experiences may result in increased psychological distress when the avoidance interferes with effective living which often happens in PTSD [14, 15]. Randomized controlled trials are currently underway to evaluate the efficacy of ACT as a stand-alone treatment for PTSD. ACT targets avoidance of thoughts, memories, emotions, and other private experiences. In PTSD, these experiences may include intrusive recollections of the traumatic event and emotional states of guilt or anger [5].

2.1.3. Mindfulness-Based Stress Reduction (MBSR)

Mindfulness-Based Stress Reduction (MBSR) is a group psychosocial intervention consisting of mindfulness meditation practice and gentle yoga stretches that has been applied within chronically ill populations including cancer, with the goal of reducing stress and symptoms of disease [16] that appear also in PTSD. MBSR promote a state of awareness of the *"here and now"* and nonevaluative cognition about the reality. Mindfulness-Based Stress Reduction programs are intended to change automatic thoughts and other cognitive processes which can decrease PTSD symptoms and increase the quality of life [17, 14] of the PTSD patients.

2.1.4. Mindfulness-Based Cognitive Therapy (MBCT)

MBCT [14, 18] is based on an integration of elements of CBT for depression [14, 19], with the components of MBSR [16]. Compared to CBT, the goal of MBCT is not to change the *content* of core beliefs or automatic thoughts, it addresses obtaining a state of *awareness* and *acceptance* of the thoughts, feelings, and bodily sensations that some experience. In other words, its emphasis is primarily on facilitating a high discomfort and promotes ways of thinking like "Thoughts are not facts" and "I am not my thoughts." Mindfulness Based-Cognitive Therapy might be a useful tertiary care program for patients struggling with PTSD and depression [5].

3. The neuroscience of mindfulness and its implications in PTSD

A systematic review of neurobiological and clinical features of mindfulness meditations [20] shows that studies using Electroencephalographic (EEG) as an objective measurement tool for observing the changes in brainwaves produced by mindfulness meditation have revealed a significant increase in alpha and theta waves during mindfulness practice. Studies using fMRI observed that mindfulness practice activates the prefrontal cortex (PFC) and the anterior cingulate cortex (ACC) and that practicing mindfulness for a long period of time produces an increased activation in attention-related cerebral areas [20].

The clinical findings show that Mindfulness-Based Stress Reduction (MBSR) is effective for different psychiatric and also for different somatic conditions for both healthy and mental disordered subjects [please see table 1], Mindfulness-Based Cognitive Therapy (MBCT) efficacy ways observed predominantly in reducing depression relapses in cases of a history of three or more depressive episodes, Zen meditation produces a significant decreases of

Outcome of interest	Vipassana	Zen	MBSR	MBCT
Psychiatric disorders				
Prevention of depression relapses in MD				++
Reduction of overall depressive symptoms in MD			+	+++
Reduction of anxiety levels in BD				+
Social phobia				+
PTSD	N			
Alcohol and substances dependence	+			
Physical disorders				
Psychological symptoms in cancer			++++	
Reduction of blood pressure		++		
Chronic pain			++	
Rheumatoid arthritis			++	
Fibromyalgia			++	
Psoriasis			+	
Multiple sclerosis			+	
Tinnitus				N
HIV			+	
Healthy subjects				
Stress	+	+	+++++++++	

MD, Major depressive disorder; BD, bipolar disorder; PTSD, post-traumatic stress disorder; MBSR, Mindfulness-Based Stress Reduction; MBCT, Mindfulness-based Cognitive Therapy; +, MM better than control condition; N, no significant difference between MM and control condition.

MD, Major depressive disorder; BD, bipolar disorder; PTSD, post-traumatic stress disorder; MBSR, Mindfulness-Based Stress Reduction; MBCT, Mindfulness-bassed Cognitive Therapy; +, MM better than control condition; N, no significant difference between MM and control condition

Table 1. Clinical findings [20]

hypertension level and the traditional meditation Vipassana [focus on the breath] shows efficacy in reducing alcohol and substance abuse in prisoners. However, given the low-quality designs of current studies, it is difficult to establish whether clinical outcomes are due to specific or non-specific effects of MM (see also table 1) [20].

The implication of amygdala as a quick way to process emotional stimuli of any type of valence is well known. Research has shown a decrease in the amygdala activation level as a response to emotional stimuli, in the moments of practicing mindfulness, after an 8-week meditation training. A recent longitudinal study by Desbordes, Negi, Pace, Wallace, Raison, and Schwartz (2012) [21], investigated the effects of an 8-week mindfulness training on amygdala activation level toward emotion-related stimuli in cases where the participants were in a non-meditative state. Participants included in the study were healthy adults and had no experience in meditation practice. The author used two types of training programs (a) Mindful Attention Training (MAT), (b) Cognitively Based Compassion Training (CBCT; based on Tibetan Buddhist compassion meditation practices) and compared the results also with an active control group.

http://dx.doi.org/10.5772/60635

As pre- and post-intervention assessment, was used an fMRI experiment. The experimenters show the participant's images with three different emotional valences (e.g., positive, negative, and neutral) when there were in a nonmeditative state. They reported a longitudinal decrease in right amygdala activation in the Mindful Attention group as a reaction to all three types of images. In the CBCT group, they reported a trend increase in right amygdala reaction to negative images, and presented a negative correlation with the depression score. The control group presented no modification in the response of the amygdala toward emotional related stimuli's. The results of this study suggest the possibility that the effect of long-term mindfulness practicing on emotions could be extended or generalized also to nonmeditative states. [21].

A recent study made at Durham VA Medical Center from Duke University, published in *Archives of General Psychiatry [22],* have observed a smaller volume of amygdala in the case of war veterans diagnosed with PTSD. Their study provides objective evidence for a positive relation between the volume of amygdala and PTSD. This result offers a promising direction of research, which has the task of establishing if a smaller amygdala is a risk factor and vulnerability to develop PTSD or if it is the other way around. [22].

Translating these findings to PTSD patients, there is a possibility that people who practice mindfulness mediation for a longer period of time could have a higher level to which their amygdala react to outside stimuli, including events with a trauma content. These results could suggest that mindfulness practice could decrease the risk of developing PTSD. An open question is if there exists a relation between the volume and the activation level of amygdala in the case of PTSD.

4. The mechanism of mindfulness

4.1. Measuring and operationalization mindfulness

Studies [23] systematically assess and compare the properties of instruments to measure self-reported mindfulness. Ovid Medline, CINAHL, and PsycINFO databases were searched for articles whose primary purpose was the development or evaluation of the measurement properties (validity, reliability, and responsiveness) of a self-report mindfulness scale [23]. They identify 46 articles that met the inclusion criteria of their study, describing 10 scales which operationalized mindfulness as a: (a) unidimensional process or (b) bi-dimensional or multidimensional process. From the unidimensional scales The Mindful Attention Awareness Scale (MAAS) was described by most studies and presented positive psychometric properties. From the multidimensional scales The Five Facet Mindfulness Questionnaire had presented highest internal consistency and construct validation [23]. From the revised scales no one had presented sufficient evidence for a significant content validity. The studies describing the mindfulness scales did not assess the level to which the measurements cover all the aspects of the mindfulness concept or the level of the comprehensiveness of the items by the subjects. One reason for these omissions could be also the differences in the scientific literature regarding the definition of the mindfulness concept. Another limitation of the validation studies for the revised scales was errors in the estimation of (a) test-retest reliability estimation, and (b) guidelines for the interpretation of scores in the cases of measurement errors were missing.

By the authors revised mindfulness measurements [23] have important differences and defining and operationalizing mindfulness, and no scale present enough content validity in order to be recommended only by their superior psychometric properties. The significant limitations identified are due to the absence of qualitative evaluations and accepted external referents to sustain construct validity. Researcher using mindfulness-based intervention programs in their clinical controlled trails studies need to be aware that based on the existing measurements it could be difficult to optimize mindfulness intervention programs [23].

The MAAS assesses awareness of present experience throughout daily life presenting a single factor after exploratory and confirmatory factor analysis [24–26]. The Five-Factors Mindfulness Questionnaire (FFMQ) [13] operationalize mindfulness using a multidimensional conceptualization, using subscales for different attention, cognitive, and behavioral processes present during practicing mindfulness, like: (a) observing, (b) describing, (c) acting with awareness, (d) acceptance without judgment, and (e) nonreactivity to inner experience. Other bi-dimensional or multidimensional mindfulness scales are: (a) The Cognitive Affective Mindfulness Scale - Revised (CAMS-R) [27], (b) the Philadelphia Mindfulness Scale (PHMS) [28], and (c) the Freiburg Mindfulness Inventory (FMI) [29]. These scales assess the level of individual's long-term awareness of the present experience/moment or in other words, mindfulness as a trait [4]. Philadelphia Mindfulness Scale [28] present two mindfulness factors: [a] tendency to be aware of the present experience over time, and [b] tendency to accept the present experience [28].

In a recent study we have analyzed the relation between the two ways of conceptualization Mindfulness: as a one-dimensional versus a two-dimensional process, respective the relationship between the mindfulness measurements and anxiety, depression, optimism, pessimism and unconditional self-acceptance. For this propose we have used The Mindful Attention Awareness Scale (MAAS) and Philadelphia Mindfulness Scale (PMS).

According to the scientific literature [13, 15, 30, 31, 36] we expected that mindfulness will correlate positively with optimism and unconditional self-acceptance and correlate negatively with anxiety, depression, and pessimism. The results confirmed our hypothesis for the one-dimensional mindfulness measurement (MAAS). The two Mindfulness measurements presented a low to medium relation ($r=.433$ at $p=.001$ between MAAS and PMI awareness, and $r=.326$ at $p=0.001$, $N=112$ between MAAS and PMI acceptance). Mindfulness measurement as a two-dimensional concept presented no relationship between: (a) mindfulness awareness and (b) mindfulness acceptance scales, respective optimism and unconditional self-acceptance. Mindfulness awareness scale (PMI awareness) presented a negative relationship with pessimism ($r=-.310$ at $p=0.001$, $N=112$) and a low positive relationship with unconditional self-acceptance ($r=.190$ at $p=0.05$, $N=112$), respective no relationship with anxiety and depression measurements. The Mindfulness acceptance scale (PMI acceptance) presented a negative relationship with anxiety ($r=.-325$ at $p=0.001$) and depression ($r=-.474$ at $p=0.01$), and no relationship with other measured variables. Besides optimism and unconditional self-acceptance, the two dimensional Mindfulness measurements PMI confirm the hypothesis.

Concluding, the main difference between the two measurements seems to be at the cognitive level, [optimism--pessimism scale, unconditional self-acceptance] suggesting one conceptualize mindfulness more as a cognitive process of attention and the other measurement more as nonevaluative detachment. Our results confirm the conclusion of the study conducted by Park, Reilly-Spong, and Gross, (2013) [23] that current mindfulness scales have important conceptual differences and important limitations and that researchers need to proceed cautiously before optimizing any mindfulness intervention based on the existing scale [23].

4.2. The Influence of Mindfulness on PTSD Cognitive Processes

4.2.1. Mindfulness, memory, and attention

A study conducted by Lykins, Baer, and Gottlob, (2012) [32] compared the results at performance-based attention tests, respective short-term and long-term memory measurements, between a group of long-term meditators and a group of persons which didn't have previous meditation training or practice. The meditators included in the study had practice mindfulness meditation in a regular way for of least 6 years. As expected, the results showed significantly higher scores at mindfulness scales for the meditator's group. The results showed little difference between the two groups regarding the performance-based tasks measured in the study. The differences between the two groups were significant only between the short- and long-term memory scores [32].

There results indicated that the two groups scored significantly differently on these measures: (a) California verbal learning test (CVLT) and (b) letter-number sequencing (LNS0. Follow-up univariate ANOVAs revealed that, as predicted, meditators scored significantly higher on two measures of short-term memory (CVLT short delay free recall, short delay cued recall) and one measure of long-term memory (long delay free recall). Contrary to predictions, they did not score higher on a second index of long-term memory (long delay cued recall), working memory, or total learning. Mean effect size for this group of variables was 0.49 [32].

No differences in sustaining attention between mindfulness intervention group and controlled groups were presented. In other studies on sustained attention, MacCoon MacLean, Davidson, Saron, Lutz (2014) [33] have done a longitudinal randomized trial comparing the study between MBSR versus active control group, which participated in a Health Enhancement Program (HEP). They have found no significant correlations between performance change and either total minutes of practice or sessions of practice from pre- to post-intervention [33]. Attentional sensitivity is not affected by mindfulness practice as taught in MBSR, but it is unclear whether mindfulness might positively affect another aspect of attention, vigilance [33].

This findings suggest that mindfulness could be used in the case of PTSD patients in at least two ways: (a) in addition to using mindfulness as a relaxation method before Prolonged Exposure [PE, 7], it may also increase the ability to recall the exposure experiences in order to consolidate the operant conditioning process, (b) for the category of PTSD patients who tend to avoid recalling traumatic events necessary for Cognitive Processing Therapy [CPT, 6].

4.2.2. Mindfulness and acceptance

In a study that analyzed the relationship between mindfulness, acceptance, and catastrophizing in chronic pain [34], the results showed a significant positive strong relation between (a) mindfulness and acceptance, r (85) = 0.52, p<0.001; (b) pain-related catastrophizing beliefs and acceptance (r (82) = 0.42, p<0.001).

These results suggest that increasing the level of acceptance could produce a decrease in the levels of pain-related catastrophizing beliefs. The findings show no relation between pain-related catastrophizing beliefs and mindfulness.

The subjective intensity of the pain experience presented a positive significant relation only with pain-related catastrophizing beliefs (r [82] = 0.40, p<0.001), suggesting that the eventual benefits of mindfulness or acceptance on reducing the intensity of the subjective pain experience intensity could mediated thought changing pain-related catastrophizing thoughts. Thus, acceptance explained an additional 12% of the variance in pain-related catastrophizing, but mindfulness was not a significant predictor of pain-related catastrophizing. This study has used the acceptance and action questioner (AAQ II) developed by Hayes [34, 35] as a measurement of acceptance and the MAAS as a measurement of mindfulness. Other studies [46] found a significant relationship between the unconditional self-acceptance and mindfulness scale MAAS (r =.31, p =.001), and between the unconditional self-acceptance and the mindfulness scale CAMS-R (r =.45, p =.001). This study has used the unconditional self-acceptance questioner (USAQ) as an acceptance measurement.

These findings suggest that acceptance is related to mindfulness, but clearly distinct from the construct of mindfulness [24, 37]. In contrast to this view other researchers present acceptance as a necessary component of mindfulness [16, 37]. This debate suggests the need for future research to study whether acceptance is a result of mindfulness or is it an independent concept.

4.3. Mindfulness versus hypnosis, traditional meditation, and relaxation

4.3.1. Mindfulness and hypnosis

Mindfulness can be easily integrated with hypnotherapy in the management of emotional disorders. Mindfulness-Based Cognitive Hypnosis (MBCH) describes an intervention framework on changing and reframing dysfunctional, irrational, and core beliefs. MBCH include the following components: (1) intention, (2) direct attention on the present moment, (3) the development of a detached attitude (nonevaluative, non-judgmental) toward the present experience, and (4) the acceptance of the reality with the entire being. In the therapeutic process all these four components are addressed and developed using different types of intervention from education and training in the prior stage of the intervention, to incorporating them into the hypnotherapy strategy [38].

Yapko (2011) [39] provides an excellent discussion on the similarities and differences between hypnosis and mindfulness and the rationale for integrating hypnotherapy with mindfulness techniques. Lynn, Das, Hallquist, and Williams (2006) [40] have proposed that "hypnosis and mindfulness-based approaches can be used in tandem to create adaptive response sets and

http://dx.doi.org/10.5772/60635

ameliorate maladaptive response sets" (p. 145). Moreover, hypnosis can be used to catalyze mindfulness-based approaches [39–41]. Hypnosis can also be used as a substitute for relaxation techniques [38]. Although most of the techniques described are scientific and evidence based, there is a need to study the effectiveness of cognitive hypnotherapy when it is combined with mindfulness [38].

4.3.2. *Mindfulness and traditional meditation*

In a recent study, the authors [42] compared how neurophysiologic (EEG, EKG) and cognitive correlates to meditative practices that use (a) focused or (b) distributed attention, from both Theravada and Vajrayana traditions [42].

The study used two ways of Theravada meditation practice:

Shamatha practice relates to training in the concentration of attention. During the practice of Shamatha, the practitioners are instructed to place undistracted attention on the object of meditation, while withdrawing their focus from other objects [42, 43]. Shamatha meditation, which is similar to the Vipassana method, uses the meditators' breath as the meditation object. So far the focus of attention/awareness moves from the breathing, the mediators are instructed to observe the new focus of their attention (beliefs, flashbacks, memories, etc.), and to move the focus of attention back to their breath [42, 44]— focused attention.

Kasina meditation is a particular type of Shamatha practice. Kasina meditation refers to objects of meditation that are typically colored disks, which differ from each other in terms of their color, size, object composition, and other properties, depending on the type of Kasina used. In the study [42], Kasina was used instead of the more popular Shamatha practice where a meditator focuses on the breath for a long period of time [44] to dissociate it more easily from Vipassana, which implements focusing on the breath [42]—distributed attention.

Both of these traditional meditation practices overlap highly with the mindfulness practice incorporated in the "third wave" cognitive behavioral psychotherapies. Focusing on the breath or on a specific object, for example, one's own hand, is also well described in accepted and dedicated therapy textbooks [15, 30].

The study also presented two steps of Vajrayana practices:

Deity meditation involves a visualization practice by generating an internal image of oneself as a supernatural being. The mediators must create an internal image full of details including: colors, ornaments, and environment in a three-dimensional way, respective body image, emotions, and feelings of the supernatural being. This image has the role to replace the perception of the real world or of the self. This visualization is the first stage of the Vajrayana meditation practice [42]—focused attention.

Rig-pa meditation is the second stage of the Vajrayana meditation practice and is develop to be complete the meditation stages [42, 45]. The main goal of the Rig-pa meditation is to develop a state of emptiness and awareness without a conceptualization of the reality. In order to transit from Deity to Rig-pa the meditators visualize the dissolution of the initial visualization. Rig-pa meditation presumes distributive attention without any focus on objects or experiences.

While Rig-pa is considered to be a meditation without an object, Vispassana is considered a meditation which is focused on an object, noticing and observing the content of attention [42, 45]—distributive attention.

This type of traditional meditation practices differ in a significant way from mindfulness meditation that is incorporated in psychology.

The results [42] show that the meditation techniques of the Theravada tradition produced an increased activation of the parasympathetic nervous system, which is an indication for a relaxation response. In contrast, the meditation techniques of the Vajrayana tradition produced an increased activation of the sympathetic nervous system, which is an indication for arousal [42]. These results also pointed out that: (a) Theravada and Vajrayana meditations are based on different neurophysiologic mechanisms, which give rise to either a relaxation or arousal response. (b) That it may be more appropriate to categorize meditations in terms of relaxation vs. arousal, rather than as focused vs. distributed attention dichotomy [42].

4.3.3. Mindfulness and relaxation training

A random controlled trail study compared the effect of mindfulness meditation versus relaxation training on distress, positive state of the mind, rumination, and distraction [46]. The relaxation training integrates primarily body awareness--based relaxation intervention: (a) autogenic relaxation, (b) progressive muscle relaxation, (c) simple breathing techniques, and (d) guided imagery to give a comprehensive course on stress reduction via a focus on bodily relaxation.

The results show a large effect sizes on reduction of distress for both meditation and relaxation (Cohen's d = 1.36 and.91, respectively), whereas the meditation group showed a larger effect size for positive states of mind than relaxation (Cohen's d =. 71 and.25, respectively). There was no significant difference between meditation and relaxation on distress and positive mood states over time. The meditation group also demonstrated significant pre and post decreases in both distractive and ruminative thoughts/behaviors compared with the control group, with mediation models suggesting that the mindfulness meditation's effects on reducing distress were partially mediated by reducing rumination.

5. Conclusions and discussions

The analyzed researches suggest that mindfulness may improve the therapeutical results and the outcome of PTSD patients. Mindfulness can be used in two ways: (a) as an emotion regulation support technique for existing empirically supported PTSD treatments, and (b) as a standalone treatment—mindfulness-based cognitive behavior psychotherapies (ACT, DBT, MBSR, MBCT, etc.).

Otherwise, the term mindfulness is used often for different meditative techniques, which are incorporated in psychology, but are differently named in the traditional meditation approaches. These facts indicate the need to use neuroscience research techniques (EEG, fRMN) to obtain a clear image of the neurophysiologic and psychological processes implicated in different types of mindfulness exercises. Based on the presented research it seems that there are different ways of conceptualizing and assessing mindfulness in measuring the efficacy of treatment, which brings us to inconsistent and incomparable results. However, before definitive conclusions can be drawn about the efficacy of mindfulness in the treatment of PTSD, further basic and applied research is needed [5].

Acknowledgements

This paper is partly supported by the Sectorial Operational Programme Human Resources Development (SOPHRD), financed by the European Social Fund and the Romanian Government under the contract POSDRU 141531.

Author details

Delia M. Podea[1,2*] and Karol J. Wild[1,3]

*Address all correspondence to: deliapodea@yahoo.com

1 "Vasile Goldis" Western University of Arad, Psychiatry Department, Arad, Romania

2 Psychiatry Department, County Clinical Emergency Hospital of Arad, Arad, Romania

3 "VasileGoldis" Western University of Arad, Psychology Department, Arad, Romania

References

[1] Post-Traumatic Stress Disorders (PTSD) [Internet] Available from: http://www.nimh.nih.gov/health/topics/post-traumatic-stress-disorder-ptsd/index.shtml [Accessed: 2015-02-02].

[2] American Psychiatric Association: Diagnostic and Statistical Manual of Mental Disorders (DSM-5®), Fifth Edition, 2013. Washington DC.

[3] World Health Organization. The ICD-10 classification of mental and behavioural disorders: clinical descriptions and diagnostic guidelines. Geneva, 1992 (http://www.who.int/classifications/icd/en/bluebook.pdf; accessed 4 January 2011).

[4] National Institute of Health and Care Excellence (NICE) 2005. [Internet] Available from: http://www.nice.org.uk/guidance/cg26/resources/guidance-posttraumatic-stress-disorder-ptsd-pdf [Accessed: 2014-11-05].

[5] Vujanovic, Niles, Pietrefesa, Potter, Schmertz: Potential of mindfulness in treating trauma reactions. 2014. [Internet] Available from: http://www.ptsd.va.gov/professional/treatment/overview/mindful-PTSD.asp [Accessed: 2014-11-04].

[6] Resick PA, Monson CM, Chard KM: Cognitive Processing Therapy: Veteran/military version, 2007. Washington, DC: Department of Veterans' Affairs.

[7] Foa EB, Hembree EA, Rothbaum BO: Prolonged exposure therapy for PTSD: Emotional processing of traumatic experiences. Therapist Guide, 2007. New York: Oxford University Press.

[8] Follette VM, Vijay A: Mindfulness for trauma and posttraumatic stress disorder. In: F. Didonna (Ed.), Clinical Handbook of Mindfulness 2009 (pp. 299-317). New York: Springer Science & Business Media.

[9] Hembree EA, Cahill SP, Foa EB: Impact of personality disorders on treatment outcome for female assault survivors with chronic posttraumatic stress disorder. Journal of Personality Disorders, 2004, 18, 117-127.

[10] Schottenbauer MA, Glass CR, Arnkoff DB, Tendick V, Gray SH: Nonresponse and dropout rates in outcome studies on PTSD: Review and methodological considerations. Psychiatry: Interpersonal and Biological Processes, 2008, 71,134-168.

[11] Becker CB, Zayfert C: Integrating DBT-based techniques and concepts to facilitate exposure treatment for PTSD. Cognitive and Behavioral Practice, 2001, 8, 107-122.

[12] Cloitre M, Koenen KC, Cohen LR, Han H: Skills training in affective and interpersonal regulation followed by exposure: A phase-based treatment for PTSD related to childhood abuse. Journal of Consulting and Clinical Psychology, 2002,70, 1067-1074.

[13] Lineham MM: Cognitive Behavioral Treatment of Bordeline Personality Disorder, 1993 (p. 3-65). New York: The Guilford Press.

[14] Hayes S, Follette VM, Lineham MM: Mindfulness and Acceptance: Expanding the Cognitive-Behavioral Tradition, 2004. New York: The Guilford Press.

[15] Hayes SC, Strosahl KD, Wilson KG. Acceptance and Commitment Therapy: An Experiential Approach to Behavior Change, 1999 (p. 3-49). New York: The Guilford Press.

[16] Kabat-Zinn J. Full Catastrophe Living: Using the Wisdom of Your Body and Mind to Face Stress, Pain and Illness, 1990. New York: Delacourt.

[17] Carlson LE, Speca M, Patel KD, Goodey E: Mindfulness-based stress reduction in relation to quality of life, mood, symptoms of stress, and immune parameters in breast and prostate cancer outpatients. Psychosomatic Medicine, 2003, 65, 571-581.

[18] Beck AT, Rush AJ, Shaw BF, Emery G. Cognitive Therapy of Depression, 1979. New York: Guilford Press.

[19] Segal ZV, Williams JMG, Teasdale JD. Mindfulness-Based Cognitive Therapy for Depression, 2001. New York: Guilford Press.

[20] Chiesa AA, Serretti A: A systematic review of neurobiological and clinical features of mindfulness meditations, Psychological Medicine, 2010, 40, 1239–1252.

[21] Desbordes G, Negi LT, Pace TWW, Wallace BA, Raison CL, Schwartz EL: Effects of mindful-attention and compassion meditation training on amygdala response to emotional stimuli in an ordinary, non-meditative state, Human Neuroscience, 2012; 6: 292.

[22] Morey RA, Gold AL, LaBar KS, Beall SK, Brown VM, Haswell CC, Nasser JD, Wagner HR, McCarthy G: Amygdala volume changes in posttraumatic stress disorder in a large case-controlled veterans group. Arch Gen Psychiatry, 2012, 69(11):1169-1178.

[23] Park, Taehwan P, Reilly-spong, Maryanne R-S, Gross, Cynthia RG: Mindfulness: a systematic review of instruments to measure an emergent patient-reported outcome (PRO), Quality of Life Research, 2013, 22(2), 2639-2659.

[24] Brown KW, Ryan RM: The benefits of being present: Mindfulness and its role in psychological well-being. Journal of Personality and Social Psychology, 2003, 84, 822-848.

[25] Brown KW, Ryan RM, Creswell JD: Mindfulness: Theoretical Foundations and Evidence for its Salutary Effects. Psychological Inquiry, 2007, 18(4), 211-237.

[26] Clarson LE, Brown KW: Validation of Mindful Attention Awareness Scale in cancer population. Journal of Psychosomatic Research, 2005, 58, 29-33.

[27] Feldman G, Hayes A, Kumar S, Greeson J, Laurenceau JP: Mindfulness and emotion regulation: The development and initial validation of the cognitive and affective mindfulness scale-revised (CAMS-R). Journal of Psychopathology and Behavioral Assessment, 2007, 29, 177-190.

[28] Cardaciotto L, Herbert JD, Forman EM, Moitra E, Farrow V: The assessment of present-moment awareness and acceptance: The Philadelphia mindfulness scale. Assessment, 2008, 15, 204-223.

[29] Walach H, Buchheld N, Buttenmuller V, Kleinknecht N, Schmidt S: Measuring mindfulness--the Freiburg mindfulness inventory (FMI). Personality and Individual Differences, 2006, 40, 1543-1555.

[30] Harris R. ACT Made Simple: A Easy-to-Read Primer on Acceptance and Commitment Therapy, 2009. Canada: New Harbinger Press.

[31] Ellis A: Rational emotive behavior therapy and the mindfulness based stress reduction training of John Kabat-Zinn. Journal of Rational-Emotive & Cognitive-Behavior Therapy, 2006, 24(1), 63-78.

[32] Lykins ELB, Baer RA, Gottlob LR: Performance-based tests of attention and memory in long-term mindfulness meditators and demographically matched nonmeditators. Cognitive Therapy Research, 2012, 36, 103-114.

[33] MacCoon DG, MacLean KA, Davidson RJ, Saron CD, Lutz A: No sustained attention differences in a longitudinal randomized trial comparing mindfulness based stress reduction versus active control. PLoS ONE 2014, 9(6), e97551. doi:10.1371/journal.pone.0097551.

[34] De Boer MJ, Steinhagen HE, Versteegen GJ, Struys MMRF, Sanderman R: Mindfulness, acceptance and catastrophizing in chronic pain. PLoS ONE, 2014, 9(1), e87445. doi:10.1371/journal.pone.0087445.

[35] Hayes SC, Strosahl K, Wilson KG, Bissett RT, Pistorello J: Measuring experiential avoidance: A preliminary test of a working model. The Psychological Record, 2004, 54, 553–578.

[36] Thompson BL, Watz JA: Mindfulness, Self-Esteem, Unconditional Self-acceptance. Journal of Rational-Emotive & Cognitive-Behavior Therapy, 2008, 26(2).

[37] Borynski M. Clarifying the Construct of Mindfulness and its Relationship to Neuroticsm [thesis]. Central Michigan University Mount Pleasant, Michigan August, 2006.

[38] Alladin A, Mindfulness-based hypnosis: Blending science, beliefs, and wisdoms to catalyze healing. American Journal of Clinical Hypnosis, 2014, 56, 285-302.

[39] Yapko MD. Mindfulness and hypnosis: The power of suggestions to transform experience, 2011. New York: Norton.

[40] Lynn SJ, Das LS, Hallquist MN, Williams JC: Mindfulness, acceptance, and hypnosis: Cognitive and clinical perspectives. International Journal of Clinical and Experimental Hypnosis, 2006, 54, 143–166.

[41] Alladin A: Experiential cognitive hypnotherapy: Strategies for relapse prevention in depression. In: Yapko M (Ed.), Hypnosis and Treating Depression: Advances in Clinical Practice, 2006 (pp. 281–313). New York: Routledge.

[42] Amihai I, Kozhevnikov M: Arousal vs. Relaxation: A Comparison of the Neurophysiological and Cognitive Correlates of Vajrayana and Theravada Meditative Practices. PLoS One, 2014, 9(7). doi: 10.1371/journal.pone.0102990.

[43] Corby JC, Roth WT, Zarcone VP Jr, Kopell BS: Psychophysiological correlates of the practice of trantric yoga meditation. Archives General Psychiatry, 1978, 35, 571–577 [PubMed].

[44] Lutz A. Meditation and the neuroscience of consciousness: an introduction. In: Zelazo PD and Thompson E (Eds.), The Cambridge Handbook of Consciousness, 2006 (pp. 499-551). New York: Cambridge University Press.

[45] Rinpoche TU. As it is. Hong Kong, 1999 (p 224). Ranjung Yeshe Publications.

[46] Jain S, Shapiro SL, Swanick S, Roesch SC, Mills PJ, Bell I, Schwartz GER: A randomized controlled trial of mindfulness meditation versus relaxation training: Effects on distress, positive states of mind, rumination, and distraction. Annual Behavior Medicine, 2007, 33(1), 11-21.

Chapter 16

Anxiety — Is There an App for That? Considering Technology, Psychiatry, and Internet-Assisted Cognitive Behavioral Therapy

David Gratzer, Faiza Khalid-Khan and Sarosh Khalid-Khan

Additional information is available at the end of the chapter

http://dx.doi.org/10.5772/60816

Abstract

Across Western countries, more than a third of people will have a mental health disorder over their lifetime; mood and anxiety disorders are the most common. The effectiveness of psychological interventions is well established. Cognitive Behavioural Therapy (CBT), for example, is as effective for mild and moderate anxiety as medications; combined psychopharmacology and CBT is superior to either modality alone, suggesting a synergistic effect. However, CBT requires a major investment of time and resources. Thus, in public systems, CBT has limited availability and is subject to long waiting times; primary-care physicians and psychiatrists may not offer CBT.

Can technology address the deficiency of psychological interventions for mental illness? Internet therapies (including smart phone apps) have been developed, offering CBT and other psychological interventions. In this chapter, we focus on Internet-assisted CBT (ICBT).

ICBT allows patients to receive ongoing CBT with easier and quicker access, at reduced cost, and with increased convenience over traditional CBT. We review evidence from randomized trials and meta-analyses, which strongly support the use of ICBT in clinical practice, especially in combination with ongoing therapist support. We consider government experimentation with ICBT, with a particular focus on Australia. We also present a case demonstrating the clinical application of ICBT. Finally, with an eye to the future, we will look at potential research questions.

Keywords: Cognitive Behavioral Therapy, CBT, Internet-Assisted CBT, ICBT, Apps, Psychological Intervention, Depression, Anxiety, Access, Australia, Sweden, United Kingdom

1. Introduction

A problem, the world over: anxiety disorders are common, with the global prevalence of such disorders estimated to be 7.3%, although that number varies highly by region [1]. Across Western countries, more than one-third of people have a mental health disorder over their lifetime; mood and anxiety disorders are the most common [2]. The World Health Organization (WHO) estimates that spending on anxiolytics alone is, on average, $94,880 USD per 100,000 people and sharply higher in wealthier countries, $315,560 USD per 100,000 [3]. There is an alternative to medications: psychological interventions are effective for anxiety. For example, cognitive behavioral therapy (CBT) is as effective as medications for mild and moderate anxiety, and there is evidence that combined psychopharmacology and CBT is superior to either modality alone, suggesting a synergistic effect [4]. CBT is based on the concept that people's thoughts, emotions, and behaviors influence each other (Beck's Cognitive Triad). In essence, the patients cannot control the world, but they can take control of how they interpret things in that world.However, CBT requires a major investment of time and resources. Thus, in public health-care systems, patients are often subjected to long wait times, and primary-care physicians and psychiatrists may not offer CBT [5]. This raises the question: can technology address the deficit of psychological interventions for mental illness? Internet therapies (including smart phone apps) have recently been developed to offer CBT and other psychological interventions for anxiety patients. In this review, we focus on Internet-assisted CBT (ICBT) for anxiety and anxiety comorbid conditions.

ICBT allows patients to receive ongoing CBT with simpler and faster access, at reduced cost, and with increased convenience over traditional CBT [6]. In this chapter, we will review evidence from the literature, including randomized control trials and meta-analyses. We will include the young literature on smart-phone apps. While additional studies are needed, the cumulative results strongly support the use of ICBT in clinical practice, especially in combination with ongoing therapist support. This chapter will also highlight governments that are embracing ICBT to better serve patients – experiments that are stretching from the Highlands in Scotland to Queensland in Australia. Overall, ICBT is a viable contribution to address the global mental health crisis.

2. Evidence for ICBT

ICBT has been the focus of much research, though the quality of these studies has varied. Early studies suffered from a lack of rigorous experimental design [7]; however, in recent years, improved study designs have generated a robust, reliable body of literature. A PubMed search with the terms "cognitive behavioral therapy" and "Internet" yielded 825 papers, covering everything from the treatment of mood and anxiety disorders to video game "addiction" and tinnitus. We chose the 40 most relevant articles related to anxiety that presented results from randomized controlled trials (RCT), meta-analyses, and reviews. We also incorporated literature on smart phone apps (apps), which is a growing, albeit young, field of study. Many well-controlled, randomized trials of ICBT were identified for various psychiatric conditions.

Although there are several types of ICBT programs, they have many common features: short-term, goal-oriented sessions that are self-guided by the patient [8], typically consisting of 8 to 12 modules [9]. There are RCTs of ICBT for various conditions; however, studies differ with respect to the kind of the control group used (e.g., waitlisted controls, placebo groups, or therapy as usual), the intensity of the online interaction between patients and therapists, the types of communication methods (such as email or text), and the format of online modules [10]. These variables make it difficult to directly compare the results of these studies, since they impact patient participation, adherence, and the efficacy of the approach. However, overall, the quality of evidence supporting integration of ICBT into clinical practice is strong for specific conditions and specific populations.

Focus on Panic Disorder and ICBT. There are a many studies considering ICBT. One of particular interest: Hedman et al. [11] performed a cohort study of panic disorder patients treated with guided ICBT through a Swedish university hospital clinic. The study had several interesting aspects. First, the hospital had created a permanent, dedicated ICBT unit to treat patients. Second, the study evaluated patients over a long period: 4.5 years. Third, patients never met their therapists, but therapists maintained an integral role in treatment (therapist-guided ICBT). Fourth, the results were robust and comparable to traditional, face-to-face CBT. And fifth, the paper was published in a prestigious journal, *Acta Scandinavica Psychiatrica.*

Patients with panic disorder were enrolled in an ICBT program that was structured as a 10-module self-help program. Each module covered specific principles of CBT treatment, such as interoceptive exposure and cognitive restructuring, and homework assignments were included. The ICBT was supported by a therapist, who monitored patient progress and provided feedback on homework with communication by email, although phone calls were included on an as-needed basis. Patients also had access to an online forum to discuss issues with other patients (though they could post anonymously). The online modules also included self-reported symptom assessments to flag patients who were deteriorating or were at risk of dropping out of the program. Following completion of the treatment program, patients could access the materials for 6 months.

Of the 570 patients included in the study, the majority completed the program (404) and a reasonable data set was generated (451 completed some form of postassessment and 156 provided 6-month follow-up data). Participants showed significant improvement in panic-related anxiety and depressive symptoms, which was maintained at the 6-month follow-up. Additionally, patients showed high satisfaction with the program. The therapists spent, on average, just 11 minutes per patient per week on patient communication (in contrast to, say, an hour per patient per week); in total, therapists spent slightly less than 2 hours per patient over the entire treatment course. The study also charted the effect size over time. Significantly higher effects were seen with patients enrolled in the program further from its inception, suggesting that the effectiveness improved as the therapists gained more experience. The effect size was equivalent to those seen in ICBT RCTs of panic disorder patients and to values estimated from meta-analyses of traditional face-to-face ICBT. Hedman et al. conclude: "As ICBT requires less resources compared with conventional CBT, the most important implication of the results of this study is that ICBT can be used as a mean to increase availability to empirically supported psychological treatments."

Larger Literature. This panic disorder study is just one example of the many ICBT studies, including well-designed RCTs and meta-analyses. ICBT programs have been developed for many common psychiatric disorders, including obsessive-compulsive disease (OCD), post-traumatic stress disorder (PTSD), depression, panic disorder, and social anxiety disorder [12], with particularly strong evidence supporting the efficacy of ICBT for the last three disorders [13]. For example, one meta-analysis evaluated therapist-guided ICBT versus face-to-face CBT (either group or individual) in a variety of psychiatric disorders, more than half of which were anxiety or anxiety-related conditions. The meta-analysis included 13 RCTs, and the results showed that there were no significant differences in effect size or adherence between ICBT and face-to-face CBT [14]. In an ICBT study for people with social anxiety disorder (therapist-guided and an RCT), patients showed significant improvement at the 1-year follow-up and the benefits were retained at the 5-year follow-up [15].

One quantitative meta-analysis evaluated the effect size of 19 Internet- or computer-based CBT trials for anxiety [10]. Reger et al. showed that ICBT patients had fewer symptoms and had moderate to large effect sizes in all clinical measures compared with placebo or waitlisted assignments. More importantly: the effect size was comparable to in-person CBT. Another meta-analysis of 23 computer-aided psychotherapy RCTs on anxiety disorders was performed [16]. In that study, Cuijpers et al. found that computer-based CBT showed a large effect size when compared to their respective controls (waitlisted, placebo, etc.), and there was no difference observed between face-to-face therapy and computer-based CBT. Another meta-analysis was performed evaluating ICBT's effectiveness in depression and anxiety symptoms [17]. Spek et al. considered 12 studies evaluating the effect of ICBT compared with controls (waitlisted, placebo, and treatment as usual). For the anxiety studies, both fixed and mixed effects analyses demonstrated high effect size for ICBT compared to controls.

So, to simplify three big meta-analyses covering 19, 23, and 12 trials (all randomized controlled): ICBT rivaled traditional CBT in benefits to patients. These data indicate that, despite requiring far less time and fewer resources, ICBT does not sacrifice quality of care. But a point of disagreement: Reger et al. showed no significant differences between patients receiving ICBT with or without therapist contact; the Culpers and Spek meta-analyses, in contrast, found a difference (small but significant in effect size). So is therapist-guided ICBT superior? More recent studies generally demonstrate improved adherence and outcomes with therapist contact (reviewed in [12]), and we will return to this debate shortly.

Physical Illness. Anxiety is frequently a comorbid condition with physical illnesses – and, potentially, a complicating factor in recovery. CBT has been shown to be effective for this population, but what about ICBT? This e-therapy has shown impressive outcomes in patients with various physical problems, such as chronic pain [18, 19] and cancer [20]. Recently, Dear et al. studied the effectiveness of guided ICBT for chronic pain in the journal *Pain* [19]. Patients were split into treatment or waitlisted control groups. The ICBT program, named Pain Course, was an 8-week long course specifically adapted for chronic pain and included five online lessons with summaries and homework. One clinical psychologist handled all the patient communication, including both weekly telephone calls (usually limited to 10-15 minutes) and emails. Interestingly, care continued after the modules were completed: the therapist made phone calls every 4–6 weeks posttreatment to evaluate the patient's progress and answer questions. This study had a remarkable 93% adherence. The treatment group had significantly better posttreatment scores on the Generalized Anxiety Disorder 7-Item (GAD-7) test, and these results were retained at the 3-month follow-up. Overall, a moderate effect size was obtained for anxiety-related symptoms. The therapist spent, on average, approximately 80 minutes per patient over the 8-week course and an additional 30 minutes in the time between the end of the course and the follow-up [19].

That result has been reproduced: in another study focused on chronic pain, ICBT-treated patients were compared to control patients who participated in moderated online discussion forums [18]. The 8-week ICBT treatment consisted of eight sections with therapist support (by email). An interesting aspect of this study: the material was partly customized, with the first and last sections identical for all patients, but the remaining six sections were individualized based on the clinical interview. Buhrman et al. reported that significant effects were observed in the Beck Anxiety Inventory scores and these effects were retained at the 1-year follow-up; however, the effect size was relatively small. In addition to anxiety improvements, the patient showed both statistically and clinically significant improvement in pain catastrophizing [18].

Similarly, feelings of anxiety, helplessness, and despair were reduced in patients with cancer using a program called Cancer Coping Online (discussed in detail later) [20]. These studies provide compelling support for ICBT as a treatment for the emotional distress caused by medical conditions.

Special Populations. A few studies have looked at ICBT for special populations, including children and the elderly. Treating children with anxiety presents unique challenges (including problems with adherence). In randomized, controlled trials, juvenile anxiety patients (ages 8 to 18) were responsive to CBT treatment, and the interventions demonstrated long-term effectiveness (reviewed in [21]). Children are also more inclined to embracing new technology; therefore, there seems to be much potential for ICBT in this population. There are few studies looking into ICBT's efficacy in children and adolescents. There are studies of BRAVE-ONLINE and MoodGym, used in primary-care and school-based settings, respectively. Both programs showed significant improvement in anxiety symptoms (reviewed in [22]). For example, one study looked at MoodGym as part of the curriculum in 30 different Australian schools. The program was presented in students' classrooms by their teachers. The authors found that there was significant improvement in anxiety symptoms among high adherence participants compared with waitlisted controls, and the effect was retained at the 6-month follow-up [23].

Another trial evaluated the ICBT program Camp Cope-A-Lot with individual CBT and computer-linked education, support, and attention (CESA) controls [24]. Camp Cope-A-Lot is a dynamic, interactive program that consists of twelve 35-minute "levels" with video game "rewards" for level completion. The first six levels are independent, and the remaining six are therapist-assisted. CESA controls included face-to-face therapist time, access to educational information, and computer access without including CBT protocols. Both individual CBT and ICBT produced significant improvements compared with controls. There was also greater therapist adherence to the ICBT protocol, and the patients showed significantly higher satisfaction with ICBT than with individual CBT.

It could be assumed that the elderly would be less receptive to ICBT because of their reluctance to embrace new technology. However, studies have shown that age is associated with higher completion in a primary-care setting [25, 26]. One paper focused on ICBT for older patients, specifically to determine adherence rates, treatment gains, and enrollment patterns for older versus younger adults [25]. The study used an unguided, 6-lesson ICBT program that incorporated homework following each lesson. Older patients were more likely to complete the program and had similar treatment gains but did not enroll in ICBT more frequently than younger adults. This indicates that ICBT is relevant and effective in older populations – but they do not seek it out. This could possibly be remedied by increasing awareness of the programs' availability.

Overall, the research strongly suggests that ICBT is an effective treatment for anxiety symptoms and requires fewer therapist resources than face-to-face CBT. A British Medical Journal editorial opined: "ICBT is effective for common psychiatric disorders, is a useful adjunct to face-to-face treatment, and has the potential to substantially increase accessibility to effective psychological treatment [13]."

3. Clinical Implementation: Australia

E-therapy is of interest to governments and government bodies; the WHO recently touted Internet-based self-management programs especially for chronic illness [27]. Given the evidence in support of ICBT, a number of national health services have rolled out government-endorsed ICBT programs. Australia, in particular, has made significant strides in developing and implementing e-mental health services, including ICBT.

In recent years, the Australian federal government has committed resources to mental health reforms (the Better Access initiative), as well as funding e-therapy projects like MoodGYM (a web-based program that is free with registration – see below). Based on the promising research in the field, the e-Mental Health Alliance was formed in 2009 to further expand Australia's e-mental health services. The justification? "It is estimated that, even with improvements in access resulting from the Better Access initiative, only about 46 percent of people with a mental health disorder accessed treatment in 2010" [28]. E-mental health is seen as a way of reaching more people in need. In the words of Mark Butler, who was the Minister of Mental Health and Ageing: "This reform agenda gives us an opportunity and presents us with a challenge: to remain alert and alive to innovative ways to further improve our mental health system. Online mental health services offer such an approach – both as an alternative, and as an adjunct, to face-to-face mental health care." The rhetoric is matched with ambitious plans to invest tens of millions of dollars over a short period of time in e-therapy, including ICBT, with a virtual clinic to provide service to 50,000 people over 5 years.

Australia is something of a hotbed for ICBT initiatives. THIS WAY UP Clinic, created through a university–hospital partnership, is one example. The e-clinic offers a number of anxiety-related courses including: Worry (for generalized anxiety disorder), Worry and Sadness (for mixed depression and anxiety), Shyness (for social phobias), Obsessions and Compulsions (for OCD), and Panic (for panic and agoraphobia). The courses are available by referral through clinic-registered clinicians – including family doctors but also mental health nurses and psychologists.

THIS WAY UP Clinic makes good use of the Internet: patients can set up an online calendar to provide email reminders; progress reports are provided to referring clinicians, by email; patients have access to "patient recovery stories"; the website is graphically pleasing and uses comic book-style lessons, with vivid colors, to explain key concepts in story form. These stories focus on fictional but realistic characters with mental health issues (a character-based approach, as opposed to the text-based approach of the Swedish panic study). In Lesson 1 on "The Diagnosis" in one course, for example, we are introduced to "a 32 year old woman called Jess" who recounts her struggles with low mood beginning a few years before, she notes: "I'd had a pretty tough year. My boss was always on my case." This caption is accompanied with a picture of Jess being criticized by her boss. She describes other stresses and then reports: "Life had lost its colour" – with a picture of her sitting on a park bench but with the colors blanched out.

Like other ICBT programs, THIS WAY UP Clinic has lessons, followed by homework with summaries of the lessons and activities to apply the newly learned skills, with patients typically completing course-work over 6-8 weeks. The programs come with a fee: $55 AUS for 90 days' access, with an additional 90 days of access upon completion. The e-clinic also features free self-help courses.

Developed in the Clinical Research Unit for Anxiety and Depression (CRUfAD) at the University of New South Wales and St. Vincent's Hospital, the courses have been the focus of much study; the CRUfAD website includes more than two dozen papers on ICBT (including a paper they suggest is in press and looks at how e-therapy is here to stay). THIS WAY UP Clinic claims strong results: according to the website, they boast a success rate of 75% for course completion and a 90% satisfaction rate. It is, as they claim, a success.

THIS WAY UP Clinic is part of a larger effort, including courses designed to teach school children about mood and anxiety disorders as part of their health curriculum (THIS WAY UP SCHOOLS). And the Clinic has also experimented with different types of service delivery. A unique focus of study: incorporating ICBT into primary care. Other countries involve mental health care directly in primary-care settings. Psychiatrists in Canada and psychologists in Norway are sometimes affiliated with family medicine clinics. Can ICBT be used in primary care, a virtual experiment in Shared Care? The idea was tried [25, 29, 30]. In one study, patients enrolled in the Worry and Sadness course and were assigned either a CRUfAD psychologist or their family doctor. Not surprisingly, the busy family physician was not quite able to motivate and encourage patients the way a dedicated psychologist could: adherence was 41% vs. 89%, respectively – though the effect size was equivalent and dropouts still showed benefit.

In a recent 5-year progress update to the Commonwealth Government and National Mental Health Commission [31], the e-Mental Health Alliance took stock of the e-mental health efforts. According to the report, THIS WAY UP is logging an average of 1,000 unique visitors per month, with 80 patients registered for the Clinic. Newby et al. [25] reported that more than 3,600 clinicians were registered with THIS WAY UP as of May 2013. The self-help program alone had over 6,000 registrations since its inception and approximately 275 registrations per month. How effective was treatment? The progress update suggests a cost of $1800 AUS for every Disability Adjusted Life Year (DALY) – to put that figure in context, interventions are generally considered cost-effective under $50,000 AUS per DALY. And THIS WAY UP's reach extends beyond the doctor's office and into the classroom: approximately 500 primary and high schools had registered to use the coursework [31]. It is apparent that in five short years, the program is being embraced by the medical community, and it is a valuable resource for the general public. This provides encouraging results for successful ICBT implementation in other countries, especially those with public health-care systems.

4. Advantages of ICBT

There are three principle advantages to ICBT: patient empowerment, increased clinical efficiency, and cost-effectiveness.

Patient empowerment. Patients have the ability to schedule their own care at any time and any location with an Internet connection [7, 16], which allows the treatment to be adjusted around work schedules and other responsibilities. And ICBT programs allow patients to acknowledge and address issues in real time rather than waiting for their next therapist appointment.

ICBT also provides a solution for geographic barriers. Patients in remote rural areas with limited access to direct patient care can benefit from ICBT. Primary-care physicians in rural areas of Scotland and Australia have been encouraged to refer anxiety patients to ICBT programs. Efforts have also been made to raise general public awareness of these programs in an effort to increase self-referrals. This strategy has proven effective in clinical trials, and rural patients showed increased adherence in some cases [19, 23, 29, 32]. In one study, rural populations in Scotland were targeted; investigators contacted 56 general practitioners for direct referrals, and also distributed posters in family medicine practices, dentist offices, and emergency departments. Among the individuals who provided pretreatment data, 74% completed treatment, and there were moderate to large effect sizes on most anxiety measures [32].

ICBT may also be well-received by patients who would not otherwise seek CBT. Individuals who are isolated due to physical conditions (pain) or psychological issues (social anxiety) can seek and receive treatment (Box 1) [6]. And ICBT may also help address the significant social stigma associated with mental health care. In a study investigating ICBT patients' attitudes to psychological treatments, up to 21% of patients expressed some form of skepticism toward psychotherapy, and up to 11% had a self-stigma ideation [33]. (It is likely that these percentages are higher in the general population.) Currently, Australia's e-Mental Health Services are trying to decrease this stigma through online health promotion and psychoeducation programs [31]. It is hoped that ICBT will help act those with negative attitudes toward therapy to seek professional treatment [34]. The Internet also provides a sense of privacy and anonymity that may also help introverted or depressed patients to be more open and receptive to treatment [7].

Box 1: Applying ICBT to clinical practice:

A 25-year-old Toronto man presents to a psychiatrist on referral from his family physician. He has a long history of low mood, and now presents with profound anxiety. Initially,he was able to work despite panic attacks and "dizzy" episodes thata neurologist couldn't diagnose. Eventually, he left his job, 7 months prior to the initial appointment. He now spends his time in his house, afraid to leave. His social circle is limited to a few high school friends. Although no past suicide attempts are reported, he expresses passive suicidal ideation. He notes that he is particularly afraid of crowds and describes ongoing anxiety about "everything." "I can't get my mind to shut off." He is very negative in his thinking, taking small issues like a disagreement with family and building them into disaster scenarios (total estrangement).

We agree to start an SSRI trial, and Seroquel to target his insomnia. He is unable to attend a CBT program through his local hospital's outpatient center because of his profound anxiety ("I don't think I can get on the bus"), but he enrolls in the ICBT research study. Through the ICBT, he learns about Beck's Cognitive Triad.

Every Tuesday, he is emailed a module, and he emails back his "homework" by the next Monday afternoon. A therapist is available to answer any questions by email and also gives email comments on his assignment. When he misses a deadline, the therapist sends a reminder email.

After completing the 6 sessions, he writes, "This is really helpful. Thank you so much." He gained insight into his cognitive errors, including his catastrophization. With the medications and the ICBT, he notes a marked reduction in depressive symptoms.

Commentary.This case illustrates how ICBT can be beneficial for moderate anxiety, in combination with psychopharmacological treatment. In this case, in-person therapy was not an option. The ICBT was immediately accessible.

Increased Clinical Efficiency. ICBT saves time and resources for health-care providers. As mentioned above, guided ICBT generally shows higher adherence than unguided ICBT. This support can include telephone calls and emails, which are less time consuming and require fewer resources than traditional CBT. Such communications can occur asynchronously, so the therapist does not have to be readily available [7]. In an RCT of face-to-face therapy versus ICBT for social phobia, the therapists spend on average 18 minutes per ICBT patients, compared with 240 minutes for face-to-face patients with no significant differences between the groups posttreatment [35].

How much training is required for a therapist who can guide ICBT? In a study on generalized anxiety disorder, the efficacy of clinicians was compared to technicians [36]. In that study, the patients were assisted by either a registered clinical psychologist or a technician with no previous psychological experience who was provided with a script. The technician gave support and encouragement, and answered questions, but was instructed not to give clinical advice. The results demonstrated that a modestly trained individual with no prior therapy or counseling qualifications could guide ICBT with similar outcomes and adherence as a clinician.

In a different study on the content of therapist interactions in ICBT, investigators analyzed 490 emails collected from patients receiving treatment for generalized anxiety disorder [37]. Preliminary content analysis identified eight therapist behaviors: task reinforcement, task prompting, empathetic utterance, deadline flexibility, alliance bolstering, psychoeducation, self-disclosure, and self-efficacy shaping. Of those, the first three were correlated with patients completing their modules. These studies, taken together, support the idea of a resource- and cost-effective treatment model with a single clinician supervising and supporting several technicians with communication scripts optimized to improve adherence. (It could be pointed out, though, that the often-used model of therapist-guided care is still much more resource-effective than traditional CBT.)

Cost-effectiveness. Several studies investigated the cost-effectiveness of ICBT. On average, the probability of ICBT as a cost-effective treatment was 57% (range 38–96%) compared with waitlisted controls (reviewed in [38]). Hedman et al. performed a cost-effectiveness analysis on data from a social anxiety disorder trial comparing in-person CBT to ICBT [39]. The data included posttreatment and 6-month follow-up evaluations, and the results showed that there was a 79.5% probability that ICBT would be efficacious at a lower cost. In addition, they reported that the societal cost was reduced by $7,046 USD for each patient. Several other studies investigating societal costs showed that for each patient who improved using ICBT, the overall societal cost was reduced by $16,000 USD to $39,000 USD compared with waitlisted controls [38]. These studies clearly indicate that there is a huge cost benefit to implementing ICBT.

Another study considered the cost-effectiveness of translating an existing (English) ICBT program into another language (Norwegian). Data showed that the cost of translating well-researched programs was roughly a quarter of the cost of developing a new one, and implementing it would result in a 21-fold return in investment based on the quality-adjusted life years gained [40]. By using existing, well-tested programs translated into other languages, health services have the opportunity to expand their programs with small investment.

5. Disadvantages of ICBT

There are three potential disadvantages to ICBT: lack of direct patient monitoring, misdiagnosis/inappropriate treatment, and accessibility issues.

Lack of Direct Patient Monitoring. A number of studies have shown that the lack of direct patient monitoring may contribute to low adherence, both in unguided ICBT and in ICBT managed by primary-care physicians [12, 25, 29]. This is a serious consideration that needs further study and is a major challenge for future program development [31].

Several studies indicated that for anxiety patients, poorer adherence is related to increased baseline symptom severity and baseline psychological distress (reviewed in [41]). For those patients that do not complete their programs, several factors contribute to their lack of adherence. The reasons vary by study, and include time constraints, lack of motivation, technical problems, lack of face-to-face therapy, preference for medication, and skepticism regarding the treatment's effectiveness (reviewed in [42]).

And while there are many reasons for nonadherence, unguided ICBT seems to have very high dropout rates. Different studies have different designs and interventions, but the pattern is clear: patients enrolled in MoodGym: 37% completed the self-directed program [43]; patients with mild panic symptoms enrolled in Don't Panic Online: 27% completed the unguided ICBT [44]; patients enrolled in This Way Up Clinic's Sadness program without therapist support: 33% completed it, compared to 77% in a clinician-assisted version [45]. Adding in the support of primary-care physicians, incidentally, helped, but not profoundly, as noted above (in the context of THIS WAY UP). Primary-care physician-guided ICBT had repeatedly achieved approximately 40–60% adherence, whereas involving a clinical psychologist-guide was something of a game-changer in terms of adherence, with rates rising to 80–90% [29, 30, 41]. (However, conflicting results should be noted. Berger et al., for example, had a unique study in that they directly compared unguided, minimally guided, and flexibly guided ICBT for social phobias, and found all three treatments to be equally effective with no statistical difference in adherence rates [46] – suggesting that other factors are at play in overall adherence, not simply whether or not the therapy involves a therapist.)

The big question is: how much therapist support is needed? Even modest therapist interaction seems to be effective. For example, Klein et al. used emails in ICBT and demonstrated that one email a week increased adherence rates in panic disorder patients, and was as effective as three emails a week [47]. And, as discussed above, this support may not necessarily need to be provided by a clinician.

Misdiagnosis/Inappropriate Treatment. Because the treatment is often based on patient self-assessment and not direct interaction, critical cues (such as a patient's voice or body language) cannot be assessed, possibly leading to misdiagnosis and inappropriate treatment as signs of comorbidity, distress, or an imminent crisis are missed. However, several studies have shown that well-crafted questionnaires are effective and may in fact highlight potentially overlooked issues (reviewed in [12]). There is also evidence that statistical prediction is superior to a clinician's judgment in diagnosis and treatment planning [48]. A recent study compared automated pretreatment assessments with clinician diagnoses for ICBT program assignment. In this study, the patients were evaluated and assigned programs for depression, anxiety, or mixed depression and anxiety. Similar outcomes were achieved with automated- and clinician-diagnosed assessments, indicating that the automated assessment was as effective as the clinician diagnosis [49]. It seems likely that this concern may be overstated.

Accessibility. Because roughly 25% of the population in high-income countries does not have Internet access [50] and up to 30% may not own a computer [51], ICBT may inadvertently select against economically disadvantaged, rurally located, or elderly patients, many of whom would most benefit from this resource. In the rural Scotland study, several laptops were provided to patients to give them access to the program [32]. This further underscores that those who benefit most may not have the resources necessary for treatment. Additionally, patients who are not technologically proficient may be hesitant about replacing in person visits with e-treatment. ICBT appears to be preferred by educated, technologically savvy patients (reviewed in [52]). To reach out to those less comfortable with technology, ICBT programs must be user-friendly to be effective and achieve a sustained response (reviewed in [51]).

When considering disadvantages, we must acknowledge that the long-term effects of ICBT have not yet been adequately studied; thus, the specific populations who will benefit and the potential adverse effects of ICBT remain to be established, especially for programs that are administered without therapist support.

6. ICBT resources available

Numerous ICBT programs are available, both web-based and app-based. But not all ICBT programs are created equal – obviously, the quality is mixed. Several ICBT programs stand out: some carry formal endorsements of government health services; some belong to clinical groups that hold hospital and academic affiliations; some have been studied in clinical trials with published results; some have been developed with larger development teams involving psychologists and psychiatrists. Fourteen anxiety and anxiety-related ICBT websites/apps are described in Table 1. We highlight a few here:

FearFighter (http://www.fearfighter.com) went live in 2005 and focuses on patients with panic and phobias. It consists of nine steps and includes activity worksheets and progress tracking. FearFighter includes video explanation of core CBT concepts. Step 6, for example, is introduced by a young (reassuring) woman who describes exposure therapy, after quickly reviewing the lessons of the past 5 steps. The approach, then, is therapist-focused, as opposed to the character-focus of THIS WAY UP or the text-based focus of the Swedish panic study. The videos include clear graphics – demonstrating, for instance, diaphragmatic breathing with illustrations of lungs and breathing techniques. Therapist support is offered by phone and in-person, but also through Skype.

FearFighter is endorsed by the United Kingdom's National Institute for Health and Care Excellence (NICE). The program can be "prescribed" by a family doctor or another health professional (and, for some English patients, the fees are then covered by the NHS), but it can also be self-referred. FearFighter has been the subject of several studies [32, 53-57] with patients typically having moderate to moderately severe symptoms at the beginning and showing improvement equivalent to the effects of traditional CBT – but the dropout rate was higher with this program. FearFighter consistently showed high patient satisfaction [57]. The program was also shown to be effective in rural areas with limited access to psychological resources [32].

Though iTunes offers many ICBT apps, the literature on these programs is limited. One study concluded that there were no outcome differences between web-based and app-based ICBT [58]. One popular app is MoodKit, developed by Pepperdine University psychologists Edrick Dorian and Drew Erhardt, which is available for a small fee. MoodKit has gathered much press and was even featured in Discover magazine. Among its various features: MoodKit offers over 200 activities in five mood-improvement categories that suggests concrete steps to improve mood, and includes examples and tips to help implement the concepts.

MoodKit includes a Thought Checker to identify thoughts that contribute to negative feelings and the situations and patterns that generate them, which allows the user to manage them. The Thought Checker also walks the user through the factors that contribute to their feelings and helps them identify alternative positive or more rational thoughts to alleviate the negative ones. The Mood Tracker charts the mood range of the user throughout the day and records their progress over time. The app has a Journal function to collate the patient's notes and comes with preformatted templates to ensure productive journaling. Many of these features can be exported for the user's personal records or can be integrated into professional therapy.

And for those with physical illness? Cancer Coping Online is being developed. This 6-week intervention program targets distress in cancer patients and includes CBT-based worksheets and immediate-feedback quizzes. The modules include topics like communicating with medical professionals and decision making, coping with physical symptoms, coping with emotional distress, interacting with friends and family, and managing life style following remission. In a pilot study, the program achieved reduced anxious preoccupation [20]. High patient satisfaction was reported. It should be emphasized that the data are small and the experimentation is very early: 10 of the 12 participants completed the full program, and the patients stated that the program was easy to use. Negative affect, hopelessness, and anxiety were reduced in patients following completion. The program has moved forward for further testing. Preliminary data from this new trial showed significant, sustained interaction effects for both cancer-specific distress and anxious preoccupation, indicating that type of ICBT may help prevent and treat the anxiety so commonly found in cancer patients [59].

ICBT programs in research trials			
Cancer Coping Online	An online program available to cancer patients to help cope with distress. The program has six modules and takes 6 weeks to complete. This program showed high patient satisfaction, relatively good adherence, and reduced negative affect, hopelessness, and anxiety [20].		
ICBT programs available[1]			
Name	**Description**	**Country availability[2]**	**Fee**
THIS WAY UP Clinic **(https://thiswayup.org.au/clinic/)**	A web-based virtual clinic designed for patients with depression and anxiety disorders. The program is endorsed by the Australian government. Patients must be referred by a clinician. This 6–8 week course includes 5 to 6 lessons. Significant reductions in psychological distress and disability have been achieved with this program [25, 26, 29-31, 60].	AUS	Yes
***Phobia Free, Stress Free* (http://virtually-free.com/)**	Apps designed for patients with panic disorder and phobias. These programs are advocated by the NHS and AnxietyUK.	INT	Yes

	They are designed to provide meditation, relaxation, self-hypnosis, and breathing techniques to treat fear, anxiety, and stress. The website claims more than 19,000 users of the apps. A new program, Agoraphobia Free, is currently in clinical trials.		
MoodKit **(http://www.thriveport.com/products/moodkit/)**	An app designed for users with mood disorders including anxiety. It includes over 200 mood-improving activities, thought modulation strategies, progress tracking features, and export capabilities to integrate with clinical treatments.	INT	Yes
Beating the Blues **(http://www.beatingtheblues.co.uk/)**	An online program designed for depression or anxiety patients. Recommended by the UK NICE. Patients must be referred by a physician for NHS coverage; it is available internationally for a fee. The program consists of eight 50-minute sessions where patients are taught to identify symptoms and set goals. Data show statistically significant improvements in anxiety and depression [61].	INT	Yes
FearFighter **(http://www.fearfighter.com/)**	An online program designed to treat patients with panic and phobia. This program is available to NHS patients in the UK (and must be prescribed by a general practitioner); it is available internationally for a fee. The program has 9 interactive steps with downloadable content, videos, and homework exercises to challenge avoidance behaviors. Patients and referring health-care providers praise its ease of use and reported a high level of satisfaction with this program [32, 54, 56, 57, 62, 63].	INT	No
MoodGYM **(https://moodgym.anu.edu.au/welcome)**	An online program developed for patients with anxiety and depression. The program is supported by the Australian government. This program consists of five interactive modules, quizzes, and homework, and has been translated into Finnish, Dutch, Norwegian, and Chinese. There are at least 600,000 registered users, and the majority of users found this program as acceptable as in-person CBT [23, 43, 63].	INT	No
Online Therapy USER **(https://www.onlinetherapyuser.ca)**	An online program focused on developing general well-being, well-being after cancer, and maternal depression. A course for fibromyalgia patients is currently in clinical trials. The program has 5 to 7 modules depending on the course and is completed in 7 to 8 weeks with weekly email therapist interactions. According to the website, 262 patients started it with 190 having fully completed the course; 96% felt it worth their time.	Sask	No
Pain Squad	An app developed to help manage pain in children with cancer. It was developed by the Hospital for Sick Children in Toronto, ON, Canada. The app helps children journal their	INT	No

(http://www.campaignpage.ca/sickkidsapp/)	pain symptoms and evaluates medications and other physical and psychological pain management strategies. Research shows high adherence among adolescents [64].		
OCFighter **(http://www.ocfighter.com/)**	An online program developed for patients with OCD. The program has 9 steps/modules with worksheets and emails containing tips. The program reduces OCD symptoms. Adherence rates are good with as little as 16 minutes of therapist support per week [65, 66].	INT	Yes
PTSD Coach **(https://itunes.apple.com/us/app/ptsd-coach/id430646302?mt=8&ign-mpt=uo%3d2)**	An app developed for patients with PTSD. Versions of PTSD Coach have been developed by the US Department of Veterans Affairs, (PTSD Coach), Veterans Affairs Canada (PTSD Coach Canada), and the Australian Government Department of Veteran Affairs (PTSD Coach Australia). The program has features for self-assessment and symptom management, includes links to support groups, and provides educational resources. The international version of this app is estimated to have been downloaded more than 130,000 times in at least 78 countries, and patients reported satisfaction, improved symptom control, and better sleep [67].	INT	No
Optimism **(http://www.findingoptimism.com/)**	An online program, app, and stand-alone software developed for people with anxiety, depression, bipolar disorder, and PTSD. The program features include tracking the user's mood to identify triggers, determining effective strategies, and developing a wellness plan. It also offers a clinician interface. According to the website, the program is used by thousands of people and mental health providers in over 80 countries.	INT	No
iCouch CBT **(http://secure.icouch.me/)**	An app developed as a companion to iCouch online therapy. The program helps the user break down incidents or situations into their base components to identify the distorted thinking and helps the user develop new, positive thoughts. Notes can be emailed to a therapist.	INT	Yes
eCBT **(http://www.mymindapps.com/)**	Several apps including eCBT Calm, eCBT Trauma, and eCBT Mood were developed for patients with anxiety, depression, or PTSD. Depending on the program selected, these apps include thought identification and challenge tools, daily and weekly assessments, and relaxation training.	INT	Yes

[1]The list of resources is not fully inclusive of all available sites or applications. Additional resources are available, some of which may be found at http://www.getselfhelp.co.uk/links2.htm.

[2]AUS, Australia; UK, United Kingdom; Sask, Saskatchewan, Canada; INT, internationally available.

Table 1. ICBT Resources

7. Challenges and future directions

Moving forward, there are a number of questions that need to be addressed. What patient-specific factors can help make ICBT successful? What about program-specific factors or therapist-specific factors? And, with the latter, what level of therapist support is optimal for completion and efficacy of ICBT? Is there a role for extra or "booster" sessions of ICBT – and how often (sessions every six months or twelve months)? Not surprisingly, others are wrestling with similar questions. The e-Mental Health Alliance has outlined its own challenges for popularizing and improving e-therapy: increasing awareness of available services and optimizing the programs to increase adherence and maximize outcomes [31].

Current evidence indicates that ICBT has tremendous potential in psychiatric practice. Studies should examine if additional types of therapy, such as pharmacotherapy, or even intermittent face-to-face therapist support are needed in combination with ICBT for optimal benefit. The literature regarding "blended treatments," a combination of both online and face-to-face therapy, is limited [68, 69]. And what about special populations? Currently, there are a limited number of studies on anxiety and ICBT in children, elderly populations, and rural settings [21, 22, 26, 32]. There is a dearth of literature on several relevant populations including minorities, the economically disadvantaged, and the poorly educated [6]. In many ways, these populations are the ideal demographics of ICBT programs, and ensuring that the programs are effective and accessible to them should be a priority.

Further research should also focus on identifying those who will benefit the most and who may actually be harmed by ICBT – such as those with serious phobias, severe depression, or suicidal thoughts. Similar to traditional CBT, ICBT is not appropriate for patients with severe illnesses, which is reflected in the poorer adherence rates [41]. Those patients with less support or those who feel isolated may react negatively to ICBT due to a lack of in-person visits. This is consistent with the self-reported reasons for noncompletion [42]. For these patients, intermittent clinical visits or support groups may be beneficial. Thus, ICBT may be better-suited for patients with mild to moderate disease and those with sufficient social support [51]. Current evidence indicates that ICBT is most effective when a) an accurate diagnosis has been made before ICBT is initiated, b) ICBT is combined with therapist support, and c) the website or app is user-friendly [52]. Regarding the software, the format, speaking voice, font, organization, and various other factors can influence the overall experience, participation, adherence, and outcomes. There is value in tailoring ICBT modules according to the needs of each patient, which may allow individualized treatment and better outcomes. As discussed above, anxiety is frequently comorbid with other disorders. While there are some studies focused on developing a single program for mixed anxiety and depression [25, 30, 58], there is room for improvement of the programs, diversification into other comorbidities, and developing alternative strategies such as a variety of modules that can be mixed and matched for each individual patient. Determining the optimal benefits of ICBT will require robust, large-scale studies with long-term follow-up. These studies would also help address whether repeated ICBT exposure at fixed intervals is necessary for optimal effects.

http://dx.doi.org/10.5772/60816

8. Conclusions

ICBT has enormous potential. ICBT offers a revolutionary approach for treating patients who suffer from anxiety or anxiety comorbid conditions while minimizing the limited resources and time of health-care professionals. There is robust evidence about its efficacy for patients with anxiety disorders. Governments are increasingly finding this treatment modality attractive in terms of both cost and efficacy. Overall, it is clinically efficient, consistent with the way patients interact with health-care providers, and empowers patients. In the Internet Age, with patients accessing health resources online, from physician ratings to medical information, this type of psychological intervention is an ideal direction for the future.

Author details

David Gratzer[1*], Faiza Khalid-Khan[1] and Sarosh Khalid-Khan[2]

*Address all correspondence to: dgratzer@tsh.to

1 Mental Health PSG, The Scarborough Hospital, Toronto, and the University of Toronto, Canada

2 Division of Child & Adolescent Psychiatry, Hotel Dieu Hospital, Kingston, and Queen's University, Canada

References

[1] Baxter AJ, Scott KM, Vos T, Whiteford HA. Global prevalence of anxiety disorders: a systematic review and meta-regression. *Psychol Med*. 2013;43(5):897-910.

[2] Pedersen CB, Mors O, Bertelsen A, Waltoft BL, Agerbo E, McGrath JJ, et al. A comprehensive nationwide study of the incidence rate and lifetime risk for treated mental disorders. *JAMA Psychiat*. 2014;71(5):573-81.

[3] Organization WH. *Mental Health Atlas: 2011*. Geneva: Department of Mental Health and Substance Abuse, World Health Organization; 2011. 82 p.

[4] Katzman MA, Bleau P, Blier P, Chokka P, Kjernisted K, Van Ameringen M, et al. Canadian clinical practice guidelines for the management of anxiety, posttraumatic stress and obsessive-compulsive disorders. *BMC Psychiat*. 2014;14 Suppl 1:S1.

[5] Kessler D, Lewis G, Kaur S, Wiles N, King M, Weich S, et al. Therapist-delivered Internet psychotherapy for depression in primary care: a randomised controlled trial. *Lancet*. 2009;374(9690):628-34.

[6] Williams AD, Andrews G. The effectiveness of Internet cognitive behavioural therapy (iCBT) for depression in primary care: a quality assurance study. *PloS one*. 2013;8(2):e57447.

[7] Andersson G, Cuijpers P. Internet-based and other computerized psychological treatments for adult depression: a meta-analysis. *Cog Behav Ther*. 2009;38(4):196-205.

[8] Australia and New Zealand Health Scanning Network. Horizon Scanning Technology Prioritising Summary. Internet delivered cognitive behavioural therapy for patients with depression In: Commonwealth of Australia Department of Health and Ageing, editor. 2009.

[9] Online Therapy User Update. March 2013. In: University of Regina, editor. 2013.

[10] Reger MA, Gahm GA. A meta-analysis of the effects of Internet- and computer-based cognitive-behavioral treatments for anxiety. *J Clin Psychol*. 2009;65(1):53-75.

[11] Hedman E, Ljotsson B, Ruck C, Bergstrom J, Andersson G, Kaldo V, et al. Effectiveness of internet-based cognitive behaviour therapy for panic disorder in routine psychiatric care. *Acta psychiatrica Scandinavica*. 2013;128(6):457-67.

[12] Andersson G, Titov N. Advantages and limitations of Internet-based interventions for common mental disorders. *World Psychiat*: official journal of the World Psychiatric Association. 2014;13(1):4-11.

[13] Hedman E. Therapist guided internet delivered cognitive behavioural therapy. *BMJ*. 2014;348:g1977.

[14] Andersson G, Cuijpers P, Carlbring P, Riper H, Hedman E. Guided Internet-based vs. face-to-face cognitive behavior therapy for psychiatric and somatic disorders: a systematic review and meta-analysis. *World Psychiat*: official journal of the World Psychiatric Association. 2014;13(3):288-95.

[15] Hedman E, Furmark T, Carlbring P, Ljotsson B, Ruck C, Lindefors N, et al. A 5-Year follow-up of internet-based cognitive behavior therapy for social anxiety disorder. *J Med Internet Res*. 2011;13(2):e39.

[16] Cuijpers P, Marks IM, van Straten A, Cavanagh K, Gega L, Andersson G. Computer-aided psychotherapy for anxiety disorders: a meta-analytic review. *Cog Behav Ther*. 2009;38(2):66-82.

[17] Spek V, Cuijpers P, Nyklicek I, Riper H, Keyzer J, Pop V. Internet-based cognitive behaviour therapy for symptoms of depression and anxiety: a meta-analysis. *Psychol Med*. 2007;37(3):319-28.

[18] Buhrman M, Syk M, Burvall O, Hartig T, Gordh T, Andersson G. Individualized guided internet-delivered cognitive behaviour therapy for chronic pain patients with comorbid depression and anxiety: a randomized controlled trial. The clinical journal of pain. 2015; 31:504-16.

[19] Dear BF, Titov N, Perry KN, Johnston L, Wootton BM, Terides MD, et al. The Pain Course: a randomised controlled trial of a clinician-guided Internet-delivered cognitive behaviour therapy program for managing chronic pain and emotional well-being. *Pain*. 2013;154(6):942-50.

[20] Beatty LJ, Koczwara B, Wade TD. 'Cancer Coping Online': A pilot trial of a self-guided CBT internet intervention for cancer-related distress. *Electr J Appl Psych*. 2011;7:17-25.

[21] Compton SN, March JS, Brent D, Albano AMt, Weersing R, Curry J. Cognitive-behavioral psychotherapy for anxiety and depressive disorders in children and adolescents: an evidence-based medicine review. *J Am Acad Child Adol Psychiat*. 2004;43(8): 930-59.

[22] Calear AL, Christensen H. Review of internet-based prevention and treatment programs for anxiety and depression in children and adolescents. *Med J Aus*. 2010;192(11 Suppl):S12-4.

[23] Calear AL, Christensen H, Mackinnon A, Griffiths KM. Adherence to the MoodGYM program: outcomes and predictors for an adolescent school-based population. *J Affect Dis*. 2013;147(1-3):338-44.

[24] Khanna MS, Kendall PC. Computer-assisted cognitive behavioral therapy for child anxiety: results of a randomized clinical trial. *J Consult Clin Psychol*. 2010;78(5):737-45.

[25] Newby JM, Mewton L, Williams AD, Andrews G. Effectiveness of transdiagnostic Internet cognitive behavioural treatment for mixed anxiety and depression in primary care. *J Affect Dis*. 2014;165:45-52.

[26] Mewton L, Sachdev PS, Andrews G. A naturalistic study of the acceptability and effectiveness of internet-delivered cognitive behavioural therapy for psychiatric disorders in older Australians. *PloS one*. 2013;8(8):e71825.

[27] Organization WH. Integrating the response to mental health disorders and other chronic diseases in health care systems. Geneva: World Health Organization; 2014. 50 p.

[28] Department of Health and Ageing. E-Mental Health Strategy for Australia. In: Department of Health and Ageing, editor.: Commonwealth of Australia,. 2012. p. 1-22.

[29] Williams AD, O'Moore K, Mason E, Andrews G. The effectiveness of internet cognitive behaviour therapy (iCBT) for social anxiety disorder across two routine practice pathways. *Internet Intervent*. 2014;1(4):225-9.

[30] Newby JM, Mackenzie A, Williams AD, McIntyre K, Watts S, Wong N, et al. Internet cognitive behavioural therapy for mixed anxiety and depression: a randomized controlled trial and evidence of effectiveness in primary care. *Psychol Med*. 2013;43(12): 2635-48.

[31] e-Mental Health Alliance. e-Mental Health Services in Australia 2014: Current and Future. 2014. p. 28.

[32] Hayward L, MacGregor AD, Peck DF, Wilkes P. The feasibility and effectiveness of computer-guided CBT (FearFighter) in a rural area. *Behav Cog Psychother*. 2007;35(04): 409-19.

[33] Moritz S, Schroder J, Meyer B, Hauschildt M. The more it is needed, the less it is wanted: attitudes toward face-to-face intervention among depressed patients undergoing online treatment. *Depr Anx*. 2013;30(2):157-67.

[34] Cuijpers P, Donker T, Johansson R, Mohr DC, van Straten A, Andersson G. Self-guided psychological treatment for depressive symptoms: a meta-analysis. *PloS one*. 2011;6(6):e21274.

[35] Andrews G, Davies M, Titov N. Effectiveness randomized controlled trial of face to face versus Internet cognitive behaviour therapy for social phobia. *Aus N Zea J Psychiat*. 2011;45(4):337-40.

[36] Robinson E, Titov N, Andrews G, McIntyre K, Schwencke G, Solley K. Internet treatment for generalized anxiety disorder: a randomized controlled trial comparing clinician vs. technician assistance. *PloS one*. 2010;5(6):e10942.

[37] Paxling B, Lundgren S, Norman A, Almlov J, Carlbring P, Cuijpers P, et al. Therapist behaviours in internet-delivered cognitive behaviour therapy: analyses of e-mail correspondence in the treatment of generalized anxiety disorder. *Behav Cog Psychother*. 2013;41(3):280-9.

[38] Hedman E, Ljotsson B, Lindefors N. Cognitive behavior therapy via the Internet: a systematic review of applications, clinical efficacy and cost-effectiveness. *Exp Rev Pharmacoecon Outcomes Res*. 2012;12(6):745-64.

[39] Hedman E, Andersson E, Ljotsson B, Andersson G, Ruck C, Lindefors N. Cost-effectiveness of Internet-based cognitive behavior therapy vs. cognitive behavioral group therapy for social anxiety disorder: results from a randomized controlled trial. *Behav Res Ther*. 2011;49(11):729-36.

[40] Lintvedt OK, Griffiths KM, Eisemann M, Waterloo K. Evaluating the translation process of an Internet-based self-help intervention for prevention of depression: a cost-effectiveness analysis. *J Med Internet Res*. 2013;15(1):e18.

[41] Mewton L, Smith J, Rossouw P, Andrews G. Current perspectives on Internet-delivered cognitive behavioral therapy for adults with anxiety and related disorders. *Psychol Res Behav Manag*. 2014;7:37-46.

[42] Christensen H, Griffiths KM, Farrer L. Adherence in internet interventions for anxiety and depression. *J Med Internet Res*. 2009;11(2):e13.

[43] Twomey C, O'Reilly G, Byrne M, Bury M, White A, Kissane S, et al. A randomized controlled trial of the computerized CBT programme, MoodGYM, for public mental

health service users waiting for interventions. *Brit J Clin Psychol*/the British Psychological Society. 2014;53(4):433-50.

[44] van Ballegooijen W, Riper H, Klein B, Ebert DD, Kramer J, Meulenbeek P, et al. An Internet-based guided self-help intervention for panic symptoms: randomized controlled trial. *J Med Internet Res*. 2013;15(7):e154.

[45] Titov N, Andrews G, Choi I, Schwencke G, Mahoney A. Shyness 3: randomized controlled trial of guided versus unguided Internet-based CBT for social phobia. *Aus N Zea J Psychiat*. 2008;42(12):1030-40.

[46] Berger T, Caspar F, Richardson R, Kneubuhler B, Sutter D, Andersson G. Internet-based treatment of social phobia: a randomized controlled trial comparing unguided with two types of guided self-help. *Behav Res Ther*. 2011;49(3):158-69.

[47] Klein B, Austin D, Pier C, Kiropoulos L, Shandley K, Mitchell J, et al. Internet-based treatment for panic disorder: does frequency of therapist contact make a difference? *Cog Behav Ther*. 2009;38(2):100-13.

[48] Meehl PE. *Clinical versus Statistical Prediction; a Theoretical Analysis and a Review of the Evidence*. Minneapolis: University of Minnesota Press; 1954, p. 149.

[49] Mason EC, Andrews G. The use of automated assessments in internet-based CBT: The computer will be with you shortly. *Internet Intervent*. 2014;1(4):216-24.

[50] World Development Indicators 2014: The World Bank; 2014. 136 p.

[51] Carlbring P, Andersson G. Internet and psychological treatment. How well can they be combined? *Comp Hum Behav*. 2006;22(3):545-53.

[52] Andersson G, Carlbring P, Berger T, Almlov J, Cuijpers P. What makes Internet therapy work? Cognitive behaviour therapy. 2009;38 Suppl 1:55-60.

[53] Marks IM, Kenwright M, McDonough M, Whittaker M, Mataix-Cols D. Saving clinicians' time by delegating routine aspects of therapy to a computer: a randomized controlled trial in phobia/panic disorder. *Psychol Med*. 2004;34(1):9-17.

[54] Gega L, Marks I, Mataix-Cols D. Computer-aided CBT self-help for anxiety and depressive disorders: experience of a London clinic and future directions. *J Clin Psychol*. 2004;60(2):147-57.

[55] Schneider AJ, Mataix-Cols D, Marks IM, Bachofen M. Internet-guided self-help with or without exposure therapy for phobic and panic disorders. *Psychother Psychosom*. 2005;74(3):154-64.

[56] McCrone P, Marks IM, Mataix-Cols D, Kenwright M, McDonough M. Computer-aided self-exposure therapy for phobia/panic disorder: a pilot economic evaluation. *Cog Behav Ther*. 2009;38(2):91-9.

[57] MacGregor AD, Hayward L, Peck DF, Wilkes P. Empirically grounded clinical interventions clients' and referrers' perceptions of computer-guided CBT (FearFighter). *Behavi Cog Psychother*. 2009;37(1):1-9.

[58] Watts S, Mackenzie A, Thomas C, Griskaitis A, Mewton L, Williams A, et al. CBT for depression: a pilot RCT comparing mobile phone vs. computer. *BMC Psychiat*. 2013;13:49.

[59] Beatty L, Koczwara B, Wade T, editors. Cancer Coping Online: Findings and lessons learned from a phase II RCT of an eHealth program for reducing cancer-distress. Clinical Oncological Society of Australia Annual Scientific Meeting; 2013; Adelaide, Australia: *Asia-Pacific J Clin Oncol*.

[60] Sunderland M, Wong N, Hilvert-Bruce Z, Andrews G. Investigating trajectories of change in psychological distress amongst patients with depression and generalised anxiety disorder treated with internet cognitive behavioural therapy. *Behav Res Ther*. 2012;50(6):374-80.

[61] Cavanagh K, Seccombe N, Lidbetter N. The implementation of computerized cognitive behavioural therapies in a service user-led, third sector self help clinic. *Behav Cog Psychother*. 2011;39(4):427-42.

[62] Marks IM, Cuijpers P, Cavanagh K, van Straten A, Gega L, Andersson G. Meta-analysis of computer-aided psychotherapy: problems and partial solutions. *Cog Behav Ther*. 2009;38(2):83-90.

[63] Schneider J, Sarrami Foroushani P, Grime P, Thornicroft G. Acceptability of online self-help to people with depression: users' views of MoodGYM versus informational websites. *J Med Internet Res*. 2014;16(3):e90.

[64] Stinson JN, Jibb LA, Nguyen C, Nathan PC, Maloney AM, Dupuis LL, et al. Development and testing of a multidimensional iPhone pain assessment application for adolescents with cancer. *J Med Internet Res*. 2013;15(3):e51.

[65] Greist JH, Marks IM, Baer L, Kobak KA, Wenzel KW, Hirsch MJ, et al. Behavior therapy for obsessive-compulsive disorder guided by a computer or by a clinician compared with relaxation as a control. *J Clin Psychiat*. 2002;63(2):138-45.

[66] Nakagawa A, Marks IM, Park JM, Bachofen M, Baer L, Dottl SL, et al. Self-treatment of obsessive-compulsive disorder guided by manual and computer-conducted telephone interview. *J Telemed Telecare*. 2000;6(1):22-6.

[67] Kuhn E, Greene C, Hoffman J, Nguyen T, Wald L, Schmidt J, et al. Preliminary evaluation of PTSD Coach, a smartphone app for post-traumatic stress symptoms. *Milit Medicine*. 2014;179(1):12-8.

[68] Mansson KN, Skagius Ruiz E, Gervind E, Dahlin M, Andersson G. Development and initial evaluation of an Internet-based support system for face-to-face cognitive behavior therapy: a proof of concept study. *J Med Internet Res*. 2013;15(12):e280.

[69] Kooistra LC, Wiersma JE, Ruwaard J, van Oppen P, Smit F, Lokkerbol J, et al. Blended vs. face-to-face cognitive behavioural treatment for major depression in specialized mental health care: study protocol of a randomized controlled cost-effectiveness trial. BMC Psychiat. 2014;14(1):290.